PSYCHOSURGERY AND THE MEDICAL CONTROL OF VIOLENCE

PSYCHOSURGERY AND THE MEDICAL CONTROL OF VIOLENCE

Autonomy and Deviance

by Samuel I. Shuman
Wayne State University

Wayne State University Press Detroit 1977

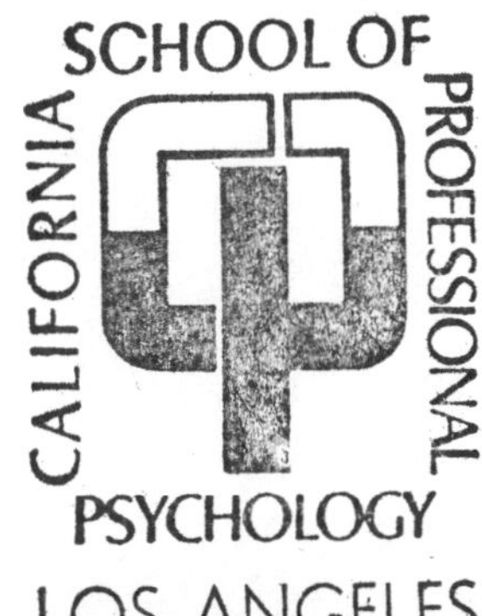

Library of Congress Cataloging in Publication Data

Shuman, Samuel I.
Psychosurgery and the medical control of violence.

Includes bibliographical references and index.
1. Psychosurgery—Law and legislation—United States. 2. Insanity—Jurisprudence—United States. 3. Informed consent (Medical law)—United States. 4. Psychosurgery. 5. Kaimowitz, Gabe, 1935– 6. Michigan. Department of Mental Health. I. Title.
[DNLM: 1. Psychosurgery. 2. Violence. 3. Ethics, Medical. WL370 S562p]
KF3827.P78S5 344'.73'041 77-23374
ISBN 0-8143-1579-8

To the Mykonos Macu Mob

Who have taught me
Different is not deviant

CONTENTS

APPENDICES

PREFACE

Throughout history "medicine" has been an instrument of social policy, and physicians have been involved in the control and suppression of social deviance. Now, because advances in medicine have created the added prospect of controlling violence or aggression by surgical and other medical procedures, there is an escalating public concern about the scientific legitimacy of such procedures and about the possible erosion of important legal rights.

This book will be concerned primarily with psychosurgery. However, much of what is said about the legal, moral, and philosophical problems raised by psychosurgery is also applicable to other biomedical techniques aimed at the control of deviance. Psychosurgery is the vehicle for our discussion because it is the most dramatic currently available biomedical technology having a potential to control deviance, and because it was the procedure involved in the Detroit psychosurgery case (*Kaimowitz vs. Dept. of Mental Health*), the most important legal controversy thus far to have considered some of the relevant questions.

The first chapter therefore describes the facts of the Detroit case, while chapter 2 deals with the difficulties interent in defining psychosurgery itself. Against this background, chapter 3 confronts what many regard as the core problem. That is, when is it scientifically correct to conclude that a given effect has been, or would be, caused by a given identifiable biomedical intervention? I try to show why, despite the obvious importance of this question, no "answer" furnishes a basis for the even more crucial question of whether or when a given biomedical intervention is justified. I then focus further attention in chapter 4 upon when and how a given procedure is justified.

I next turn to the large social and legal questions about brain manipulation. Chapter 5 discusses the reasons for widespread concern about psychosurgery, and examines the nature of expert medical testimony and its relevance to the regulation of medicine. Chapters 6 and 7 deal with different aspects of the relationship between behavior control techniques and freedom of thought. In chapter 6 I analyze Professor Michael Shapiro's arguments developing the First Amendment basis for resisting psychosurgery; chapter 7, on informed consent, deals with what some regard as a key concept for future legal and social developments involving human beings as subjects in biomedical research. The material here suggests that despite the advantages in a requirement for informed consent, there are still good reasons for not overemphasizing consent in deciding whether a subject may be an appropriate member of a research population.

Chapters 8 and 9 deal with some broader philosophical aspects of the psychosurgery problem. In these chapters I am concerned not only with psychosurgery but also with the full range of biomedical and behavioral techniques by which people can be manipulated. My concern is with the wider theoretical problems of induced normalcy that arise when "mechanical" technologies replace the usual socialization processes. In these chapters I also consider the reasons for, and possible consequences of, relying upon allegedly value-neutral medical science as the appropriate mechanism for identifying deviance.

As will be clear from what follows, I am aware of the fiction about neutrality, even for such allegedly value-free activities as "pure science," and I can hardly pretend to exhibit even equal "purity" while engaged in such value-laden activities as law and social philosophy. However, I have tried to make my own prejudices obvious while not deliberately selling either the use or the wholesale rejection of psychosurgery or alternative scientific behavior manipulation techniques. I add this comment because I served as counsel for respondent-defendants (the doctors) in the Detroit psychosurgery case, and did so not just because the doctors had a right to hire me, but rather because I was, an am, generally sympathetic to the position they represented in that matter.

If, despite the sometimes heavy subject matter, this book is still readable, much of the credit goes to Dr. William D. Darby and Dr. Sherwyn Carr, who provided valuable editorial assistance. I am also grateful to Mrs. Sara S. Hartman for helpful comments on some of the early chapters, to Mrs. Maria B. Shuman for help in preparation of the index, and to Mrs. Iona Morrison and the secretarial staff of the law school for considerable help in readying the manuscript for the publisher.

Chapter 1

THE DETROIT PSYCHOSURGERY CASE*

In the spring of 1972, the Lafayette Clinic of Detroit proposed a study on the effects of medical or surgical treatment of patients committed to the Michigan hospital system because of severe recurrent aggressive outbursts. The medically treated group was to receive the antiandrogen cyproterone acetate while the surgical patients were to have depth electrodes implanted in order to determine their suitability for amygdalotomy. The surgical aspect of the project was largely influenced by Drs. Vernon H. Mark and Frank Ervin, who had suggested correlations between spontaneous, uncontrollable aggression and electrical abnormalties in the limbic system, particularly the amygdala.[1] Partial destruction of the amygdala reportedly eliminated episodic aggressive outbursts without serious damage to cognitive or personality functions. The choice of medical or surgical treatment was left to the individual patients, who were provided with either option as well as with the right to refuse participation.

Candidates for this research were selected on the following bases:

(1) aged twenty-five or older
(2) male
(3) resistant to treatment with conventional methods and

*This chapter is based upon a summary of the case prepared in collaboration with my colleague Dr. Elliot Luby.

committed to a state hospital for over five years for predominantly aggressive behavior

(4) possessed of full scale I.Q. over 80

(5) manifesting no paranoid ideation

(6) manifesting no schizophrenic signs or symptoms

(7) having history of multiple aggressive outbursts with or without releasing agents or associated sexual behavior

(8) possessed of ability to remember acts of violence and some capacity for remorse

(9) possessed of sufficient cognitive competence to understand the procedures of depth electrography and stereotactic surgery so that informed consent would be possible

(10) having voluntary informed consent from relatives or guardians

These criteria were considered necessary to establish chronicity and potential for recurrence of violent behavior while excluding paranoid and schizophrenic disorders which probably would be uninfluenced by the surgery.

A comprehensive, organic psychological test battery was to be administered before and after surgery or drug maintenance, while behavioral observations, periodic neurological examinations, and electroencephalography would determine the effects of these approaches upon recurring violent behavior and possibly help identify undesirable side effects accompanying the treatments.[2]

A two-stage consent procedure was proposed for those patients deemed suitable for surgery. An initial consent was to be obtained for depth electrography. If abnormal electrical activity was found in the amygdala, the significance of such data was to be explained to the patient and a second consent requested for a definitive amygdalotomy. In the absence of severe abnormality the implanted electrodes were to be removed and the patient discharged from the project or, if he desired, placed in the medical treatment group. It was, of course, the patient's prerogative to withdraw his consent at any time during the research and return to his referring hospital.

In addition to the Lafayette Clinic peer review human research committee, two other clinic committees were created to safeguard the subjects. A medical review board, consisting of a psychiatrist, a neurosurgeon, and a neurologist, was convened to insure that prospective subjects really fit the demographic and symptom profile outlined in the proposal. A second human rights group, consisting of a clergyman, a lawyer, and a citizen representing the community, was to interview each subject to assure that his civil rights were protected and his consent sufficiently informed.

In the spring of 1972 it was assumed that a research pool of some 300 patients would be available, most of whom were hospitalized at an institution for the criminally insane at Ionia, Michigan, and diagnosed as sexual psychopaths. However, gradually, and unknown to the primary investigators, the State Director of Mental Health had discharged all but fifty of this group by June 1972, and then further reduced this population to fourteen by March 1973. The reduction of the criminal sexual psychopath population was caused by the Michigan State Legislature's repeal of the statute under which these persons had been committed and by the state's willingness to assume the risk because of New York's favorable experience with the release of the Baxtrom group.[3]

In November 1972, the Lafayette Clinic's initial subject was chosen after careful chart review. This thirty-six-year-old-man, confined in a state institution for the criminally insane under the criminal sexual psychopath statute, had allegedly strangled to death and then raped a young nurse while an involuntary patient in a state hospital under treatment for sexually disturbed aggressive behavior. His offenses also included voyeurism and a breaking and entering in which he attacked a sleeping girl with a croquet stick. The alleged murder occurred during a two-week period of growing tension in which the subject felt he was going to lose control. While such surges of tension had frequently occurred and on one occasion had been treated with electrotherapy, these tense periods were usually precipitated by disappointment. Just prior to the alleged murder, for example, the subject lost his job in the hospital kitchen and was denied the privilege of going to a football game. According to the state hospital record, at that time he got "such a drive and urge that he could not control himself." As a child he had been described as hyperactive and hard to manage. When he was two his mother contracted tuberculosis and he had to be placed in a foster home. At about the same time he developed measles with a possible encephalitic component. The record suggests that a succession of foster home placements was necessary because of his defiance, stubbornness, tantrums, and cruelty to animals. He was finally reunited with his parents at age eight.

Confinement to Ionia from 1954 to 1972 did not necessarily help the subject. Since detailed records were not kept, it is impossible to document accurately his behavior or his responses to the limited therapy available. He had homosexual relationships and later occasional sexual contacts with women. In 1969 psychological testing showed that fully a third of his responses reflected poorly controlled aggressive and sexual impulses. He was described as an "affectively labile individual who expresses his emotions in a somewhat explosive manner." Despite the release of large numbers of criminal sexual psychopaths, officials were reluctant to discharge this man because of concern about his being potentially dangerous. As late as July 1972, he told an Ionia psychiatrist that "he had periods which he could not control. He felt that his head was swelling and he became flushed. At this point he felt that he could not control his behavior and he usually went to his room. He says he knows these episodes come on rather frequently."

In November 1972, he was transferred to the Lafayette Clinic to determine his suitability for depth electrography. A surface electroencephalogram was interpreted as showing moderate intermittent bitemporal slowing. He was placed in a mixed ward under close supervision and actively mingled with women for the first time in eighteen years. His passivity and docility were so impressive that the clinic's staff could hardly believe that he might have once committed murder. A female laboratory technician found him attractive, gentle, and kind, and became involved in an intimate relationship with him before their liaison was discovered and discouraged by a staff psychiatrist. Soon the manifestations of paroxysmal tension described at Ionia became apparent at the clinic. This tension had a physical rather than a psychological character, a paroxysmal quality, and was responsive to frustration and disappointment. These "surges" of tension made it impossible for him to sustain effort in any activity and caused him to be physically ill. Despite the sensitiveness of his position, he made overt sexual overtures to several female patients, frequently grabbing and touching them. He requested a pair of panties from one woman and was found masturbating in his room with them.

A final series of psychological tests revealed "a striking lack of impulse control and a low tolerance for frustration. . . . in any situation providing anger, he would be quite unlikely to control ensuing impulses toward aggression." The major behavioral themes from his history and the clinic's five-month observation period were: (1) severe defect in impulse control; (2) inability to develop close human relationships; (3) polymorphous expression of sexuality including homosexual and heterosexual activity, voyeurism, fetishism, and exhibitionism; (4) minimal capacity to endure disappointment; (5) paroxysmal waxing and waning of a painful physical tension; and (6) charmingly superficial and shallow manner of relating to others.

In February 1973, attorney Gabe Kaimowitz, representing the Medical Committee for Human Rights, brought suit to release John Doe on a writ of habeas corpus, charging that he was being illegally detained in the state hospital system under a criminal sexual psychopath statute repealed by the Michigan legislature in 1968, and as a result, being denied accepted medical treatment which might lead to regaining his liberty. In addition, it was alleged that the subject was not fully informed of the risks inherent in the clinic's research, that his parents were not consulted, and that the state legislature was not fully informed that psychosurgical procedures were contemplated when the grant request was submitted. Doubts about the scientific validity of the research were also raised in Kaimowitz's brief filed before Judge Horace M. Gilmore of the Wayne County Circuit Court. Because of the significance of the trial for psychosurgical research, as well as for research on involuntarily detained subjects, Judge Gilmore agreed to hear the matter with Judges George E. Bowles and John D. O'Hair in an unusual three-judge panel, and allotted fifteen days for the presentation of evidence and argument. Judge Gilmore appointed Francis A. Allen and Robert A. Burt of the University of Michigan Law School to represent John Doe and allowed Charles R. Halpern and Alix Sanders of the Center for Law and Social Policy to participate as an Amicus representing the American Orthopsychiatric Association.

For some years prior to this trial, I had been associated with the Lafayette Clinic as professor of forensic psychiatry. In view of my involvement with the clinic and familiarity with its procedures and personnel, Michigan Attorney General Frank Kelley permitted me to represent the clinic and the individual staff physicians named in the complaint. Mr. Thomas R. Wheeker of the attorney general's office joined me as counsel representing the clinic and the state Department of Mental Health.

At a pretrial meeting all the attorneys agreed that two questions should be answered by the court. As the court stated in its opinion:

> (1) After failure of established therapies may an adult or the legally appointed guardian, if the adult is involuntarily detained at a facility within the State Department of Mental Health, give legally adequate consent to an innovative or experimental surgical procedure on the brain, if there is demonstrable physical abnormality of the brain and the procedure is designed to ameliorate behavior which is either personally tormenting to the patient or so profoundly disruptive that the patient cannot safely live or live with others? (2) If the answer to the above question is yes, then is it legal in this state to undertake an innovative or experimental surgical procedure on the brain of an adult involuntarily detained at a facility within the jurisdiction of the State Department of Mental Health, if there is demonstrable physical abnormality of the brain and the procedure is designed to ameliorate behavior which is personally tormenting to the patient or so profoundly disruptive that the patient cannot safely live or live with others?

When the trial opened John Doe's attorneys sought his release by arguing that the law under which he had been committed was invalid, inasmuch as it was a denial of equal protection under the law to this particular class of subjects. The panel quickly ruled that Doe's detention was illegal because the criminal sexual psychopath law was unconstitutional. The State refused to pursue civil commitment and Doe was released. However, the trial nonetheless proceeded, since all counsel, except the Attorney General, agreed that there remained important questions that the court should consider.

During the fifteen-day trial an enormous amount of complex and often contradictory scientific evidence was presented. The scientific witnesses opposing psychosurgical intervention, Dr. Ayub Ommaya of the National Institute for Neurological Diseases and Stroke, Dr. Andrew Watson of the University of Michigan, Dr. Peter Breggin of the Washington School of Psychiatry, and Dr. Paul Lowinger, a psychiatric consultant to the Lafayette Clinic, marshalled numerous arguments to convince the court that the research should not proceed. They all attacked the methodology of the protocol because of an insufficiency of control groups. Dr. Ommaya stated that depth electrography was a dangerous procedure of minimal diagnostic value and that no correlation had ever been established between electrical abnormalties in the brain and such complex human behavior as a coordinated aggressive outburst. He described amygdalotomy and all psychosurgical procedures as nonspecific, sedating, and destructive of affective and intellectual functions and attacked clinical results based on the quantity of brain tissue removed rather than the area of brain excised. He testified that further research on animals was needed before humans were exposed to such a major brain operation.

Dr. Watson declared that the clinic's criteria for surgical selection constituted a sociological profile rather than a recognized medical syndrome. He went on to urge that all therapeutic possibilities of a less intrusive and irreversible nature had not been exhausted inasmuch as the patient had not had access to an experienced and competent psychotherapist. Although he examined John Doe over a five-hour period, Dr. Watson neither subjected the patient to any psychological testing nor examined the results of previous testing reports. In addition, Dr. Watson did not consult the Lafayette Clinic's charts or reports on the subject's closely observed ward behavior. Solely on the basis of his interview, Dr. Watson claimed that John Doe lacked the symptoms which the contemplated psychosurgery purported to treat. He considered the subject's history of aggression to have been overdrawn, and laid great stress upon the fact that there had been no overt aggressive acts during Doe's eighteen years at Ionia.

In summary, the plaintiff's attorneys claimed: (1) amygdalotomy was a dangerous, intrusive surgical procedure; (2) the Lafayette study was methodologically flawed because it was poorly controlled; (3) selection criteria constituted a sociological profile rather than a recognized medical syndrome; (4) important preliminary animal work remained to be done; (5) although depth electrography carried significant danger of mortality and morbidity, it would, at best, produce information of doubtful value; (6) no correlation had been established between either surface or depth electrical abnormality and complex aggressive behavior; (7) John Doe had an insignificant history of aggression following commitment to Ionia; and (8) conventional therapies such as psychotherapy had not been exhausted through eighteen years of hospitalization. For these reasons the court was asked to forbid the brain surgery as a matter of common law medical malpractice. The case cited was *Fortner v. Koch,* where the Michigan court recognized "the fact that if the general practice of medicine and surgery is to progress, there must be a certain amount of experimentalization carried on; but such experiments must be done with the knowledge and consent of the patient or those responsible for him and must not vary too radically from the accepted method of procedure."[4]

Plaintiff's interpretation of the *Fortner* ruling as it applied to this case was that the risks of depth electrography and amygdalotomy were considerable as regards both mortality and morbidity and that their potential benefits were clearly uncertain. Accordingly, the court was asked to rule that under *Fortner* this experiment was impermissible even with subject consent because it varied too radically from accepted therapeutic procedure. In addition, if the experiment represented an extreme instance of what is legally permissible human research in the general population, then it was wholly inappropriate for an involuntarily detained population. Quite apart from and in addition to the malpractice arguement, issues were raised as to the violation of the constitutional prohibition on cruel and unusual punishment and the fundamental right to privacy. If the state can compel a committed patient to undergo therapy, does the state also have the right to command submission to psychosurgery? Is there duress when such a patient gives knowledgeable consent? It was argued that confinement is so inherently coercive that a committed patient can never provide an adequately informed consent. Such a person is so much at the mercy of his "jailers" that he will accede to any procedure to gain their approval. His privileges, comforts, and, in the final analysis, freedom, are at the whim and discretion of his institutional physician-managers. How can he bargain with them as an equal from a position of such powerlessness?

Amicus based the concept of informed consent on three criteria—competence, knowledge, and voluntariness. Because of institutional pressures on the involuntarily detained, competence is diminished, knowing is not based upon full and objective information, and voluntariness is an impossibility. Amicus again emphasized that amygdalotomy is dangerous, intrusive therapy of uncertain results and therefore either inappropriate or harmful medical care for involuntarily detained subjects. Plaintiff's lawyers' analogy of psychosurgery to expatriation was partly based on the opinion of Mr. Justice Brennan in *Trap v. United States:* "Nevertheless it cannot be denied that the impact of expatriation . . . may be severe. Expatriation in this respect, constitutes an especially demoralizing sanction. The uncertainty, and the consequent psychological hurt, which must accompany one who becomes an outcast in his own land must be reckoned a substantial factor in the ultimate judgement."[5] Thus, subjection to experimental brain surgery described as having destructive impacts upon emotion, cognition, and the total personality would constitute cruel and unusual punishment and would contravene the constitutional right of privacy recently confirmed by the Supreme Court to invalidate state laws compelling women to bear unwanted children.[6]

The subject's withdrawal of consent once his legal status had been changed was also emphasized by plaintiff's witnesses. This action of John Doe was confirmation, plaintiff's psychiatric witnesses insisted, that one state of mind existed in a coercive institutional confinement and another when the subject was free of institutional controls. His informed consent had not been the act of a man seeking medical gain, who cognitively and emotionally understood the research in which he was to participate, but an inmate's desperate attempt to gain his freedom after eighteen years of imprisonment. Amicus counsel argued that the First and Fourteenth Amendments prohibit experimental psychosurgery on involuntarily confined mental patients. The First Amendment protects both the communication and the generation of ideas and the Fourteenth Amendment applies the guarantees of the First Amendment to the states. From such reasoning it was claimed that state-supported psychosurgery constituted an unwarranted interference with the brain functions mediating the communication and creation of ideas.

Defense counsel argued that informed consent is often largely symbolic since patients or research subjects are seldom fully informed or free from the doctor's suggestion or persuasion. Although this symbolic act acknowledges the patient's humanity and allows for his participation in the research adventure, the transference relationship between the sick, dependent patient and the authoritative, parental physician is never a partnership of equals and consequently consent is really the product of an assumptive system which views the physician, rather than the patient, as "knowing best." According to defense counsel, the difference between free and detained men as regards their competence to offer consent is therefore not legally significant. Indeed, the involuntarily detained patient in an understaffed state hospital may be less influenced by his physician than the patient at liberty with greater access to his private practitioner.

It was then argued that legally adequate consent cannot be determined by category or status but should instead be decided on a case-by-case analysis of the physician-investigator's behavior and the procedures used to obtain consent from the individual patient. Doctrinaire approaches which exclude entire classes of subjects from a particular experimental therapeutic intervention disenfranchise and deny civil rights in an arbitrary and capricious manner, particularly where there is no rational or scientific basis for such decisions. Despite involuntary detention, patients differ in character structure, and the assumption that all are equally vulnerable to institutional coercion in a matter as serious as psychosurgery was contradicted in this case by an unsolicited letter from thirteen Ionia inmates who wrote to the court about not wishing to serve as subjects for the Lafayette Clinic experiments. Defense counsel also argued that depriving institutionalized persons of any opportunity to consent denies their essential humanity and that the informed consent issue was but the tip of a philosophical iceberg about how the law may function to protect the liberty of individual citizens from technological advances which can be used to manipulate and control human behavior. Furthermore, counsel asked why behavior control, by altering the brain's gross structure, is ultimately more insidious or destructive of freedom than control by drugs, control by disease, or control by imparting values through psychotherapy.

The defense called nationally prominent neurological and neurosurgical witnesses, Dr. Richard Walker of the University of California at Los Angeles Medical School, Dr. Ernst Rodin of the Lafayette Clinic, and Dr. Earl Walker of the Johns Hopkins Medical School. Their testimony affirmed the value of both surface and depth electrography; indeed, depth electrography and coagulation of the amygdala were characterized as relatively safe procedures. It was pointed out that the risk-benefit ratio of these procedures had already been established by thousands of depth electrode implantations and at least 500 amygdalotomies done all over the world. A thorough review of the literature pertaining to those procedures was then presented to contradict Dr. Ommaya, the plaintiff's neurosurgical witness. His credibility was questioned because his expertise was outside the area of electroencephalography. The criticism that the Lafayette Clinic's research protocol lacked adequate controls was countered by demonstrating to the court that much clinical research uses the patient as his own control to compare variables before and after an experimental intervention. The importance of animal models of disease was minimized by pointing out the species difference between man and animals and the virtual impossibility of creating animal models for certain human behavior disorders.

Defense witnesses agreed that specific correlations between limbic electrical discharge and coordinated aggressive behavior are not well established. They pointed out, however, that people who commit aggressive crimes have an unusually high incidence of abnormal surface electroencephalograms,[7] that the relationship between disturbed brain function, limbic electrical discharge, and aggressivity has been extensively investigated with human subjects, and that the results reported in the world medical literature warranted consideration of a psychosurgical intervention in the proper cases. Finally, Dr. Rodin, the clinic's major investigator, testified that his research proposal exceeded Department of Health, Education, and Welfare (HEW) requirements for the protection of human subjects. The subjects' parents had been involved and two additional committees had been established to insure that the subjects fit protocol criteria and that their rights were protected.

While the full opinion is found in Appendix B, the following are the major findings and holdings of the court:

> (1) We start with the indisputable medical fact that no significant activity in the brain occurs in isolation without correlated activity in other parts of the brain.
>
> (2) Psychosurgery should never be undertaken upon involuntarily committed populations, when there is a high-risk low-benefit ratio as demonstrated in this case. This is because of the impossibility of obtaining truly informed consent from such populations.
>
> (3) Violent behavior not associated with brain disease should not be dealt with surgically. At best, neurosurgery rightfully should concern itself with medical problems and not the behavior problems of a social etiology.
>
> (4) Psychosurgery is clearly experimental, poses substantial danger to research subjects, and carries substantial unknown risks. There is no persuasive showing on this record that the type of psychosurgery we are concerned with would necessarily confer any substantial benefit on research subjects or significantly increase the body of scientific knowledge by providing answers to problems of deviant behavior.

(5) Psychosurgery flattens emotional responses, leads to lack of abstract reasoning ability, leads to a loss of capacity for new learning, and causes general sedation and apathy. It can lead to impairment of memory, and in some instances unexpected responses to psychosurgery are observed.

(6) Generally, individuals are allowed free choice about whether to undergo experimental medical procedures. But the State has the power to modify this free choice concerning experimental medical procedures when it cannot be freely given, or when the result would be contrary to public policy. For example, it is obvious that a person may not consent to acts that will constitute murder, manslaughter, or mayhem upon himself. In short, there are times when the State for good reason should withhold a person's ability to consent to certain medical procedures.

(7) We do not agree that a truly informed consent cannot be given for a regular surgical procedure by a patient, institutionalized or not. The law has long recognized that such valid consent can be given. But we do hold that informed consent cannot be given by an involuntarily detained mental patient for experimental psychosurgery. . . .

(8) To be legally adequate, a subject's informed consent must be competent, knowing, and voluntary.

(9) Involuntarily confined mental patients live in an inherently coercive institutional environment. Indirect and subtle psychological coercion has profound effect upon the patient population. Involuntarily confined patients cannot reason as equals with the doctors and administrators over whether they should undergo psychosurgery. They are not able to voluntarily give informed consent because of the inherent inequality in their position.

(10) The keystone to any intrusion upon the body of a person must be full, adequate, and informed consent. The integrity of the individual must be protected from invasion into his body and personality not voluntarily agreed to. Consent is not an idle or symbolic act; it is a fundamental requirement for the protection of the individual's integrity.

We therefore conclude that involuntarily detained mental patients cannot give informed and adequate consent to experimental psychosurgical procedures on the brain.

(11) The State's interest in performing psychosurgery and the legal ability of the involuntarily detained mental patient to give consent must bow to the First Amendment, which protects the generation

and free flow of ideas from unwarranted interference with one's mental processes.

To allow an involuntarily detained mental patient to consent to the type of psychosurgery proposed in this case, and to permit the State to perform it, would be to condone State action in violation of basic First Amendment rights of such patients, because impairing the power to generate ideas inhibits the full dissemination of ideas.

Chapter 2

THE MEANING OF PSYCHOSURGERY

Definitional fiat will not dissipate the moral and philosophical uncertainties surrounding the use of psychosurgery. However, the lack of some reasonably clear understanding about what is meant by psychosurgery can only add to the opacity thus far effectively insulating the subject from rational analysis. The problem is exacerbated by those who use euphemisms to identify what they do in performing psychosurgery. In May 1974, *Psychology Today* reported (without any source for its data) that "an estimated 500 to 700 people a year undergo brain surgery aimed at controlling their behavior."[1] If this is an accurate estimate, it would hardly be surprising to find many different names for what is done since there are so many different kinds of "behavior" which one might wish to control. Among the circumlocutions currently used to identify these behavior-controlling procedures are "psychiatric neurosurgery," "mental surgery," "sedative surgery," "functional neurosurgery," and "behavioral surgery," as well as the more familiar "psychosurgery."

Definitions of Psychosurgery

Mark and Ervin's *Violence and the Brain* (1970) precipitated much of the contemporary concern about psychosurgery because the authors seemingly implied that psychosurgery may be an efficacious way to diminish significantly violence in contemporary

American society.[2] More recently Mark, in "Brain Surgery in Aggressive Epileptics" (1973), an article written together with the philosopher Robert Neville, states: "For purposes of this discussion, psychiatric neurosurgery will be taken to comprise various techniques for placing destructive lesions in the brain, but not including electrode implantation."[3] What is interesting about their definition is that it is so *un*interesting. Indeed, rather than elucidating what could be meant by psychosurgery, this definition seems designed to cut off real inquiry into what the authors are talking about. They might as well have said "psychosurgery" (or their euphemism) is a certain technique in brain surgery. Indeed, the very poverty of their "definition" makes it provocative because one naturally wants to know not only what but why so much has been left out. As we shall see, neither question is very difficult to answer.

Neville, writing alone in 1974, points out: "Popular definitions begin by saying that psychosurgery is neurosurgery performed with the intent to cure psychiatric illness. It is very difficult, however, to find pure intentions." Because of this difficulty, Neville suggests that "it may be considered desirable to limit the term 'psychosurgery' to operations on 'healthy' brain tissue and to consider operations on epileptic or damaged brains to be within the general classification of neurosurgery, whatever the intention." For reasons to be advanced, I concur in this suggestion, although Neville rejects it because "it might give psychosurgeons license to perform whatever procedures they desire on brains in which they can find some abnormality." He therefore concludes, as have most nonmedical writers, that "psychosurgery should be understood as including all neurosurgery that has direct psychological effects."[4]

It might be helpful to know why Neville thinks it less difficult to discover direct effects than pure intentions, even if it is easier to agree on the effects of a surgical procedure than to agree on the intentions of the surgeon. It should be noticed, however, that at least for some people it will be no easier to agree on effects than on intentions as regards surgical procedures on the brain. Indeed, the most controversial aspect of the scientific literature about psychosurgery relates to the so-called side effects of surgical procedures on the brain; requiring *direct* effects as decisive criteria hardly constitutes an advance over definitions rejected because of reliance on pure intention. This is why I applaud Neville's suggestion that the term "psychosurgery" be limited to designating brain surgery on healthy tissue, rather than adding any requirement about effects, intentions, or purposes.

Nonmedical writers, and many medical ones, tend to make psychosurgery synonymous with brain surgery where the purpose or intention is to affect behavior by bringing about psychological changes. Thus George J. Annas and Leonard H. Glantz, two lawyers knowledgeable about health law, decare that " 'pyschosurgery' will be used to mean any procedure that destroys brain tissue for the *primary purpose* of modifying behavior."[5] Stephan Chorover, a psychologist who has written extensively and critically about psychosurgery, believes "psychosurgery may be defined as brain surgery that has its *primary purpose* the alteration of thoughts, social behavior patterns, personality characteristics, emotional reactions, or some similar aspects of subjective experience in human beings."[6] Chorover's definition echoes that of Dr. Bertram S. Brown, director of the National Institute of Mental Health (NIMH), who defines psychosurgery "as a surgical removal or destruction of brain tissue . . . with the *intent* of altering behavior, even though there may be no direct evidence of structural disease or damage in the brain."[7] Not without justification (although there may be differences between primary purposes and intentions), Chorover regards these two definitions as essentially the same since Brown hedges on the potentially crucial distinction between intending to alter behavior by psychosurgery *only* when there is no "direct evidence" of pathology and doing so "even though" there be no such evidence.

With the elimination of any requirement that a procedure will be psychosurgery only if there is no pathological tissue, Brown's "intention" definition, Chorover's and the lawyers' definitions, and Neville's "direct effects" definition all become functionally equivalent to Mark's and Neville's nondefinition of psychosurgery as "various techniques for placing destructive lesions in the brain." Each of these supposed definitions makes it all but impossible to distinguish any surgical destruction of brain tissue from psychosurgery.

Interestingly, Dr. Peter Breggin, a psychiatrist who has been the most vociferous and often the most extreme and hostile critic of psychosurgery, has tendered an initially more sophisticated definition than those of supposedly more neutral lawyers, psychologists, and doctors. Testifying before the same congressional committee which heard Brown give his definition, Breggin defined psychosurgery as destruction of "normal brain tissue to control the emotions or behavior or, a diseased tissue when the disease has nothing to do with the behavior . . . the man is trying to control."[8] Thus Breggin leaves open the possibility that destruction of some diseased brain tissue, even if the primary purpose or intention is to control behavior, may not be psychosurgery. However, this greater subtlety vanishes when one realizes that the surgical destruction of brain tissue will not be psychosurgery only if the diseased tissue has "nothing to do with the behavior . . . the man is trying to control." Yet since Breggin defends the extreme integrationist brain theory, according to which each part of the brain affects every other part, it is virtually impossible to consider the most minuscule amount of brain tissue as having nothing to do with behavior. Consequently, Breggin's definition of psychosurgery also reduces to destruction of brain tissue to control behavior and like those considered above, offers no criterion to distinguish psychosurgery from any brain surgery which involves tissue ablation.

In a 1974 publication, Mark distinguishes the "classical" and the "expanded" senses of psychosurgery.[9] The former is characterized by "operations on the frontal lobes or their connections . . . in patients with no known brain disease," while the latter includes "any neurosurgical operation that affects human behavior, even if the patients being treated have obvious brain disease." In terms of this distinction, all of the definitions considered above (including that of Mark and Neville) embody the expanded sense of psychosurgery and, as such, can logically furnish no criterion to distinguish surgical brain lesions from psychosurgical ones. By contrast, the classical sense of psychosurgery, like that first proposed and then rejected by Neville in his 1974 article, furnishes the criterion that psychosurgery is brain surgery in the absence of brain damage, brain disease, or pathological brain tissue.

Legislative Definitions of Psychosurgery

It is worth noticing how the newer, expanded "nondefinition" definition of psychosurgery has fared in the hands of those who have legislated about psychosurgery. Two enacted statutes, one federal and one state, deal with psychosurgery, and at least two other relevant legislative proposals have received substantial attention. The National Research Service Award Act of 1974 contains a very important provision which empowers the commission created by the act to, among other things, study the use of psychosurgery in the United States over the five-year period preceding December 1975. The statute provides:

> For purposes of this paragraph, the term "psychosurgery" means brain surgery on (1) normal brain tissue of an individual, who does not suffer from any physical disease, for the purpose of changing or controlling the behavior or emotions of such individual, or (2) diseased brain tissue of an individual, if the sole object of the performance of such surgery is to control, change, or affect any behavioral or emotional disturbance of such individual. Such term does not include brain surgery designed to cure or ameliorate the effects of epilepsy and electric shock treatments.[10]

The enacted Oregon statute (1971) for the regulation and control of psychosurgery defines that crucial term as:

> any operation designed to irreversibly lesion or destroy brain tissue for the primary purpose of altering the thoughts, emotions or behavior of a human being. "Psychosurgery" does not include procedures which may irreversibly lesion or destroy brain tissues when undertaken to cure well-defined disease states such as brain tumor, epileptic foci and certain chronic pain syndromes.[11]

Part (1) of the federal statute is the classical definition of psychosurgery while part (2) reflects the expanded sense. What is interesting about part (2) is the effort to avoid a nondefinition by injecting the requirement that "the sole aspect" of the surgery be to control behavior. However, as pointed out above, primary purpose, pure intention, or direct effects, when joined to the expanded sense of psychosurgery, really add no operationally significant standards, principles, or policies for distinguishing psychosurgery from any other brain surgery. The multiplicity of different words used to create the appearance of the same criterion should be enough to suggest that the effort is likely to be misguided. This should be especially clear when all the concepts used are as intrinsically vague and ambiguous as "purpose," "intention," "effect," or "object." Modifying these terms by "primary," "pure," "direct," or "sole" only makes them obscure and opaque.

The first sentence of the Oregon statute also exemplifies the expanded sense of psychosurgery, relying upon the by now familiar device of requiring that the "primary purpose" of the surgery be to alter behavior. The second sentence does not water down the first by restoring the classical sense of psychosurgery, yet it is clear that a gesture is made toward such a definition. Almost everyone who criticizes psychosurgery tries to save surgical treatment of brain tumor and epilepsy from inclusion within "psychosurgery." As I will try to show, there is an intrinsic inconsistency between these saving provisions and the expanded definition of psychosurgery because of the impracticality of distinguishing brain tissue destruction which is psychosurgery from that which is not by relying upon an operationally ineffective and unmanageable criterion, such as the presence of "well-defined disease states." The functional utility of "disease state" is about as great as that of "purpose," "intent," "effect," or "object," and the concept of a "well-defined disease state" is about as lucid as "primary purpose," "pure intention," "direct effect," or "sole object."

The largely unsuccessful legislative struggle with the definition of psychosurgery is further illustrated by several proposals considered in the Ninety-Third Congress.[12] Indeed, it was largely in response to such proposed legislation that the commission mentioned above was created to study current psychosurgical practices. In H. R. 5371 psychosurgery was defined as "brain surgery . . . performed" for the:

> (A) modification of thoughts, feelings, actions, or behavior rather than the treatment of a known and diagnosed physical disease of the brain;
>
> (B) modification of normal brain function or normal brain tissue in order to control thoughts, feelings, action, or behavior; or
>
> (C) treatment of abnormal brain function or abnormal brain tissue in order to modify thoughts, feelings, actions, or behavior when the abnormality is not an established cause for those thoughts, feelings, actions, or behavior. Such term does not include electroshock treatment, the electrical stimulation of the brain, or drug therapy, except when substances are injected or inserted directly into the brain tissue.[13]

Once more we find that the purpose for which the surgery is performed determines whether the surgery falls within the definition. We again confront essentially paradoxical principles for distinguishing psychosurgery from brain surgery which is not psychosurgery because the distinguishing criterion presumes a distinction which, if it can be said to obtain at all, can be found only at the most artificial level. Clause (A) makes the difficulty particularly apparent. Indeed, only if there could be "a known and diagnosed physical disease of the brain" which had absolutely no connection with or effect upon "thoughts, feelings, actions or behavior" would it even begin to make sense to talk about the purpose for which the surgery is performed as a basis for distinguishing psychosurgery from other brain tissue destruction. Moreover, even if one rejects the extreme brain integration theory (no bit of brain is unrelated to any bit of behavior), it is highly improbable that there can be a diagnosable, physical brain disease entirely unconnected with thoughts, feelings, action, or behavior. Consequently, if the purpose of the surgery is to treat a brain disease, this necessarily implies that the physician can be presumed to know the surgery will affect behavior or feelings. Unless one wishes to argue that the known, inevitable consequences of a purposeful act are nonetheless unintended, it would seem necessary to conclude that surgery initiated to treat a physical brain disease is also surgery which must necessarily modify thoughts, feelings, or behavior.

The difficulties with the definition proposed by H.R. 5371(A) become even clearer when clause (C) is read in connection with (A). Clause (C) implies that the surgery is *not* psychosurgery even if the purpose is to modify thoughts, feelings, or behavior so long as the "treated" brain tissue is abnormal and "an established cause" for the thoughts, feelings, or behavior. Thus, if brain site X is the established cause for ear scratching behavior, and even if the subject's ear scratching is entirely normal, it would not be psychosurgery to destroy tissue at site X if it is abnormal tissue. However, (A) is apparently intended to prevent such a result by its implication that psychosurgery would not treat abnormal brain tissue which is the established cause of ear scratching unless such action is also treatment of a "known and diagnosed physical disease of the brain." Read together, (A) and (C) imply that brain surgery is not psychosurgery if its purpose is to treat abnormal brain tissue or an abnormally functioning brain whose abnormality is a known and diagnosed physical brain disease. Thus interpreted, (A) and (C) are at least more straightforward than as written. Clearly, however, there are still important unresolved difficulties. Can abnormal tissue alone be a known and diagnosed brain disease? Conversely, can an abnormal brain function be a known and diagnosed brain disease in the absence of evidence of any abnormal tissue? Is abnormal tissue or abnormal function a symptom or cause of brain disease? Are these phenomena separately or together the disease itself?

Clause (B) in H.R. 5371 reflects the classical sense of psychosurgery while clause (C) is another way of avoiding the nondefinition consequence inherent in the extended sense of psychosurgery. Here, rather than determining pure intentions or direct effects, we are required to distinguish established causes from other kinds of causes. While I suspect that there is not much difference in the degree of obscurantism among "purposes," "intentions," "effects," "objects," and "causes," the concept least likely to provide a manageable basis for distinguishing psychosurgery from other brain tissue destruction is that of "established cause." However, for reasons considered more fully elsewhere, one can agree that, despite its obscurities, the notion of established cause may be the most generally accepted criterion for justifying surgical intervention on the brain or elsewhere.

In connection with this notion of "established cause," consider the definition of psychosurgery contained in a 1974 Massachusetts bill introduced in order to regulate the use of psychosurgery. In writing about this legislation, Massachusetts Senator Atkins and his legislative assistant state that psychosurgery "is defined as neurosurgery designed primarily for altering behavior or for relieving pain for which no organic cause is evident, by destruction of brain tissue, whether such tissue is demonstrably pathological or not."[14] Here the cause need not be established if the surgery is neurosurgery but not psychosurgery; rather, the cause must be evident, as well as organic. One need not be familiar with Kant, Hume, contemporary epistemologists, or philosophers of science to appreciate that there are deep obscurities about causation, let alone about the more specialized meaning of an "established" or "evident" cause. However, despite the difficulties which surround the notion of causation, it may be that we will be unable to find a more serviceable criterion for justifying surgical intervention. What make the criterion of causation more obscure and difficult when applied to brain surgery, rather than to surgery elsewhere, are the vestiges of mind-body dualism which induce us to seek a causal connection between both the surgery and the surgically altered tissue system and the altered tissue system and the thoughts, actions, and behavior "connected" with it.

The Shapiro Definition of Psychosurgery

Obviously there is much to be said about causation as a criterion for justifying psychosurgery or any surgery. However, as I shall consider causation elsewhere, I should here like to discuss in detail a definition of psychosurgery suggested by Michael H. Shapiro in his article "Legislating the Control of Behavior Control: Autonomy and the Coercive Use of Organic Therapies" (1974).[15] Despite the generally high analytical sophistication shown throughout this important article, Shapiro underestimates the importance of carefully defining psychosurgery. He does, however, devote a two-and-a-half-page footnote to the definition and suggests that "Defining *psychosurgery* poses some difficulties." He offers what he calls a "lexical" definition of psychosurgery as brain surgery initiated "principally for purposes of altering or controlling mentation and behavior, whether or not such mentation and behavior is associated with 'mental disorder,' or with 'diseased' portions of the brain."[16] Although cognizant of serious difficulties, particularly in connection with the surgical treatment of temporal lobe epilepsy, Shapiro seems to accept this statement as a suitable working definition of psychosurgery. I find his formulation seriously misleading and indeed intrinsically circular so long as the "whether or not" clause is included. It is also vague because of the essential imprecision involved in the notion of being "associated with" mental disorder or disease. Moreover, just as a matter of the mechanics of definition, it seems rather strange to characterize such a heavily loaded definition as "lexical." Indeed, Shapiro's "lexical definition" is philosophically interesting primarily because it is something more than just a lexical one.

The circularity of Shapiro's definition stems from the fact that if the surgical target is mentation or behavior, whether or not associated with disease or disorder, then the entire possible universe of mentation or behavior is covered by the definition. Consequently, Shapiro could just as well say that psychosurgery is brain surgery designed to alter or control *any* mentation or behavior. This restated definition at least makes it clear that any brain surgery is psychosurgery unless the "principally for purposes" clause is deliberately interjected to create a metaphysical escape mechanism. The only way to avoid reducing Shapiro's definition to "any brain surgery is psychosurgery" is by playing games about the principal purpose of a surgical intervention. One wonders whether the test is the principal purpose of the surgeon, the neurologist, the psychiatrist, the patient, his family, or the official position of relevant professional societies. What criteria distinguish "principal" from other purposes? Although it may seem naive, is not the "principal" purpose always to make the patient "better," and if so, does not the test become simply whether or not the patient improves? Moreover, if the purpose is always to make the patient better, then whether or not he is made better, is not any brain surgery initiated to make him better necessarily psychosurgery?

Much of Shapiro's definitional struggle arises from an exaggerated emphasis upon aggression or violence as the primary target for psychosurgery. Indeed, the California organic therapy statute, with which Shapiro was associated and with which he deals in his article, is permeated by the same unwarranted identification of psychosurgery with the control of violence.[17] Of course, there are good reasons for some people to be misled into making this correlation—the book by Mark and Ervin, the alleged potential of psychosurgery for solving the crime problem, and the alleged violent crime of the subject in the Detroit psychosurgery case.[18] However, despite an understandable temptation to fuse psychosurgery and the control of violence, one of the single most important needs surrounding the regulation of psychosurgery is to recognize the wide divergence of available procedures and the equally wide scope in patterns of behavior or mentation other than violence which may be the target of such procedures. Should a surgical procedure on the brain be subject to the same regulations as one for the control of alleged violence if the "prinicipal purpose" is to affect a handwashing obsession? I am not suggesting that the answer is clearly pro or con, but it seems that the identification of psychosurgery and the control of violence distorts the problem and thereby generates additional confusion in an area already sufficiently obfuscated.

I hope my concern with greater specificity about the meaning of psychosurgery is not misinterpreted as a plea for the unregulated, free resort to brain surgery. Aspirin and hair transplants are also readily available, but neither should be recommended for that reason alone. Just as a blanket recommendation for or against aspirins or hair transplants would be grotesquely inappropriate and unscientific, so too is a blanket prohibition of all psychosurgery for any type of case unscientific and grotesque. As is almost always true with any medical intervention which is not a fraud, selection of the appropriate patient by accurate diagnosis and evaluation is the crucial factor in determining the propriety of any intervention. Indeed, the most serious aspect of the unregulated use of psychosurgery by private clinicians (often unchecked even by a restraining institutional affiliation) is what may aptly be called the "knee-jerk diagnosis" syndrome.

This syndrome is by no means unique to surgeons, let alone neurosurgeons. It afflicts medicine in general and is the source of frequent criticisms levelled at the medical profession. While the patient's selection of doctors is almost always haphazard, the doctor's selection of patients is not—although it is often the result of knee-jerk diagnoses. The knee-jerk diagnosis is characterized by a lack of precision, and may be illustrated by the complaint that eighty percent of all patients who see a urologist come away (even if they didn't arrive) with a urinary problem, eighty percent of all who consult a proctologist have hemorrhoidal problems, and eighty percent of those who consult a surgeon can benefit from a surgical intervention. If, however, the patient consults a psychiatrist his condition will benefit from drugs without surgery, and if he sees a psychoanalyst, then time and talk, without either drugs or surgery, will cure the problem at its cause, rather than mask the symptoms. The situation is exacerbated by the specialist's inference that if a patient consults him, then the problem is located within his field of special competence, even though the specialist is often consulted in order to ascertain whether, in fact, the problem is within his field.

A Proposed Operational Definition of Psychosurgery

The common temptation to identify psychosurgery with the control of violence is the reason that Shapiro's lexical definition ends up meaning that all brain surgery is psychosurgery. If, instead of his "whether or not associated with mental disorder or disease" clause, he had restricted the range to surgical intervention in the absence of " 'diseased' portions of the brain" (that is, if he had preserved the classical sense of psychosurgery), he might have provided a reasonably workable, noncircular standard for distinguishing some brain surgery from the entire universe of brain surgery. In other words, using his language, the lexical definition ought to be that psychosurgery is surgery on the brain principally for the purposes of altering or controlling mentation and behavior, where such mentation and behavior is not associated with "diseased" portions of the brain. As already indicated, I find the notions "principal purpose" and "associated with" obtuse and cumbersome, and therefore tender the following as a better working standard for distinguishing psychosurgical procedures from the more general class of brain surgery: Psychosurgery is surgery on the brain for the purpose of altering or controlling behavior not caused by diseased tissue in the brain. Perhaps a better, but more cumbersome, definition would see psychosurgery as *brain surgery initiated because biomedical specialists such as surgeons, neurologists, and psychologists recommend the procedure, and believe it will favorably affect the patient's disposition to desist from "objectionable" (abnormal) behavior in cases where there is an absence of demonstrable evidence of any diseased brain tissue which is believed to bear a neurological, causal relationship to the objectionable disposition.* Hereafter, I shall refer to this as the operational definition of psychosurgery. In my opinion, the single greatest difficulty about psychosurgery, and brain surgery in general, arises from the problem of "neurological causation." Shapiro tries to blunt this difficulty by using the notion "associated with," but I see no strategic gain in that move and therefore would continue to use the conventional language of causation, although fully cognizant of the real problem masked by reliance upon the concept of cause.

It may be helpful to consider why the causation connection is crucial in avoiding the improper identification of psychosurgery with the control of violence. The causation issue may be the core problem about psychosurgery in the same way that it may be the core problem in discussions of nicotine and lung cancer, or motorcycle crash helmets and the reduction of serious injuries. But just as any answer to the causation questions about lung cancer or motorcycle injuries does not dispose of the legal or moral issues about smoking or helmets, so too any answer about neurological causation would fail to determine the social propriety or desirability of psychosurgery for all cases. Why then insist that causation is *the* core problem? It is simply because no rationally attractive decision about psychosurgery can be made until there is greater clarity about what constitutes a causal connection in this neurological context; when we know what we mean, we can at least look for confirming or disconfirming evidence of what is meant by such a connection. If it is agreed that neurological causation is only regularity of coincidence, then the *minimum* knowledge condition for a possibly rational decision will be available. Regularity of coincidence means that in a patient sample large enough to be statistically significant the postsurgical changes are sufficiently similar to warrant the use of the procedure when the given kind of change is desired. If people regularly take aspirin when they have a headache and the headache goes away, they could plausibly argue that when they want a headache to go away they are warranted in taking aspirin. Whether we want to refer to this relationship between aspirin and reduction of headache as causal is not a matter of biology or medicine, but rather a matter of psychology and its parent discipline, philosophy.

If the relevant specialists concur that destruction or ablation of tissue in the temporal lobes is generally followed by reduction in the frequency or severity of epileptic seizures, then to say that such brain surgery causes improvement is only a telescoped way of making the following set of statements:

(1) patients with a certain medical profile are suitable candidates for such surgery
(2) neurosurgeons who use this procedure for such patients are not acting in violation of their professional responsibilities
(3) patients who fulfilled the appropriate profile and who

> nonetheless did not obtain the expected (usual) improvement, would not prevail were they to initiate a malpractice action (presuming there were no promises, there was consent, no negligence, etc.)—that is, the doctors would not have been guilty of legally actionable negligence in recommending or carrying out the procedure.

To say that the procedure is warranted, or that the doctors were justified in recommending or carrying out the procedure is another way of saying that, as a minimum, the causal relation between the procedure and the postprocedure changes is believed to obtain. "Believed to obtain" means or implies that the doctors will not be subject to professional discipline or legal action; that is, if called to account before a specialty board or a court, the doctors will prevail. This may seem like an excessively functional, operational and pragmatic view of causation. However, I am concerned only with causation in neurology—even though the model is more generally applicable in medicine. In addition, one must bear in mind that this "sense" of causation is expected to function in the most mundane and pragmatic context, that of establishing financial liability. It is not likely to be an equally useful model in explaining relationships among subatomic particles or galactic phenomena.

Temporal Lobectomy as Psychosurgery

The reference to brain surgery for temporal lobe epilepsy was not a random example, for the classification of temporal lobectomy is a real sandtrap for any definition of psychosurgery. In the Detroit psychosurgery case, the court in its opinion characterized this procedure as "established therapy," and therefore not psychosurgery; even such extremist critics as Breggin try to avoid including temporal lobectomy within the definition of psychosurgery. More moderate critics such as Shapiro and the NIMH have also tried to keep temporal lobectomy from falling under the psychosurgery label. In its 1973 statement, the NIMH defines psychosurgery as the "surgical removal or destruction of brain tissue or the cutting of brain tissue to disconnect one part of the brain from another with the *intent of altering behavior.* Usually it is performed in the absence of direct evidence of existing structural disease or damage in the brain."[19] In this definition "intent" functions like Shapiro's "prinicipal purpose," and this definition dodges the causation problem by using "intention" language; however, the evasion is of little avail. The notion of demonstrable physical evidence used in my proposed operational definition is in this definition served by the notion of direct evidence.

The sandtrap of temporal lobectomy brings out the futility of trying to avoid the causation problem by using intention language. The following is a report on the views of Drs. William H. Sweet, Mark, and Ervin and their Neuro-Research Foundation in the NIMH statement:

> If an apparent focus (in the brain) of seizure activity is found, and if this seizure activity appears to correlate with outbursts of aggressive behavior, then a small lesion may be made to destroy tissue at the seizure focus. . . . Whether or not this surgical procedure constitutes "psychosurgery" as defined . . . [above] is debatable. Although the surgery is done to treat aggressive behavior, it is *primarily intended* to stop the seizure activity of the brain.[20]

As I suggested in connection with Shapiro's definition, much difficulty arises from exaggerating the connection between aggression and the use of brain surgery. Temporal lobectomy is *not* done only or primarily because of aggressive behavior "correlated" with seizure activity. The Neuro-Research Foundation position seems flatly wrong and seriously misleading in holding that "the surgery is done to treat aggressive behavior." Because of this mistake this definition resorts to the metaphysics of primary intent (as if the notion of intent alone were not already sufficiently opaque). Just as there was no strategic gain in Shapiro's use of "associated with" to avoid confronting the causation issue, so there is no gain in the NIMH ploy of "correlated with." If a serious definitional effort is to be made, there is simply no way to avoid the core causation problem as the temporal lobectomy case makes clear.

There have been approximately 1,500 temporal lobectomies performed in the past thirty years and there is simply no empirical evidence to support the position that in a substantial number of cases, let alone a majority, the patients were appropriate candidates for the procedure because of "correlated" aggressive behavior. There is, of course, the possibility that "aggressive behavior" here means the physical movements of the epileptic while in a seizure state, rather than assaultive behavior directed against another person or against something ("unconscious" or not). If so, then by definition an epileptic seizure would necessarily involve aggressive behavior and its treatment would "mean" treating aggressive behavior. However, this intrinsically tautological formulation cannot be what is intended by the Neuro-Research Foundation. Furthermore, the report on epilepsy and violence sponsored by the National Institute of Neurological Diseases and Stroke (NINDS) states: "the best generalization is that violence and aggressive acts do occur in patients with temporal lobe epilepsy but are rare, perhaps no higher than in the general population."[21]

Had an effort been made to unpack the notion of aggressive behavior, it would be easy to see how the definitional sandtrap is created by presuming an intimate connection between brain surgery and the control of aggression. Even in the operational definition of psychosurgery recommended above, there is sufficient difficulty in deciding whether temporal lobectomy is psychosurgery. Under that definition, even if the seizure state is taken to be "objectionable behavior," there would still be the very difficult question of the causal relation between specific brain tissue (diseased or not) and the disposition to suffer seizures. There is also the still more obscure matter of whether the brain tissue believed to be causally related to the seizure is also causally related to any overt bodily movements (other than the twitching)—that is, whether there is a causal relation between that tissue and the aggressive "behavior." Even the NIMH publication states that there remains "some question as to whether seizure activity in the brain is *directly responsible* for, or even *correlated* with, aggressive behavior."[22] It is important to recognize that a possible correlation between seizure activity and aggressive behavior is a very different question from whether temporal lobe surgery is generally or frequently undertaken to cure violence.

Mark, Sweet, and Ervin may be correct in stating that "the most common focal cerebral disorder thus far identified which is associated with poor impulse control and violent or destructive behavior is the one which also gives rise to temporal lobe epilepsy."[23] However, the possibility that some reasonably distinct anatomical brain structure may be involved in more than one type of abnormal "behavior"—(A) poor impulse control, (B) violence, or (C) epilepsy—in no way establishes that there is some necessary relationship between any two of these behaviors. To establish such a relationship requires showing that there is a statistically significant correlation between, for example, the incidence of epilepsy and the occurrence of violence; but there simply is no such correlation. Consequently, all that the doctors have told us is that the same anatomical structure is associated with (A), (B), and (C), and not that (C) causes either (A) or (B). Indeed, the doctors have not even shown that the same structures are associated with (A), (B), and (C), but only that the same focal cerebral disorder is thus associated. It requires a considerable jump to go from "same disorder" to "same anatomical structure." But even if it were shown that the same structure was associated with (A), (B), and (C), to argue on this basis that there is a causal connection would be like arguing that since the same anatomical structure (my right hand) is associated with writing behavior and head-scratching behavior, writing therefore causes head scratching!

We have seen how Shapiro and the NIMH avoid or dull the bite of the causation issue in the Neuro-Research Foundation position by invoking the notion of "correlation" and how, in dealing with temporal lobectomy, this led to the further dodge of "primary intention." Thus, the reader is offered a choice of falling back on correlation or, instead of intention, seeking clarity through the notion of responsibility. In the latter event, instead of primary intention, he can rely upon the greater illumination which supposedly flows from the notion of direct responsibility. It seems to me that direct versus indirect responsibility is, at the very best, a metaphysical metaphor, rather than a descriptive, prescriptive, or evaluative concept. The operational definition of psychosurgery at least makes it reasonably clear that the relied-upon notion of causation is prescriptive. The effort to avoid the inevitably prescriptive character of the sense of causation relevant to medico-legal analysis or definition of psychosurgery, when coupled with the exaggerated emphasis upon psychosurgery to control aggression, accounts for most of the difficulties in the NIMH and Shapiro definitions.

The seizure or the seizure state, under the operational approach to psychosurgery, is not regarded as behavior, let alone objectionable behavior; therefore brain surgery initiated to prevent or diminish seizure activity could not be psychosurgery, whether or not there was demonstrable physical evidence of a neurological causal relationship between diseased brain tissue and the "disposition" to seizure activity. It may well be that in the absence of a proper neurological and psychological work-up and evaluation, any nonemergency brain surgery would be wrong. It may even be argued that any nonemergency brain surgery would be wrong if there were not "demonstrable physical evidence" provided by a depth or at least a surface electroencephalogram (EEG). But to use a definition of psychosurgery which could lead to the conclusion that any wrong brain surgery is psychosurgery creates the impression that all psychosurgery is bad brain surgery. This is not the place, nor am I competent, to canvass the question of whether it would be wrong for a neurologist to recommend or a neurosurgeon to initiate a temporal lobectomy on the basis of an epileptic heritage and without any EEG evidence. Based on the material with which I am familiar, I would venture that there are appropriate cases for brain surgery to treat epilepsy even though there is no supporting EEG evidence. However, my point is simply that not every piece of bad brain surgery is therefore psychosurgery; nor should all cases of brain surgery which involve diagnostic methodologies that do not rely upon, or even utilize, demonstrable physical evidence simplistically be classed as psychosurgery.

One major problem surrounding the question of demonstrable physical evidence of a neurological causal relationship is that surface EEG recordings alone are likely to be inconclusive and depth recordings may involve a surgical procedure no less invasive than that required for stereotactic tissue destruction. Therefore, depth EEG is not likely to be utilized until there is sufficiently good evidence to warrant the invasive surgery itself. But in that event, it could be argued that if the evidence *is* good enough, why subject the patient to two surgical procedures on the brain? One way of minimizing this problem is for the neurosurgeon to take depth recordings from the target site immediately prior to destructive surgery. Thus, when the patient is in surgery for the tissue destruction, the depth EEG recording would be made. The development of new kinds of wire inserts fine enough for the painless and almost always damageless multiple insertions necessary for proper remote depth recordings with electrical stimulation of the brain (ESB), but heavy enough for the electrical destruction of tissue, may make an important contribution to the resolution of this "legal" problem. With such wires, which can be left in place long enough for full recording, the surgeon would not have to subject the patient to two procedures since the wires already at the target site could be utilized for the tissue destruction if the EEG depth recordings support the decision to proceed.

The Shapiro Definition and Temporal Lobectomy

As I noted, Shapiro's lexical definition of psychosurgery is capable of covering all brain surgery, and it is therefore hardly surprising that he must construct a monster to deal with temporal lobectomy. However, his approach is much more helpful and illuminating than the overly broad position of the Neuro-Research Foundation. He points out first that alleged aggressive behavior "may in fact not be 'behavior' at all, but non-conscious, non-volitional movements (although clearly not 'seizures' or 'convulsions')."[24] Thus, we know that he is not relying upon a possible tautology (epileptic state is seizure state; seizure state is aggressive behavior) to show that temporal lobectomy for epilepsy is intended or primarily intended to treat behavior. Although Shapiro is chiefly concerned with the particular California statute, his way out of the temporal lobectomy trap is to consider each case separately, and for him the question of whether a given procedure is psychosurgery turns upon the following criteria: (1A) whether the patient suffers from some form of epilepsy that is likely to lead to grand mal seizures; or (1B) whether the *dominant* component of repeated violent "conduct" is in fact nonconscious and uncontrollable; (2) whether the seizures or outbursts are caused by "identifiable dysfunction at a clearly identified locus in the brain"; and (3) whether the surgical or ESB procedures were "reasonable therapeutic techniques to undertake in controlling the effects of the disease."[25] If all three criteria are satisfied, then surgery on the brain results in excising a clinically identifiable "disease entity"; any other case is psychosurgery.

Criterion (1B) is included because of Shapiro's preoccupation with using brain surgery to control violence, and it is this concern which makes him stumble into otherwise avoidable metaphysical quicksand. Shapiro's definition contains not only a distinction between primary and secondary intention (if not also tertiary), but also a distinction between dominant and recessive (?) components of not conduct, but "conduct." If (1B) was not already an operationally impossible criterion, one must also recognize that the component identified as dominant is "in fact" nonconscious *and* uncontrollable! Just what kind of standard "in fact" is supposed to create is exceptionally obscure. In addition, the double requirement of nonconscious and uncontrollable generates an enormous set of complexities. In what sense are some (dominant) components of conduct or "conduct" controllable, but nonconscious? Are conscious components controllable (for (1B) purposes) if the patient must regularly take drugs or if he can be externally manipulated by remote ESB telemetry?

Shapiro's criteria for separating some temporal lobe surgery from the psychosurgery category only become realistic and operational if (1B) and the "outbursts" alternative in (2) are dropped. In that event, his criteria begin to resemble the operational definition of psychosurgery tendered above. Shapiro's thus reformulated functional definitional test differs from his "lexical" definition of psychosurgery, for instead of primary intention, in the crucial place (2) relies upon causation to decide whether the surgical treatment of the seizure is psychosurgery. Shapiro's test of "identifiable dysfunction at a clearly identified locus in the brain" may be a bit rigid, but at least it is manageable, unlike the primary intention test.

It is also worth noticing that in (3) Shapiro relies upon a test of reasonableness and that reasonableness here is very similar to the notion of "warranted" relied upon above to explicate the meaning of causation utilized in my operational definition of psychosurgery. Thus as Shapiro's lexical definition becomes functional, it becomes increasingly similar to the operational definition of psychosurgery. This is not by way of criticism, since at the very outset Shapiro warns us that what he tenders is a lexical definition. Apparently, in this context "lexical" stands for a definition which, if not opposed to, at least is far from any definition which can be utilized to decide cases. In other words, "lexical" here means "not functional." The Neuro-Research Foundation position, reflecting neither the deliberateness nor the sophistication of Shapiro's lexical formula, illustrates a not very successful compromise between lexical and functional definitions. Indeed, if the NIMH did not hedge in its second sentence, it would be very close to the proposed operational definition.

Shapiro's reasons for avoiding a functional formula like my operational definition are quite clear. As already mentioned, his lexical definition is found only in an elaborate footnote at the beginning of a long article concerned with developing a First Amendment argument against coerced organic therapies and protecting freedom of mentation. It is this legal and indeed legalistic concern with the freedom of mentation which forces Shapiro into his lexical definition with its reliance upon principal purpose and its unfortunate clause about "whether or not such mentation and behavior is connected with 'mental disorder' or with 'diseased' portions of the brain."[26] The nonfunctional, unrealistic character of his definition of psychosurgery and the inconsistencies which it can generate are illustrated when, late in his article, he again discusses temporal lobe epilepsy. Although he here refers to ESB, the argument would be unchanged if the reference were to surgery.

> Why is it unjust to compel effective, non-intrusive therapy, which restores functionality and autonomy? Psychiatrists are wont to tell tales of patients who were in some way coerced or duped into such therapy and, after having been restored to health, offered their profuse thanks to the therapists, expressing dismay at their earlier "misjudgment." All this makes for a rather compelling scenario favoring coerced therapy because, by hypothesis, the proposed therapy is substantially non-intrusive.[27]

He adds in a footnote:

> If control of temporal lobe epilepsy by the use of ESB techniques developed into a sound, established procedure, it might, despite the considerable physical intrusion involved, fail to generate any changes in mentation or "behavior." The therapy would thus not be "psychotropic" and would simply not be covered by the first amendment. That is, *if* the therapy's effects were indeed precisely limited to the control of brain activity not amounting to mentation, producing no significant psychic side effects, then mind/behavior control would not be involved.[28]

I shall refer to his argument as the "precision fallacy." Before considering it, however, I wish briefly to comment upon Shapiro's use of rule-utilitarianism to answer the "compelling scenario."

After quoting from a leading philosophic text that "the rule-utilitarian view . . . 'holds that we should not judge the rightness of [an] act by *its* consequences but by the consequences of adopting the *rule* under which the particular act falls,' "[29] Shapiro adds:

> Suppose we shift the analysis away from the discrete case of compelled therapy posted as a paradigm, and consider the effects of permitting the state to adopt a *rule* or maintain a *practice* of *institutionalized* substitution of judgment for persons ill but nevertheless competent to make decisions about their therapeutic affairs. It may be that the existence of this rule or practice would be more productive of evil than of good. It would be hard indeed to verify this, for it requires an inquiry into whether an on-going policy of institutionalized substitution of judgment would tend to erode values of personal autonomy, and to generate over-reaching by the state in forcing therapies over competent protest. If, however, an empirical inquiry did not yield a conclusion that a finely tailored rule permitting coerced non-intrusive therapy for competent subjects would have such adverse consequences, then perhaps the per se rule is wrong.[30]

What I find so interesting about this argument and about Shapiro's related "precision fallacy" is what may be called the "funnel phenomenon." It is experienced when one is surprised because what comes out at the bottom of the funnel is what was put in at the top. This is particularly manifested in Shapiro's rule-utilitarian and precision arguments by the way in which the right hand gives and the left hand takes away. In Shapiro's last quotation the first three sentences use rule-utilitarianism to justify a per se ban on psychosurgery while the fourth shows that the same theory could justify some state-coerced organic therapies. In other words, if the rule put in at the top of the funnel is not "finely tailored" it cannot be surprising if what comes out at the bottom is the objectionable practice justified by the inadequate rule. The significance of the rule-utilitarian theory to a per se ban on psychosurgery is whether a rule can be manufactured which will justify a practice of using psychosurgery for some cases where the practice is not constitutionally or otherwise objectionable. What I find unconvincing in the current state of affairs is the wholesale ban on psychosurgery for given cases or populations before any serious attempt has been made by any responsbile group to formulate any, let alone any tested, rules for the private, clinical use of psychosurgery procedures. Shapiro's argument roughly amounts to saying that the importance of protecting freedom of mentation at this time requires the *per se* prohibition of psychosurgery, at least for "coerced populations." The danger of this no-rule rule is illustrated by the way in which he deals with the surgical or ESB treatment of temporal lobe epilepsy.

Shapiro's precision argument is that "if the therapy's effects were indeed precisely limited to the control of brain activity not amounting to mentation . . . then [mentation] control would not be involved."[31] Before showing the "fallacy" in this argument the curious formulation he relies upon is again worth noticing, for whenever one encounters such clearly overloaded, antinominalistic formulations, it is appropriate to wonder why more direct language was rejected. Why does the effect of the therapy have to be not merely limited, but "indeed limited"; and if that is not enough, what does "precisely" add to the already overloaded locution? Why, instead of requiring that the effects be limited to the control of brain activity other than mentation, does Shapiro require that the brain activity not "amount to" mentation?

The reason for such semantic overloading is not hard to find. By using "indeed precisely" and "amounting to," Shapiro is trying to disguise the precision fallacy which would be obvious were he to say simply that ESB or surgical control of temporal lobe epilepsy would be "psychotropic" rather than psychosurgery only if they became established techniques and did not "generate" changes in mentation or behavior. Since mentation includes "loosely any mental functioning or activity" other than "regulation of the body's autonomic functions,"[32] it would be virtually impossible to find cases where ESB, let alone surgery, has affected some control of "brain activity" in the temporal lobe where that control did not also inevitably affect "any mental functioning or activity." The fallacy then is that at the top of the funnel we put in a definition of mentation which covers any mental function or activity, and yet we are to be surprised when, at the bottom, everything which comes out is found to be mentation; unless, of course, it is "indeed precisely limited" to something "not amounting to mentation." Shapiro does not even say "something not amounting to mentation," but refers to "brain activity not amounting to mentation,'' despite the fact that *any* and all brain activity has already been included in the definition of mentation! Apparently there is both brain activity and something which amounts to, but is not, brain activity. In addition to the metaphysical puzzle of differentiating principal from other purposes, we must also be vexed by the equally mysterious distinction between brain activity and something which amounts to, but is not, such activity. Indeed, both metaphysical puzzles are connected and the resulting muddle is largely due to Shapiro's exaggerated concern about using psychosurgery to control violence.

I have contrasted several quite different definitions of psychosurgery in order to lay a foundation for a rational attack upon the problems surrounding the use of ''such'' procedures. Surely the beginning of wisdom in this matter requires an elucidation of ''such'' procedures. The NIMH definition appears inadequate because it dodges crucial issues, while Shapiro's definition is dysfunctional because it is overloaded with unnecessary obscurities introduced to achieve preconceived goals, which in turn reflect a greatly exaggerated concern for the relation between ''such'' procedures and violence, rather than recognizing the broad spectrum of target objectives for ''such'' procedures. The operational definition, on the other hand, is more serviceable for developing solutions to the relevant problems because it does not cover up the hard questions, nor begin from an entrenched value base reflecting a distinct position regarding possible solutions.[33]

Chapter 3

CAUSATION

It would be presumptuous if I thought I could improve upon Hume or go beyond those contemporary epistemologists who have sought to analyze induction and deduction, as well as universal and dispositional properties, in order to untangle the nest of puzzles which makes up the philosophical causation problem. My objectives must be considerably more modest. I only want to indicate why it has often been suggested that the core problem in any effort to regulate psychosurgery is "causation," and what this means. In addition, I will sketch how causation really functions in medicine and what this implies for the regulation of psychosurgery.

Change versus Cause

The basic presumptions in medical practice are that there is order in nature, that man is a natural phenomenon, that when a man is unhealthy he suffers a *dis*-order, and that it is not chance but cause which is operative. Were our faith in chance greater than our faith in cause, we might still have doctors, but we would not have medical science. This is why scientific medicine, as distinguished from folk medicine or witchcraft, ought not to use regularly a procedure that "works," unless the mechanism by which it works is understood.[1] In this context "to understand" implies something as to the state of knowledge about the structure or physiochemistry of the relevant organs and how the procedure causes the change. That is, enough (or at least something) is known about what happens to the structures or processes when the procedure is followed. The absence of such knowledge would warrant saying as does Peter Steinfels: "How drugs work to produce their effects is sometimes not yet understood by the experts." However, he also points out that psychosurgery is a "dramatic and visible technique . . . [which] however ill understood by the laymen, [does] at least satisfy a lingering desire for some proportionate and evident link between cause and effect."[2] We want to question whether the link is any more evident when a pill is popped into a patient's mouth or when electric current is passed through a wire placed inside his brain.

To suggest that there is a more evident causal link between the effect and medical procedure X than between the effect and procedure Y implies that more is known about the mechanism by which X changes anatomical structures or physiochemical processes than about the mechanism of Y. In deciding which medical procedure should be used it is clear that knowledge of the mechanism is not the only or even the primary criterion. Were the contrary so, aspirin would be subjected to a greater attack than psychosurgery, and the practice of medicine would be very different from what it is. It is true, however, that knowledge of the mechanism may be crucial in deciding whether a procedure is experimental; however, here again, as with aspirin and many other drugs, the absence of such knowledge by no means bars elevation of a procedure from experimental to standard. Indeed, it is conceivable that if we knew more about the mechanism by which some behavior modification drugs work we might be much less sanguine about them, and perhaps even more suspicious about their use than about psychosurgery. Since such drugs are generally believed to produce only relatively short-range, reversible effects, they are usually preferred to psychosurgery. However, even less is actually known about the structural and physiochemical changes induced by most behavior-control drugs than about the effects of psychosurgery. Thus the preference for chemotherapy over psychosurgery is due ultimately not to respect for the admonition, "Physician, at least do no harm," but rather to the more mystical belief that in choosing between necessary evils, the hidden may be preferable to the known. Such a choice makes good sense on psychological and other tactical grounds, even if not always on that of practicing medicine scientifically. Prominently displayed on the front cover of the HEW publication *Psychosurgery: Perspective on a Current Issue* is the admonition that "People don't ask for facts in making up their minds. They would rather have one good, soul-satisfying emotion than a dozen facts."[3] I would suggest that ignorance has been and is often the best of such emotional reasons.

In suggesting that knowledge about structure and physiochemical processes is the criterion for understanding scientifically how a procedure works, an important but unstated value judgment has been made. I will not attempt to defend this judgment, but it should be explicitly noted because it underlies the analysis which follows. While I believe that it is a presumption likely to be shared by nearly everyone reading this chapter and that it is one of the dominant, probably nearly universal presumptions of our age, it is nonetheless still a presumption. This widespread belief posits that physiological medicine (structure and process) is scientific because statements about deliberate changes in the physiological "order" of human beings are: (1) intersubjectively communicable and (2) subjectable to appropriate ("public") confirmation procedures. Clearly much could be said about what being scientific means in this sense, or about why understanding how a procedure affects structure or function is more scientifically important than knowing what works. However, I shall make no effort to defend the currently prevalent conception of scientific medicine against voodoo or witchcraft; indeed, I only want to indicate that this conception is presumed in the discussion which follows.

Intersubjective Communicability

If intersubjective communicability is a minimum condition for scientific understanding in medicine, it is hardly astonishing that there has been so much concern about psychosurgery. Nor is it any wonder that much concern has centered upon the alleged causal relation between the surgical intervention and the sought or claimed behavioral modification. The multiple locutions used to state, indicate, infer, or suggest actual or possible causal or "cause-like" connections between lesions and behavior sufficiently suggest that even the experts may lack scientific understanding of the mechanisms which supposedly obtain. If the core problem in the regulation of psychosurgery is the causation issue, then the most notorious aspect of that issue concerns the connection between psychosurgery and the control of violence. I shall, therefore, use the work of Mark and Ervin to illustrate how intersubjective communicability relates to a supposed causal connection between psychosurgery and violence control. It is appropriate to use their work since they initiated the modern controversy over psychosurgery and violence with *Violence and the Brain,* and have maintained an interest in the subect. However, since their book was published in 1970, I will only call attention to the several different ways its authors characterize the relation in question, and then concentrate upon the most recent (1973) statements of Mark, the neurosurgical member of the team. In the book the authors state that the brain *controls* behavior and that the brain *governs* behavior.[4] It is therefore not surprising to have Mark also state that brain malfunction *causes* violent behavior and that brain disease is *related,* or *linked,* to violence. In 1973 the linkage metaphor is again invoked by now insisting that (1) "there is *solid* medical evidence to link aggressive behavior to focal brain disease."[5] In the same publication a new locution is introduced, for (2) "it is clear that violence is sometimes a *function* of brain abnormalities."[6] Mark relies upon a third locution for what I suppose is one and the same idea: (3) "medical procedures like neurosurgery should be used only when behavior is abnormal, and bad, as the *result* of an abnormality in the brain."[7] In a somewhat expanded version of this article appearing in the *Journal of the American Medical Association (JAMA),* Mark (together with Neville) repeats (3), only now puts it this way: (4) "Medical procedures as drastic as neurosurgery should be used only when behavior is abnormal, and bad, *primarily* because of an abnormality in the brain."[8] In the *JAMA* article there is yet another formulation: (5) "We would have no problem with an abnormal brain that did not *produce* abnormal bad behavior."[9]

In the same article Mark and Neville write that those who see only the relevance of environmental factors: (6) "believe that brain function or dysfunction is not an important *determinant* as far as abnormal behavior is concerned."[10] Because I am interested in causation language, we will not consider the interesting possibilities which might obtain among "brain disease" in (1), "brain abnormalties" in (2), "an abnormality in the brain" in (3) and (4), and "an abnormal brain" in (5). (One wonders whether a tumor on the brain is "an abnormality in the brain," let alone "an abnormal brain," even if it is a "brain disease." Or, on the other hand, if a child prodigy in mathematics has "an abnormal brain," does he therefore have "an abnormality in the brain," let alone a "brain disease"?) The more immediate questions concern the relations among "link," "function," "result," "because," "produce," and "determinant." Are all or any of these synonyms for some sense of "cause"? Is there even some reasonably clear family resemblance (in the sense of a "complicated network of similarities, overlapping and criss-crossing"[11]) among them? If there is a link between A and B, does it mean that A is a function of B, or B of A? If A is a function of B, does it mean that B is the result of A, or A of B? If A is the result of B, does it mean A produces B or that B obtains because of A? There is such a thicket of thorny problems here that one wonders why the authors did not use the straightforward notion of cause throughout. Could they have believed they were illuminating the notion of a causal relationship by using terms like "link" and "result," instead of cause?

Of course, one should not think that Mark and Ervin deliberately avoided "cause" because of its deeply problematical character. On the contrary, in addition to the above six substitutes for "cause," their articles also abound in cause language: (7) "any thorough investigation of abnormal, violent behavior should look not only to the environment for causes, but also to the brain itself;"[12] (8) "the most frequent occurrence of brain dysfunction in violent behavior is in brain poisoning, the most serious and ubiquitous of which is caused by alcohol."[13] While (7) and (8) are fairly straightforward uses of "cause," although I strongly suspect that in (7) the word means something like Hume's "constant conjunction," whereas in (8) it does not,[14] the following cases are even more troublesome: (9) "Our worry is with the behavior directly and with the brain only as a cause or condition of the behavior;"[15] (10) "Our claim is that psychiatric neurosurgery to control violence should be limited to cases where the primary cause of the violence is the brain dysfunction."[16] However, the most disturbing, and at the same time possibly the most illuminating, formulation is the following:

> (11) Obsessive-compulsive neurosis, for instance, is so well accepted as a pathological behavior that when its underlying brain cause is discovered it may well be agreed to be abnormal itself. Radical po-

> litical behavior, by contrast, though intensely not desired by some people, is not agreed by the medical community to be pathological; even if its connections with certain brain functions were established, we would be slow to say those functions were themselves abnormal or pathological.[17]

This last formulation is so disturbing and yet illuminating for three reasons: (1) it makes overt what is frequently covert—that the medical "community" determines pathology; (2) the characterization of brain cell activity as normal or not may well be a function not of the perceived brain chemistry, but rather of the behavior associated with (caused by) the cell activity; and (3) the alleged normalcy of the caused behavior may require that the cell activity be regarded as normal regardless of the abnormality of the actual brain chemistry.

Causation Language and Psychosurgery

In the first six instances cited where words other than "cause" connote something about a possible causal connection, I wondered if there was some reasonably clear family resemblance among the six notions of "link," "function," "result," "because," "produce," and "determinant." In suggesting that these notions connote something about the possible causal connection, I seem to be answering in the affirmative. That is, for the authors, those six words *as embedded* in the above six statements appear to share some connotative or evocative power. The idea the words tend to connote or evoke is that of some relationship between lesion (L) and behavior (B); however, the present question is not if there is *some* relation between L and B, but whether a *causal* relation exists between them. Of the six terms, "link" is the least connotative of a causal relation, and one is only tempted to see some causal connection in (1) because of the idea that there is "solid medical evidence" linking L and B. In other words, because (1) tells us that its author believes that the appropriate model for scientific medicine is the physiological (structure-process) model, and because this idea implies a procedure is scientifically appropriate if how it works (its mechanism) is known, then the "solid medical evidence" reasonably leads us to infer that the linkage between L and B shows how L affects B, and not merely that L does affect B. Similar contextual reconstruction or elaboration makes it easier to see that each of the other five words is intended to connote not merely a relation but some causal relation between L and B. Let us grant that, with suitable contextual elaboration, all six words share a family resemblance in connoting something about a causal relation, but do they also *connote* something about the same sense of causation?

Answering the last question is difficult because the eleven statements make it very clear that no consistent sense of causation is used. "Link" in (1), particularly in connection with the idea of "solid evidence," seems closer to the "constant conjunction" sense of cause. That is, the evidence reveals that when there is L, then regularly there is B. It is this sense of statistical correlation which seems intended by the president of the International Society for Psychiatric Surgery, Dr. William B. Scoville, when he urges that at present "psychiatric surgery" should not be used (12) "to control aggressive behavior unless *accompanied* by proven mental symptoms."[18] This conjunction sense of cause also seems intended by Stephan Chorover, writing in *Psychology Today,* who focuses not upon "the legal and ethical issues raised by the use of psychosurgery as a treatment for violence," but instead "upon its purported scientific basis."[19] He takes this basis to be (13) "whether psychosurgery is a therapeutic procedure in which specific benefits for the patient *reliably follow* the production of brain lesions."[20] Thus, for L and B to be causally linked, or for B to be accompanied by L, or for B reliably to follow L, suggests that if there is a shared sense of causation, it is the sense of a constant conjunction of statistical significance.

We must consider whether this sense of causation suffices if the agreed medical model for scientific understanding is physiological. That is, can we say we have understood scientifically the mechanism by which a lesion in the amygdala effects a diminution in uncontrollable violence if all we know is that L and B are regularly linked or accompanied, or that B reliably follows L? It seems to me that the answer is clearly no. However, and this is most important, this negative answer does not constitute even a necessary, let alone a sufficient, reason for a negative response to the following, very different question: should a medical procedure be regarded as experimental, or as nontherapeutic, or as not to be recommended, if the mechanism by which it works is "understood" only in the causal sense of constant conjunction? If the negative answer to the first question about scientific understanding compelled a negative answer to the second medical practice question, then possibly most of modern medical practice would disappear, a consequence important enough to deter acceptance of "scientific understanding" of the mechanism as a necessary condition for the standard use of a procedure.

However, before further considering this matter, let us see whether there is some other sense of causation common to the family-related "cause" words used above. "Determinant" in (6), "result" in (3), and possibly "primarily because of" in (4) suggest the causation notion of necessary condition. This is a very weak and strained sense of causation when compared with the more usual definition of cause in terms of sufficient (and not merely necessary) conditions. In (6) the writers clearly do not suggest that brain dysfunction is the sufficient condition for abnormal behavior; rather it is "*an* important determinant." That is, at most they suggest that dysfunction is a necessary condition for abnormal behavior, a very dubious suggestion without a good deal of amplification about the meaning of "abnormal." Statement (3) is considerably more obscure than (6) as to whether "an abnormality in the brain" is a sufficient condition for "abnormal, bad behavior." However, modifying "because" with "primarily" in (4) suggests that an abnormality is neither the sole nor sufficient cause of abnormal behavior, and that the intended causal connection is, at best, a necessary condition. Given this weakest sense of "cause," the first question is whether a medical specialist would be practicing scientific medicine if he recommended a brain lesion because whenever there is abnormal, bad behavior, there is abnormality in the brain? The answer becomes obvious when we ask whether a medical specialist would be practicing scientific medicine if he recommended cutting off the oxygen supply because whenever there is abnormal, bad behavior, the subject is breathing? Thus it is obvious that knowledge of merely necessary conditions does not constitute a scientific understanding of how a mechanism works. Again, we must not conclude that a negative answer to the question about scientific understanding automatically or necessarily warrants a negative answer to the very different question about medical practice: is a procedure experimental, nontherapeutic, and not to be recommended if the mechanism by which it works is "understood" only in the "causal" sense of necessary conditions?

Before we turn our attention to the relation between scientific understanding and the practice of medicine, let us consider the last two causation family words used in the above statements. While there is obscurity surrounding "function" in (2), or "produce" in (5), these uses may be quite illuminating. The idea is that (2) brain abnormalties or (5) abnormal brains (2) produce violence or (5) abnormal bad behavior, or that (2) violence or abnormal behavior is a function of such brains. Apparently, as here used, if X is a function of Y, then Y produces X (5), and also if Y produces X, then X is a function of Y (2). Together (2) and (5) imply that X is a function of Y if, and only if, Y produces X. This use of "function" and "produce" is probably fairly grammatized and consistent with prevalent practice. For example, hard work and intelligence *produce* success and success, in turn, is a *function* of hard work and intelligence. However, what sense of causation is connoted by these formulas? Clearly, it cannot be that of constant conjunction, for there are too many cases where success is not a function of either hard work or intelligence, let alone both.

Many philosophical games could be played with "success" and "intelligence," but I think the point is made. Indeed, (2) does not claim that there is a constant conjunction between violence and brain abnormalties but only that the former is *sometimes* the function of the latter. Moreover (5) strongly implies that at least sometimes an abnormal brain (the child prodigy in mathematics?) does not produce abnormal, bad behavior. Thus it is clearly not the constant conjuntion sense of causation which is implied by "function" and "produce."[21] Nor would it appear that the stronger sense of causation as a set of sufficient conditions is connoted by "function" or "produce." Hard work and intelligence are not the sufficient conditions for success; indeed, they are not even necessary conditions. (If marrying the boss's daughter does not qualify as a counterexample, since that might show intelligence, then winning in the state lottery will do.) Thus in (2) and (5) the constant conjunction sense of causation is not operative as it is in (1), (12), and (13), nor is the very weak sense of a necessary condition working in (2) and (5) as in (3), (4), and (6). Finally, (2) and (5) do not rest upon "cause" as a set of sufficient conditions. Are (2) and (5) then outside the causation word family and saying something entirely different from the other statements? I think rather that they connote something about causation not found in the other statements.

In (2) and (5) causation becomes a "differential condition"—a circumstance which, though neither necessary nor sufficient, nonetheless produces an event because, given the presence of the necessary conditions, it makes the difference. The best available analysis of causation in the work of Mark and Ervin is John D. Hodson's:

> When Mark and Ervin describe the results of an ablation which has eliminated violent behavior on the part of its recipient, they are, perhaps, entitled to speak of the removed organ as causally related to the behavior, but only in the sense of a necessary condition. The organ may be necessary for the occurrence of the behavior and, if so, this would explain why its removal resulted in the elimination of the behavior. However, the organ itself, as opposed to its removal, would not in this instance be a differential condition. We find the latter, differential, condition in the instance of the artificial stimulation of the brain which produces violent behavior. Here, the occurrence of the artificial stimulation makes the difference in the occurrence of the behavior. But the artificial stimulation may not be viewed as a necessary condition because the behavior could have been caused by some normal stimulant. Accordingly, since Mark and Ervin are using two senses of "cause," and since the two senses are not coextensive, a question must be raised about the concept of causality employed when it is claimed that brain disease causes violent behavior.[22]

It is this differential condition sense of causation which colors (2) and (5), where the quite grammatical use of "function" and "produce" operates in statements which may support those who defend the use of psychosurgery to control violence "caused" by brain dysfunction (abnormality). But how does this sense of causation compare with the direct causation statements (7), (8), (9), (10), and (11)? While, as with (1) through (6), there is no consistent sense of causation in (7) through (10), let me suggest the sense which I think is operative in these statements so that we may concentrate upon (11). In (7), where brain and environment are said to cause abnormal, bad behavior, the probable sense is conjunction of instances or statistical significance. Statement (8) is actually quite a syntactical curiosity. In its two sentences, there are two causation words used (one twice) and a translation into straightforward cause language would be: "Brain poisoning caused by alcohol is the most frequent cause of brain dysfunction which causes violent behavior." The statement only would make good sense if the differential condition sense were operative, for alcohol is neither necessary nor sufficient for brain dysfunction unless any process abnormality equals brain poisoning, and brain dysfunction is neither necessary nor sufficient for violent behavior. Thus (8) confirms the belief that the differential condition sense of causation renders least ambiguously any grammatically correct causal claim about violence control and psychosurgery.

Statements (9) and (10) are hardly paradigms of clarity, but their difficulties do not arise from an uncertainty about the sense of causation. In (9) the authors are worried about "behavior directly," and about the brain as "only a cause or condition of the behavior." In (10) they claim that psychosurgery should be used to control violence only where brain dysfunction is the "primary cause" of the violence. Although these statements are comprehensible only if the differential condition sense of causation is operative (indeed, (9) speaks of "*a* cause or *condition*"), the interjection of the notion of "primary" in (10) suggests that another sense is also relevant there. However, making sense out of Mark's and Neville's cause and "cause family word" statements is hard enough without also trying to figure out what language game they are playing with the notion of primary (and therefore secondary, if not also tertiary) cause. In the most meaningful interpretation of (10) it would be fair to construe "primary cause" as "the differential condition." Thus translated, (10) would claim that psychosurgery to control violence should only be used where the conditions necessary for violence are present but the cause is neither differential conditions: (a) natural provocation; (b) normal aggression; (c) disastrous childhood; nor (d) (__________); but rather only when the cause is differential condition (n) brain dysfunction.

While (10) begins to be understandable when one can conceive of the kind of evidence which might substantiate its claim, it is because we have some understanding of what is claimed that (11) is both disturbing and illuminating. Statement (11) contrasted obsessive-compulsive neuroses with radical political behavior and questioned whether the latter could be regarded as caused by abnormal brain function if the former was. The statement is important because we have assumed that medicine to be practiced scientifically must use procedures whose physiological effects are understood. A procedure is justified only when it will remove or prevent a physiological abnormality, and the mechanism by which this effect is caused is scientifically understood only when the changes effected in structures or processes are known. We learn from (11), however, that the physiological propriety of the intervention is not decisive, but the plurality of suffrage by the "medical community" is. Indeed, the authors are perfectly frank in adding: "In the long run, there is no guarantee at all, and no protection in clinging to the physiological bias of scientific medicine, that society will not take whatever means are available to do whatever it wants."[23] Their justification for "clinging to the physiological bias" is an apparent belief that such a bias deters the development of "political medicine."

As will become clear in my concluding chapters, I share their antipathy toward the expansion of political medicine. Nonetheless, it is important to see that relying upon the differential-condition sense of causation in constructing and utilizing the psychological model for "scientific" medicine is a political and not a scientific decision. Statement (11) makes this quality clear despite deep and, I think, necessary obscurities in the statement itself. A more direct formulation of (11) could be: (14) if the differential condition for certain behavior is an identifiable specific structure or process in the brain, then, in accordance with the requirements of scientific medicine, deliberate and known changes effected in that structure or process may be a scientifically proper way of causing the behavior to change. This revised formulation avoids the political medicine problem by leaving the characterization of the relevant behavior untouched in favor of making only the relevant scientific claim. No claims are made about whether the behavior is abnormal, or, if abnormal, whether it ought to be changed. It is by treating as fungible the two different questions of how and whether behavior can be scientifically changed that the core problem of causation and psychosurgery becomes unmanageable. I do not wish to imply, however, that if the two questions are separated the core problems are then easily answerable or even answerable at all. I would also not maintain that there is sufficient evidence to support the statement made in (14) on the question about cause and psychosurgery.

The Causal Relation Between Brain and Behavior: The Symmetrical Brain Function Hypothesis

Although some esoteric philosophical theories about behavior may maintain that no causal relation between the brain and at least some behavior exists, I presume it is generally agreed that the brain "governs" behavior and that behavior is the "product" of brain "function." However, we need carefully to evaluate the claim in the antecedent clause in (14) that the differential condition (cause) for specific violent behavior is some identifiable, specific brain structure or process. I shall refer to this theory as the *localization hypothesis*. It should be noticed that (14) goes on to claim that if its hypothesis obtains, then deliberate changes in the identified structure or process may be scientifically proper ways of changing the related behavior. The localization hypothesis is thus the antecedent, and the deliberate change hypothesis the consequence, of the claim made by (14). It is essential to remember, however, that confirmation or acceptance of the localization hypothesis does not imply or require acceptance of the deliberate change hypothesis, and, conversely, that acceptance of the deliberate change hypothesis does not demand confirmation or acceptance of the localization hypothesis. Indeed, this latter proposition aptly characterizes the position of neurologists, psychiatrists, and neurosurgeons like Mark and Ervin, who believe that a deliberate change in a structure or process is *the* proper way to change specific behavior.

While Hodson was concerned primarily with causation as the concept was employed in the Mark and Ervin book, his analysis of the supposed connection between violence and the brain has more general applicability. Hodson argues, on the basis of what they have themselves said about tissue ablation, that Mark and Ervin can claim that removed tissue is a necessary condition for violent behavior, but they cannot suggest that the tissue itself (as distinct from its removal) is a differential condition.

> It seems clear that if "cause" is understood in the sense of a necessary condition, it will not support the causal claim in question. If this claim is asserting that brain malfunction is necessary for violent behavior, then not only is there no reason to believe it, there is also empirical evidence against it, since persons without brain disease

might, under certain circumstances, engage in violence. On the other hand, the understanding of causality as differential condition accords adequately with the claim that brain malfunction causes violent behavior, since we are then asserting that brain malfunction makes the difference between the occurrence and nonoccurrence of the violent behavior. . . . Apparently, [the Mark and Ervin] claim is based on observations of the effects of artificial stimulation of the brain. They show that it is possible to produce attack behavior through the stimulation of certain areas of the brain and to stop attack behavior through the stimulation of other nearby areas. Interesting though it may be, this in no way establishes a connection between brain *malfunction* and violent behavior, for the same result might be produced through normal stimulation. Such observations, at best, show that the stimulated areas of the brain are causally related to the occurrence of the behavior, perhaps as necessary conditions. . . .

[Mark and Ervin] told of the cases of Mary C., Clara T., Thomas R., and Julia S., all of whom have exhibited violent behavior and are said to have brain malfunctions. In each case, the patient underwent stereotactic surgery, in which part of the amygdala (a lobule of the cerebellum) [*sic*] was destroyed. After the surgery, the occurrence of violent behavior was either reduced considerably or eliminated entirely. However, in each of the cases cited, *the brain malfunction which the patient had before the surgery was observed to remain after the operation.* Mark and Ervin note this result in each case with some regret, but they are "gratified" that the violent behavior has been eliminated. This seems a rather casual response to a result which, as I shall argue, shows that their technique amounts to no more than the "treatment" of violent behavior instead of brain disease, and which, therefore, renders the justification in question inapplicable. . . . Thus, while the argument in question calls for the elimination of violent behavior through the removal of the disease which causes it, stereotactic surgery does indeed eliminate the violent behavior, but *not* through the removal of the disease. Stereotactic surgery, therefore, cannot be defended by the argument, despite appearances to the contrary, because it does not involve the treatment of the brain disease. The only "malfunction" eliminated by that procedure is the violent behavior.

We may see the importance of this fact about stereotactic surgery through a comparison of that procedure with one which would be defensible by the argument in question. One procedure which might serve us here is the surgical removal of a brain tumor. Assuming that there is a noncontroversial criterion for the presence

> of a brain tumor, and given a tumor which causes violent behavior, a surgical technique which removes that tumor is defensible by the argument because the violent behavior would be eliminated through the removal of the disease which caused it. In terms of the analyses of causality mentioned above, the removal of a brain tumor which causes violence would be the removal of the differential condition for the violence. The stereotactic surgery described by Mark and Ervin differs significantly from this procedure. Since the brain malfunction remains after the surgery, the differential condition for the violent behavior has not been eliminated. Instead, stereotactic surgery prevents violent behavior through the removal of what appears to be merely a necessary condition for its occurrence.[24]

According to Hodson, since Mark and Ervin have confused the treatment of violent behavior with the treatment of brain malfunction, they cannot claim anything as sweeping as (14), but only that, in some cases, psychosurgery can remove a necessary condition (but not the cause) of violent behavior. While this is a generally convincing critique of the claim by Mark and Ervin to anything like (14), we must consider if the same argument, when not limited to *Violence and the Brain,* defeats either (14) or the localization hypothesis.

There are two important legs to Hodson's argument: (A) establishing a connection between brain function and specific behavior (violent or otherwise) does not establish a causal connection between brain malfunction and that behavior and (B) if the brain malfunction (disease) remains after the surgical removal of brain tissue, then that disease could not have been the differential condition (cause) of the behavior which disappeared or improved after the surgery. While (A) attacks the antecedent of (14), the localization hypothesis, (B) strikes at the consequent of (14), the deliberate change hypothesis. (A), however, is not an attack upon the localization theory (specific behavior is caused by identifiable, specific structures or processes), but rather an assault upon the extension of that theory: if specific behavior normal X is caused by specific structure Y, then specific behavior, abnormal X, is caused by the malfunction of Y. In other words, (A) denies the theory (15) that if, for example, normal aggressivity is a function of the amygdala, then abnormal aggressivity must also be controlled by the same structure. Mark and Ervin advance no evidence to support (15); indeed, their four reported cases are counterexamples of (15) because the malfunctions continued after the specific behavior was changed. However, the ideological thrust of Hodson's first criticism (A) goes beyond the Mark and Ervin experience.

Let us apply (A) to a "favorable" hypothetical case.

Case 1: P has a history of abnormal, bad aggression. On the basis of psychiatric evaluation, psychological testing and neurological evaluation, P is subjected to depth EEG studies involving ESB with remote telemetry. These EEG tracings are interpreted as supporting the prior evaluation of P as suffering from some malfunction in the amygdala, and on the basis of the EEG data, the specific site in the amygdala is identified as the target for the stereotactic ablation. After surgery, P is no longer abnormally aggressive and further testing shows no remaining EEG patterns in the amygdala which are interpreted as abnormal.

Case 1 thus differs from the cases cited by Mark and Ervin in that surgery either "corrected" the malfunction or "cured" the disease, or at the very least, the malfunction or disease no longer persists after the intervention. Criticism (A) is still applicable because Case 1, a decided counterexample, does not defeat (A), but instead provides evidence that localized brain function is symmetrical; that is, if normal X is a function of structure Y, then abnormal X is also. It could still be argued that Case 1 is of no help since the electrical stimulation of the diseased amygdala tissue by itself could have cured P even without the surgery. However, enough instances like Case 1 in their relevant respects would diminish, if not defeat, the plausibility of nonsurgical explanations about the "cure" for the disease; that is, the behavior was caused by the malfunction. One must realize that even when thus favorably interpreted, Case 1 and other similar cases do not establish the theory of symmetrical localized brain function (if good X is a function of structure Y, then bad X is also), but at best establish or support *only* the *different* theory that bad X was a function of X. Indeed, since destroyed brain cells are not regenerated, there is obviously no way to show that the "corrected" structure causes the now normal (specific) behavior. All one knows is that other structures, free of the malfunctioning one, cause the now normal behavior—a very different and more modest thesis than that of symmetrical localized brain function.

I have continually referred only to brain structure and not to physiochemical processes in the brain because at this time, the use of psychosurgery to control behavior could not possibly rest upon a theory of localized brain function when the function is a process. In any event, I know of no justification for the use of psychosurgery based on a theory of localized brain process.

How does (A) affect the claim made by (14)? If the symmetrical localized brain theory is impeached, is the claim of (14) imperiled? It is clear that (A), even if valid, does not affect (14) because the latter is not dependent upon how the specific behavior is characterized. In other words, (14) does not rest upon the symmetry hypothesis but only upon the localization theory. Statement (14) claims only that if X is a function of Y, then changing Y may be a proper way of changing X. This argument does not require showing that Y causes normal X and therefore that abnormal Y causes abnormal X; normal and abnormal are not relevant to this hypothesis and thus a sufficient collection of cases like Case 1 would substantiate the claim of (14). Statement (14) is entirely consistent with the belief that if the malfunctioning, diseased structure (the part of the amygdala in Case 1) is removed, then the rest of the brain will function normally and "cause" normal behavior.

The Causal Relation Between Brain and Behavior: The Localization Hypothesis

If Hodson's criticism (A) was an attack upon the symmetrical brain function hypothesis, then (B) is an assault upon the localization hypothesis itself. Criticism (B) claims that if the malfunction continues after surgery, but the abnormal behavior does not, then the malfunction could not have been the differential condition (cause) of the behavior. This argument is difficult to grasp because what is meant by *the* malfunction or *the* disease which is the abnormal behavior's alleged cause needs to be clarified. If a malfunction has consequences (C 1), (C 2), and (C 3), and, if after some treatment of the malfunction, (C 1) has disappeared but (C 2) and (C 3) remain, can we say that *the untreated* malfunction was not the differential condition for (C 1)? It seems to me that (B) fails to recognize that the malfunction which Mark and Ervin report as persisting after surgery is not *the* (untreated) malfunction which obtained when there was abnormal behavior. Indeed, in a certain logical sense, the postsurgery malfunction could not possibly be the presurgery malfunction since unregenerative malfunctioning brain tissue was destroyed. Thus, lacking considerable rehabilitation through construction of a particular conception of malfunction or disease, (B) does not require abandoning the claim advanced by (14).

This concern about *the* malfunction or disease raises another important question about (14) because its claim rests squarely on the localization hypothesis; indeed (14)'s claim is weakened, if not defeated, by those who support what may be called the *generalized brain function hypothesis*. According to this theory, *the* malfunction or disease which causes abnormal behavior cannot be localized in any identifiable specific structure or process because abnormal behavior is caused by a malfunctioning, diseased brain. Thus, one cannot simultaneously support (14) and the generalized brain function hypothesis.

Is it useful to consider whether the localized brain function theory is "right?" Or, as is usually the case with polar extremes, do both brain function theories exacerbate rather than illuminate the problems? Both theories have been around for a long while. The "first published account of psychosurgery in 1891 by Dr. Gottlieb Burckhardt, who supervised the Insane Asylum in Préfargier, Switzerland," justified brain surgery on psychiatric patients on the theory that " 'our psychological existence is composed of single elements, which are localized in separate areas of the brain.' "[25] To know that both theories are old and hotly defended is not very helpful, for as any amateur historian of science will attest, neither durability nor popularity are very reliable measures of the utility or power of a theory. Consequently, instead of debating which theory is right or better, it is more helpful to "localize" our inquiry by rigorously identifying the contexts within which we will use either theory. Let me illustrate "localizing the context" by an example from a recent review of a number of books in neuropsychiatry:

> it is becoming increasingly possible to conceive how personality and brain function are connected. It seems clear that the brain works much more as a whole than was previously realised. When brain maps were first made, it was thought that, as these became more accurate, function could be more and more closely pinpointed. Brain maps are still essential; and nothing alters the fact that if a "stroke"

> deprives the left motor cortex of its blood supply, the patient will suffer paralysis of his right arm and leg. But, when consideration is given to the "higher" functions of cerebral activity, it is clear that the brain acts as a whole and that pin-point localisation is an insufficient explanation.[26]

In other words, the localization hypothesis suffices for some purposes but not for others and as an explanation of how personality or character affects physiological brain function, the localization hypothesis is probably irrelevant given our current knowledge. However, it does not therefore follow that this hypothesis is inadequate if the context of inquiry is whether an amygdalotomy should be considered. The localization hypothesis may be inadequate for this purpose too. If so, this is not because it is inadequate in some other context.

Although I shall return to this important point, let me initially generalize about what it means for the localization hypothesis to be adequate or inadequate. For scientific medicine (and science generally), "causal relations can be regarded as the elements (the 'alphabet' in Bacon's phrase) out of which scientific explanation is composed. . . . Causes are the primitive empirical ingredients out of which more comprehensive explanations are constructed."[27] And since "every cause-effect relation implies a system of laws, a theory, . . . one might expect 'the' cause of a given effect to change with the state of knowledge about it . . . [and]. . . . This is usually the case."[28] The specific brain structure or process is no more the "real" cause of abnormal behavior than is the whole brain, for there are no real causes in this abstract, universal sense: "There are [rather] only models of the world that are more or less adequate according to general scientific criteria, which will include notions of predictiveness, simplicity, generality, etc."[29] Thus, we should regard the localization hypothesis as an intellectual device which makes a certain sphere of activity more manageable, one whose utility resides in its furnishing a mechanism for generalizing about a specific range of experiences which makes possible more accurate predictions within that field.

Among those standards used to judge the utility of any scientific theory, predictiveness is probably the most important and is clearly paramount in the practice of medicine. Thus in assessing whether the local or the general brain function theory is "right," one must specify the context and purpose of the inquiry. Our purpose then is to discover if there are cases where a neurosurgeon is justified in destroying specific brain tissue believed to be the differential condition (cause) for specific behavior. Within the limited context of our present concern about abnormal, aggressive, or violent behavior, (14) may be attractive because the localization hypothesis, though a less powerful general explanation of behavior than the generalized brain function hypothesis, is based upon a comprehensible, simpler model of brain function which makes possible the most accurate predictions as to the consequences of certain interventions. The claim made by (14) can thus be subjected to some reasonable confirmation procedure and so become at least scientifically respectable, which would not be possible if it could be neither disconfirmed *or* confirmed. While not arguing that amygdalotomy to control violence is justified, or that any other specific psychosurgical procedure is warranted, I *am* saying that neither the generalized brain function hypothesis nor shotgun attacks upon psychosurgery which argue general brain function defeat the claim of (14). I should also like to note that while the localization hypothesis and the consequent claim made by (14) are subject to disconfirmation, such disconfirmation has not yet been furnished. As a necessary corollary, it is important to remember also that while confirmation has not yet been furnished, such confirmation is neither logically nor empirically impossible.

Chorover's discussion of psychosurgery in a recent issue of *Psychology Today* illustrates, through its imprecision, the shotgun attack based on general brain function:

> In 1937, Heinrich Klüver and Paul C. Bucy reported that they had destroyed the temporal lobes and parts of the limbic system in rhesus monkeys. After the operations, they observed striking derangements in the behavior of the monkeys. . . .
>
> The "Klüver-Bucy syndrome" demonstrated that temporal lobe structures are involved in a wide range of behavioral activities. Its dramatic features soon induced other investigators to pursue similar studies. For our purposes, the most important subsequent discovery was that in many species, several of the more severe emotional aspects of the syndrome could be produced by lesions restricted to one part of the limbic system, the amygdala.
>
> The results of these animal experiments suggest that no single part of the limbic system is concerned with only a single aspect of

> behavior. They should make us skeptical about the claim that specific therapeutic effects are attainable by destroying the amygdala or various other parts of the limbic system.[30]

Even though the article appeared in a quasi-popular publication, it is certainly reasonable to expect that, before we are told of animal experiments suggesting the unsoundness of the localization hypothesis, we should learn: (1) why the experiments on animals are relevant; (2) whether any of the animal work involved very small amygdala lesions, and if such lesions were also the cause for general deterioration; (3) if there is any work on humans involving comparably restricted amygdala lesions (e.g., comparing the effects of a 5 percent destruction in man and animals); and (4) whether the reported work on humans suggests that the results obtained with animals will also obtain in humans. It is worth noticing that Elliot S. Valenstein, who has made the most careful review of the psychosurgery literature, answers the most important question, the fourth, in the negative. His research indicates that stereotactic destruction of amygdala tissue in humans has *not* been followed by development of the Klüver-Bucy syndrome.[31]

More important than Chorover's factual omissions is the curiously illogical character of his conclusion. Even if there were good reasons for believing that "no single part of the limbic system is concerned with only a single aspect of behavior," why would it therefore follow that we should be skeptical "about the claim that specific therapeutic effects are attainable by destroying the amygdala?" At most, the antecedent clause should make us skeptical about specific effects which have no adverse or unwanted side effects, but not about some specific effects being attained. For example, it may be the case that abnormal aggression can be significantly diminished or prevented by ablation of certain amygdala areas, but that the patient will also lose his natural sexual aggressivity. Thus, ablation in the specified place has a specific effect, and so the animal work which might warrant rejection of the localization hypothesis does not *therefore* warrant rejecting the claim that specific behavior can be changed by specific brain lesions.

It is possible that by "specific therapeutic effects" Chorover means that the consequences of that intervention will be diffuse. This is the so-called "side effects" question, and what the writer contends (if this is what he means by "specific effects") is that any intervention will have some side effects (in addition to the specific effect) which are not specifiable. This is a controversial and complex issue, and although he has introduced the subject of side effects, Chorover has not dealt with it.

Apart from the imprecise statement of his argument, and the dubious logic of its conclusion, there are still more important reasons for rejecting Chorover's analysis. If our purpose is "to discover whether there are cases where a neurosurgeon would be justified in destroying specific brain tissue because it is believed to be the differential condition (cause) for specific behavior," then Chorover's shotgun argument furnishes no help at all. Although we have frequently come to this justification or medical practice question only to defer analysis, and must do so again, let me suggest a small part of what such an analysis involves and why the shotgun argument is useless. Let us assume that in addition to the intended (predictable) specific effect of the tissue destruction, there are also some diffuse, unspecifiable effects. How does this predictable consequence help in deciding whether the intervention is unjustified? The predictable specific effect may be intensely desired by the patient, and besides it is possible that unspecifiable mechanisms in the brain may compensate for the destroyed tissue.[32] In addition, the unpredictability of some specific side effects does not necessarily imply that no prediction can be made about the patient's general postsurgery condition. Finally, there is hardly conclusive evidence that the unpredictable, specific side effects are all bad or that the brain as a whole will be worse off. Chorover may be right in urging that "many psychosurgeons continue to ignore [the fact that 'no brain activity occurs in isolation, without correlated activity in other regions'] in favor of a pretentious and extreme doctrine of brain localization."[33] But is it not equally true that many psychosurgeons favor a pretentious and extreme doctrine of generalized brain function? The point is that without any elucidation of what it means for such theories to be "pretentious and extreme," we really know nothing about why such theories are unattractive. Chorover furnishes no means to discriminate between localization or generalization theories which are pretentious and extreme and those which are not; consequently, his analysis furnishes no help in dealing with the medical practice-justification problem.

Psychosurgery: Curing the Cause or Removing a Symptom?

Before directly confronting the justification problem, we need to consider whether specific tissue destruction cures the cause of a specific "related" behavior or merely removes a symptom. This is indeed a philosophically murky puddle, the water of which has been vigorously stirred by Wittgenstein, particularly in the *Blue Book* (1933–34):

> Let us introduce two antithetical terms in order to avoid certain elementary confusions: To the question "How do you know that so-and-so is the case?", we sometimes answer by giving '*criteria*' and sometimes by giving '*symptoms*.' If medical science calls angina an inflammation caused by a particular bacillus, and we ask in a particular case "why do you say this man has got angina?" then the answer "I have found the bacillus so-and-so in his blood" gives us the criterion, or what we may call the defining criterion of angina. If on the other hand the answer was, "His throat is inflamed," this might give us a symptom of angina. I call "symptom" a phenomenon of which experience has taught us that it coincided, in some way or other, with the phenomenon which is our defining criterion. Then to say "A man has angina if this bacillus is found in him" is a tautology or it is a loose way of stating the definition of "angina." But to say, "A man has angina whenever he has an inflamed throat" is to make a hypothesis. . . . Doctors will use the names of diseases without ever deciding which phenomena are to be taken as criteria and which as symptoms; and this need not be a deplorable lack of clarity. For remember that in general we don't use language according to strict rules. . . . [34]

Commenting upon the passage, Charles S. Chihara and J. A. Fodor offer the following explanation of the difference between "criterion" and "symptom":

> [A] symptom is "a phenomenon of which experience has taught us that it coincided, in some way or other, with the phenomenon which is our defining criterion" (BB, p. 25). Though both symptoms and criteria are cited in answer to the question, "How do you know that so-and-so is the case?" (BB, p. 24), symptoms, unlike criteria, are discovered through experience or observation: that something is a symptom is not given by the rules of the "language-game" (not deducible from the rules alone).[35]

They add that despite "this important difference between criteria and symptoms, the fact remains that Wittgenstein considered both symptoms and criteria as 'evidences.' "[36] Rogers Albritton makes the same point in his well-known essay, "On Wittgenstein's Use of the Term 'Criterion' ": "one may sometimes answer the question 'How do you know that so-and-so is the case?' quite as irreproachably by 'giving symptoms' as by 'giving criteria,' and this is what Wittgenstein thinks as far as I can find."[37] He continues:

> Criteria are for [Wittgenstein] primarily criteria that men "accept," "adopt," "fix," "introduce," and "use" or "apply" in connection with their use of certain *expressions*. If anything is the criterion of X and therefore a logically necessary and sufficient condition of X, it is because (in some sense of "because") men agree in certain *conventions*. ("Here we strike rock bottom, that is we have come down to conventions.")[38]

Wittgenstein's point, when applied to whether psychosurgery cures causes or removes symptoms, is that no real or right answer exists. Since his use of "criterion" is much like the sense of cause as the set of necessary and sufficient conditions, what Wittgenstein argues is quite clear. "Doctors will use the names of diseases without ever deciding which phenomena are to be taken as criteria and which as symptoms."[39] Albritton adds: "We are unable clearly to circumscribe the concepts we use, not because we don't know their real definition, but because there is no real 'definition' to them."[40] In other words, whether X is the necessary and sufficient condition, the criterion or the cause for Y is a matter "founded on a definition" or "founded on convention."[41] Thus, whether psychosurgery only cures causes or only removes symptoms is a question whose answer is not determined by the structural or biochemical phenomena of brain function; rather, the answer depends upon what we mean when we use or apply the word "cure." Because Wittgenstein's general operationalist theory of language makes clear that these are appropriate inquires, anyone approaching the medical practice-justification question must consider the ramifications of "used or applied." By whom, under what circumstances, and for what purpose?

The most important single concept which concerns Wittgenstein in all three parts of the *Philosophical Investigations* is "understanding,'' and in analyzing that concept he elucidates what is meant by ''meaning.'' A. M. Quinton, describing Wittgenstein's analysis, points out: ''The fundamental point of [his] new theory of meaning is that the meaning of a word is not any sort of object for which the word stands. . . . [Instead] to talk about the meaning of a word is to talk about the way in which it is used. To say of a man that he has learned or understands the meaning of a word is simply to say that he has learned or understands how to use it, that he has become party to a certain established social convention.''[42] Quinton's interpretation makes ''meaning'' clearer than does Wittgenstein, who however makes it quite apparent that he is concerned with language as an operation. ''Language is an instrument. Its concepts are instruments.'' ''To understand a sentence means to understand a language. To understand a language means to be master of a technique.'' ''Every sign by *itself* seems dead. *What* gives it life? . . . In use it is *alive*. Is life breathed into it there?—Or is the *use* its life?''[43]

The suggestion that usage determines meaning and understanding is important to our concern about psychosurgery. ''[T]o imagine a language means to imagine a form of life,'' and, if use is the source of meaning and understanding, then ''what has to be accepted, the given, is—so one could say—*forms of life*.'' ''Let the use of words teach you their meaning.''[44] The important thing to remember in looking for meaning or understanding is the *fact* that ''*this language-game is played*.''[45] Consequently, whether A understands or knows the meaning of X means finding out if A plays ''this language-game'' and seeing how A uses X in fact. As Quinton puts it:

> [Wittgenstein] sums up his theory of meaning by saying that the language games, within which alone words have meaning, are forms of life, modes of activity governed by systems of rules. . . . To understand something is to be able to apply it. . . . An image or formula as it stands can be interpreted or understood in different ways. Only its publicly observable application can show if the interpretation made of it is the correct one. Essentially the same argument is applied to the concept of meaning something by a word. What a man means by a word is not a private experience, in particular it is not an image which is itself a symbol that can be meant, i.e., used, in very different ways. The meaning a man attaches to a word is only to be discovered by considering the things to which he applies, and from

> which he withholds, the word and the verbal contexts, the statements and arguments, in which he employs it. [Wittgenstein] concludes that language is an essentially social phenomenon. The making of noises does not become linguistic utterance unless it is governed by rules, unless there is an applicable distinction between the correct and mistaken use of words.[46]

P. F. Strawson makes the same point:

> [Wittgenstein] begins with the point that the fundamental criteria for whether someone has understood an expression lie in the application which he makes of it. . . . So the production of the picture or paraphrase, though normally (and rightly) enough to satisfy us, is not the final test: *that* resides in the application.[47]

Thus:

> The criterion for the learner's having understood the rule aright is his application of it. But not *any* application (anything that could possibly be represented as an application of the expression of the rule) will do. It must be the *correct* application. But what are the criteria for correctness? Here again one is inclined to answer that the correct application is the one that was meant: and this answer may once more give us the picture of all the steps being somehow covered in advance by the act of meaning. This idea is *very* compelling. For does not the *sense* of the rule (of the expression) determine what is to count as the correct application of it? . . . Natural, but of course wrong: (or at least misleading). The criterion for the correct application of the rule is *customary practice* . . . the customary practice of those who have received a certain training; the way we are taught to use the rule and do always use it.[48]

How is all this discussion of language any help in deciding whether psychosurgery cures the cause or only removes a symptom? From it we get the very important idea that any justification for thinking, saying, or acting as though psychosurgery cures the cause (or only removes a symptom) is discovered by seeing what, in fact, people do; indeed, one of the major strands in Wittgenstein's theory of meaning or understanding is that "what people accept as a justification—is shown by how they think and live."[49] "Our mistake is to look for an explanation where we ought to look at what happens as a 'proto-phenomenon.' That is, where we ought to have said: *this language-game is played.*"[50] Two sections later, he adds: "Look on the language-game as the *primary* thing. And look on the feelings, etc., as you look on a way of regarding the language-game, as interpretation."[51]

Thus we want to find out how "cause" and "symptom" are used and applied[52] by those who have learned this "psychosurgery language-game," which in turn means identifying the relevant population and context ("What is happening now has significance —in these surroundings. The surroundings give it its importance"[53]). Let us contrast different situations and surroundings to illustrate how the appropriate population and context determine this language-game's relevance to the claims made about psychosurgery; that is, let us see how we might test the claim made by (14). In considering the following illustrations, we must bear in mind that: (1) despite important intrinsic differences between causes as matters of definition and convention and symptoms as matters of experience, both can serve as "evidence;" (2) whether X is accepted as a criterion for Y or as a symptom is not a matter of logic, but of experience and linguistic history; and (3) understanding is shown by correct application and correct application is a function of how those indoctrinated into this language-game think and live in a given "surrounding." In connection with (2) we must avoid conceptualizing an artificial, isolated system and concentrate instead on one where the contextual variables are taken into account because: "it is impossible to isolate all the contextual variables that might affect a given causal relation. At some point, the search for contextual variables must be given up, presumably when a 'satisfactory' degree of reliability in the relation has been attained."[54] It is this inevitable arbitrariness in giving up the search for contextual variables which partly accounts for Wittgenstein's insistence that whether X is a criterion or symptom of Y is a moot point. J. E. R. Staddon summarized Wittgenstein's position by noting that the "separation between cause and context is often quite arbitrary: it is a matter of convenience what we consider as cause and what context. . . . In practice, it is usual to consider as a possible cause of a particular effect just the restricted property of the environment to which we happen to be attending, and which is accessible to our manipulation. Everything else is lumped together as context."[55]

The following account and illustrations should be considered with these factors in mind, as they bear on the medical practice-justification question:

> One interesting case of confused causation is the modern epidemic of lead poisoning. For years we clinicians were faced by retarded epileptic children with high serum lead values, and we concluded that the child's symptoms were due to or caused by the circulating lead. We were overjoyed to have another treatable disease. Chelating agents removed much of the lead, the child improved, and we happily sent him home. We were chagrined when he returned with an even higher serum lead level, but we concluded that he had had another attack of the disease. We took years to realize that our medicine was good, but our thinking was bad. The elevated serum lead in these children was one aspect of the pathogenesis of the disease, but it was not "the cause." We had to go one step farther. The cause of lead poisoning in children is peeling lead paint. That is the cause that must be removed. The removal of the lead from the serum is not an attack at the disease's cause or even an attempt to control the disease's progress, because as soon as the child is released to his unchanged environment, the disease continues. Our faulty identification of the cause of lead poisoning has resulted in the ludicrous attempt of the medical profession to leech the lead from peeling paint by using the human body as a carrier. Our FDA-approved chelating agents do not work on walls; we therefore allow children to eat the paint so that we can remove the lead from the children's circulation, where our wonder drugs work so well.[56]

Illustration A: The Cause of Lead Poisoning

Context 1: At the annual meeting of the National Medical Association, the invited speaker says: "After three years of intensive work, the research team at Super University, working under a grant from HEW, has conclusively shown that circulating lead causes the high serum lead values found in retarded epileptic children."

Context 2: At the annual meeting of the National Pharmaceutical Manufacturers Association, the invited speaker says: "I am happy to report that chelating agents have been developed which produce lower serum lead values."

Context 3: At the annual meeting of the National Paint Manufacturers Association the invited speaker says: "A concerted effort must now be made to develop a new paint base because we now know that lead-base paints cause retardation in children."

In each context, there is no doubt that the invited speaker knew the meaning of "cause" (or "produce") and that the audience clearly understood what was said. "Cause" in each context obviously means something quite different, but nonetheless each audience knew what to think and do in their professional lives. Doctors should check lead serum levels in retarded children. Drug company detail men should tell doctors about their medicines for curing lead poisoning, and paint manufactures should try to make lead-free paint.

In the next three contexts, is it equally clear that each invited speaker knew the meaning of "cause," or that his audience understood what he meant?

Context 4: At the annual meeting of the National Industrial Economics Association, the invited speaker says: "It costs four times as much to produce lead-free paint as that which contains a lead base, and it is this cost differential which causes lead poisoning."[57]

Context 5: At the annual meeting of the National Association of Child Social Workers, the invited speaker says: "The affluent will not tolerate peeling paint so we see that it is poverty which causes lead poisoning."

Context 6: At the annual meeting of the National Association for Adult Education, the invited speaker says: "It is the lack of education about the significance of peeling paint which causes lead poisoning."

What distinguishes the first three from the last three contexts as to how "cause" was correctly used, applied, or understood by speaker or audience? In addition to increasingly metaphorical, nonstandard uses, and increasingly heterogeneous audiences, the last two contexts were so unspecific, the "surrounding" so indefinite, that the context did not make clear the relevant contextual variables. Or, put differently, even though there need not be a lamentable loss of clarity because of arbitrariness about criterion (cause) or symptom, or the lack of a sufficiently homogeneous population and sufficiently specific context, there is no shared language-game, and hence no shared form of life.

Let us consider, for example, the degree of audience homogeneity and context specificity presumed by statements such as:

(1) "Who could have dreamt a generation ago . . . that advances in chemotherapy and other therapeutic procedures would create [cause] a new staphylococcus pathology?"[58]

(2) "The issues posed by the physician-induced [caused] condition known as tardive dyskinesia can no longer be ignored."[59]

(3) "We see mental distress as a reaction to the world. We reject the proposition that the source [cause] of distress is inside the person's brain."[60]

These, like any other noises which function as language, presume an audience homogeneity which assures technical competence in playing the relevant game, and a context specificity sufficient to assure that the rule-competent audience knows which game to play. Knowledge of a game's rules does not guarantee that one will automatically play the right game. If, while playing baseball, your child breaks a window next door, and your neighbor subsequently approaches swinging a baseball bat, you do not expect to play baseball, even if you know all that game's rules. Conversely, even if one knows which game is to be played, whether that knowledge is implied or otherwise acquired from context specificity, he is not assured of playing the right game. If you see your neighbor swinging a baseball bat and he calls you over, you may well understand that you have been invited to play the game, but, lacking knowledge of its rules, you will still be unable to play, even though the homogeneity presumed or required to play this particular game is neither moral, political, nor social, but simply competence as to a playing technique. The language-game, however, *is* a form of life, and whether there is a shared technique because of shared values or vice versa, is similar to the criterion-symptom dilemma. It is a moot question whether shared values are a symptom of shared language-game competence or whether such competence is a symptom of shared values. In trying to decide the medical practice-justification question an arbitrariness in labeling symptom and criterion is not critical; however, this lack of precision does not imply that there is no need to ask whether tissue destruction removes a symptom (a necessary condition) or a cause (the differential condition). It is, therefore, not idle metaphysical speculation to try and diminish the arbitrary distinguishing of cause from symptom by clarifying the use, role, function, or application of the relevant words and concepts. For the medical practice-justification question any diminution in arbitrariness will affect the decision as to whether there are cases where psychosurgery is justified.

Making the same point in his illuminating article, "The Medical

Model: Its Nature and Problems," Robert Veatch uses what he regards as a "standard classification of the total realm of human behavior" and divides "behavior into organic, psychological, social, and cultural sub-systems."[61] He then concentrates upon the organic subsystem which is generally regarded as the basis for scientific medicine (I referred to the physiological [structure-process] model, but in this context the two terms are probably identical.) Veatch shows that the "notion of organicity as an essential element of the medical model" is confusing because the "appropriateness" of the medical (organic) intervention is questionable at the four different stages where such intervention might be relevant. The stages he distinguishes are "the deviant behavior itself, the response (treatment), the proximal cause and the ultimate cause."[62] The core of his argument suggests that, given our present state of knowledge about the brain, any diminution in arbitrarily saying psychosurgery removes only a symptom (or cures only a cause) will not materially influence the legal or moral response to the medical practice-justification question.

Veatch elaborates his four stages in a discussion of drug addiction:

> a. *Behavioral Stage*. Taking narcotic addiction as our model, we shall see that the confusion about organicity (and, therefore, about the appropriateness of the medical model) begins at the level of the deviant behavior itself. What is the behavior (symptom) which arouses our interest in narcotic addiction? On the one hand, there are clearly organic symptoms experienced by the addict in withdrawal —nausea, vomiting. . . . Yet narcotic addiction also produces psychological symptoms —euphoria, craving, feelings of dependency. Perhaps the social and cultural impact arouses the most interest, however. The narcotic addict's symptoms, albeit derivatively, include social impact which is economic and political. . . .
>
> b. *Response Stage*. At another stage, that of response to the deviant behavior, narcotic addiction may be classified as organic. The addict may be maintained on maintenance doses or brought down on gradually declining doses of narcotics. . . . But other forms of response are possible to these doubtful illnesses, including jail, social and psychological manipulation, preaching, moral exhortation, and peer group pressure. On the other hand, clearly nonsomatic forms of social deviancy can be controlled by the use of organic agents. . . .

> c. *Proximal Cause State*. The contrast between an abortion for socio-economic reasons and one for "medical" reasons such as a cancerous uterus indicates the third stage of sub-system analysis. In the abortion for the cancerous uterus the cause of the "problem" is also organic. In narcotic addiction, the cause of the deviant behavior may also be seen as organic. There certainly are organic changes in the body when one is addicted. . . . We need to distinguish between the immediate causes of addiction, which are at least partially organic in character, from earlier causes. Let us use the terms proximal and ultimate causes.
>
> d. *Ultimate Cause Stage*. Even if the proximal or immediate cause of addictive behavior is organic, which it may well be, it is still an open question whether the earlier or "ultimate" cause is organic. There are at least three addiction theories proposed today. The psychological theories are based on the belief that there are "addiction prone personalities." . . . Sociological theories place causation in the surrounding environment of the addict. . . . A third theory of causation is biochemical. While holders of all theories are willing to concede that the proximal cause of addiction has a biochemical component, holders of the biochemical causation theory place organic chemical factors in a much more central place. . . . If, however, one were to argue that there are anatomical or biochemical predisposing factors which lead certain individuals to addiction —say by the presence of aberrant enzymes or biochemical ratios —then organic causation would be ultimate in the sense in which we are using the term. There are analogous causation theories for homosexuality and schizophrenia. Narcotic addiction is organic at the level of ultimate cause only according to the biochemical causation theory.
>
> The confusion over the placing of narcotic addiction into the medical model on the dimension of organicity is thus seen. It is only ambiguously organic at each of the four stages of analysis: behavior, response, proximal, and ultimate cause.[63]

Veatch elaborates this analysis by showing how confusedly organicity is applied to heart attacks, alcoholism, and homosexuality, and then makes two interesting comments about the psychosurgery problem:

> The relationship between organicity and non-voluntariness is important. There is quite clearly an association between a belief in organicity and non-voluntariness. If behavior is "in the chemistry," we are convinced it is not in the control of the will.[64]

> There are (or at least theoretically may be) deviances which are considered non-organic in ultimate and proximal cause as well as in behavior, yet susceptible to chemical, surgical, or other medical "treatment" (response). We know, with a degree of certainty, that amygdalotomy will control violent behavior while we may not be certain that the "cause" of the behavior is somatic.[65]

On the basis of this analysis of the causation problem the following conclusions seem warranted:

(1) "Differential condition" and "causing" in the claim made by (14) are grammatically correct in the language-game which medical doctors and scientists play.

(2) Those who say that psychosurgery can cure the cause of certain specified, abnormal behavior use and apply the notion of "cause" correctly and their statements will be correctly understood by anyone who has mastered the technique of the medical science language-game.

(3) Those who say psychosurgery removes only a symptom and does not cure the cause also correctly use and apply the notion of "cause" and will be understood correctly by anyone who has mastered the technique of the medical science language-game.

(4) "Psychosurgery can cure the cause of specific abnormal behavior" and "psychosurgery cannot cure the cause of specific abnormal behavior (but can only remove a symptom)" are inconsistent because the use and application of "cause" is grammatically correct in both statements.

(5) The philosophy of science currently furnishes no generally accepted "form of life" which can serve as the necessary and sufficient condition (the criterion) for the use or application of the notion of cause so that either of the above uses is ruled out. In other words, the currently appropriate language-game which has institutionalized the "correct" usage of "cause" in contexts such as those here relevant, will not alone enable us to decide whether it is justified to ascribe the concept of cure to a psychosurgical intervention.

(6) Therefore, any decision as to whether there are cases in which psychosurgery is justified will not be based on the intervention's curing the cause of the unwanted behavior or merely eliminating or improving that behavior.

(7) Nor will this theory, even if it is agreed that environmental

stress causes abnormal behavior such as violence, determine if there are cases where psychosurgery is justified. Indeed, given this theory, the major question becomes: are there cases where psychosurgery is justified for the removal of a symptom?

(8) Even if we accept that "experiments with rodents have indicated that crowding and stranger contact tend to have powerful effects upon aggressive behavior, drug toxicity, endocrine function, and biogenic amine function,"[66] and that similar relationships probably obtain in humans (and that, therefore, even on the organic, physiological model for scientific medicine, the abnormal structure or process is caused by environmental stress),[67] we still cannot determine whether there are cases where psychosurgery would be justified for the removal of the environmentally caused organic symptom.

Perhaps the last four points can be summarized this way:

(9) Acknowledging linguistic convention determines whether A justifies the ascription of B, and that when such justification obtains A functions as a criterion for B, can we conclude that (A), demonstrable evidence of malfunctioning brain tissue, is a criterion for (B), abnormal violence? It seems perfectly clear that at the present time there is no linguistic convention which justifies the use of (A) as criterion for (B).

(10) While there is no linguistic convention justifying (A) as criterion for (B), there is an open question as to whether (A) is a symptom of (B), and this relation is determined not by linguistic convention but by empirical evidence (which here means statistically significant correlations).

(11) Whether psychosurgery is justified as a cure for abnormal violence after other procedures have been tried can be decided on the grounds that (A) is a symptom of (B), if it is, because symptoms count as evidence which justifies, even though not as good evidence as criteria.

(12) Finally, history, not logic, determines whether (A) is a criterion or a symptom of (B).

Chapter 4

JUSTIFICATION

Justification of a Medical Practice

If the proper use of concepts critical for medical science will not enable us to decide when psychosurgery is justified, does it mean that psychosurgery cannot be justified? This would seem to be the logical result of the "scientific" shotgun argument against psychosurgery. However, before I consider the implications of that argument, let me briefly look at the "unscientific" shotgun argument which posits that a medical intervention is justified only if the "ultimate" cause of a biological disorder is biological. The most important difficulty in this argument is its lack of any scientific procedure for deciding why, when, or how any cause is "ultimate"; and, as a result, accepting the unscientific shotgun argument leads one to the logical conclusion that *no* biomedical intervention is ever justified. For example, since there is evidence that season of birth and marriage may have "causal" relations to mental illness,[1] the unscientific shotgun argument could be the basis for rejecting any biomedical intervention directed at the correction of such illness. Moreover, since injuries occasioned by a suicide attempt may not be biological, a biological intervention to treat such injuries would clearly be unjustified; in fact, the biological treatment of injuries suffered as a result of any accident other than a "biological accident" is unjustified. The unscientific shotgun argument thus "proves" too much and is simply irrelevant to any rational procedure for deciding when if ever psychosurgery may be justified. The word "rational" is important here because the unscientific shotgun argument may reflect the emotional stage of argument reached when the "answer" is "I don't care what you say," and when that stage is reached the issue no longer concerns decision making because a universally applicable (if irrational) dictum has been invoked. A reliance upon an ultimate cause as the basis for decision is usually a signal that the "I don't care" stage has been reached.

Is the scientific shotgun argument more rationally attractive? The "scientific" basis for this thesis frequently rests upon an argument constructed along the following lines:

(1) Any scientifically acceptable decision procedure for determining the propriety of a specific biomedical intervention should rest on demonstrable causal relationships
(2) The most appropriate causal relationships obtain between: (a) the physiological function of tissue systems and the identifable intervention, and (b) the tissue system and measurable, or at least observable, physical behavior
(3) If physical behavior is not *caused* by a specific identifiable tissue system, then that tissue system does not *cause* that behavior
(4) If an identified tissue system is not the cause of specific physical behavior, then that tissue system is not *causally connected* to that behavior
(5) If a tissue system is not causally connected to some specific behavior, then it is not scientifically justifiable to manipulate biomedically the tissue system in order to effect that behavior

While there may be some good reasons for accepting steps (1) and (2), the rationale for doing so may only reflect historically current attitudes about what it means to be scientific.[2] However, I have showed previously that there is no comparable basis for the acceptance *or* rejection of steps (3) and (4), and that consequently (5) is not the logically necessary conclusion to the argument. The "scientific" shotgun thesis thus reduces to the idea that there can be *no* justification for biomedically manipulating a tissue system which is not causally connected to the observed behavior. It is the imperialism of this argument which is most objectionable: if the paradigm model for scientific justification is not applicable, then there is no justification! If such paradigmatic rigor were applied to everything physicians do, much if not most medical practice would be unjustified! Two moral lessons may be drawn here: either (A) most of what doctors do is scientifically unjustified, or (B) most of what doctors do in treating patients, because it is scientifically unjustified, ought not to be done. However, I am here concerned with whether there is some unscientific justification for permitting or expecting doctors to practice as they do when such procedures are scientifically unjustified, and if so, whether this same justification may be extended to psychosurgery. The crucial question is: what language-game are doctors, patients, and society playing when they act upon their beliefs that what the doctor did was justified?

When this belief is shared by doctor, patient, and society, we have the easiest game to identify. The patient willingly pays his bill and recommends the doctor to his friends. The doctor is proud of what he did for the patient, and in appropriate situations may publicize his act. Society shows its acceptance of the treatment as juystified by what it does not do. Although an occasional prize or honor may be awarded, society's more commonly acquiescent response can be inferred from the doctor's not being condemned or having his license challenged.

The more difficult games surrounding biomedical justification arise when the three relevant entities do not share the belief that what was done was justified. It is relatively easy to characterize what happens when the doctor and society share such a belief but the patient does not. More difficult cases arise when the patient believes a procedure is justified, while doctors and society disagree, a situation that raises difficult questions about paternalism. Even more vexing issues about paternalism arise when the patient and his doctor support, while society opposes, what has been done. Perhaps the most perplexing questions come up when the patient, his doctor, and doctors in general agree, but society does not. The current debate about psychosurgery comes closest to the situation in which the patient and his doctor agree, and at least some significant elements in society do not.

The relevant language-game in such a case is one in which the patient and his family are satisfied with what has been done and pay the bill. Because of the disorders for which psychosurgery is invoked, the patient is unlikely to recommend the surgeon to his friends and so "satisfied" customers are likely to fade away. However, such patients occasionally surface in a public debate about psychosurgery. On one such occasion, Dr. Hunter Brown of California, a neurosurgeon who does psychosurgery, arranged for Dr. Peter Breggin to interview some of Brown's patients. Breggin was unable to shake these patients' belief in what had been done and was therefore reduced to arguing that if the patients only knew more, they would see that such surgical procedures were unjustified.

In this case, the games between patients and doctor and between patients and critic are quite clear. The patients pay, the doctor proudly publicizes (as may the patient), and Breggin questions their judgment. This would seem the conventional response to differences in belief; however the intensity and extent of the attack upon psychosurgery is unusual. Breggin and others have sought federal and state legislation to prohibit psychosurgery—even if the patient and his doctor deem such an intervention justifiable. This proposed legislation would penalize acting on the belief that any specific condition justified a psychosurgical procedure, and according to this language-game, "justified" could never apply to any psychosurgical intervention. Clearly then the crucial question is how society should mandate on the justifiability of psychosurgery and upon analysis this larger question is seen to contain several different questions.

Question 1: Should society ever mandate on any intervention which the patient and the doctor believe justified? Is more harm done when society acts to protect the individual from what it perceives to be health frauds? A careful analysis of current Food and Drug Administration (FDA) regulations on the introduction of new drugs will disturb anyone who naively believes that an unregulated pharmaceutical industry would inflict more harm than good.[3] In this connection, it is important to bear in mind that rejecting the idea that society should legislate to protect individuals from wanted, but possibly dangerous or fraudulent, health "cures" does not imply that society should have no system (e.g., courts, arbitration, insurance) whereby those negligently or otherwise wrongly injured by fraudulent or dangerous "cures" may be "made whole" again.

Question 2: If the risks which accompany the free market mechanism in the health field are believed to be too great, how should society decide when to intervene by issuing a mandate which will fix the games to be played? To a considerable extent the public reaction to psychosurgery has been the result of Breggin's attack, which found its way into the *Congressional Record.* To many doctors, this is objectionable because Breggin's admittedly unscientific analysis of the relevant literature[4] is not how the medical progress game should be played, since the political decision makers and the public lack the necessary medical expertise and do not listen to and learn from those who have it. Instead, such decision makers characteristically, and perhaps even properly, respond to what they perceive to be felt anxieties and necessities, and in doing so minimize their personal responsibility for biomedical decisions by appearing to rely upon relevant medical expertise.

Question 3: If a decision to intervene has been made, how should the required legislation be created? Even if one assumes that a legislature embodies collective social wisdom, is social wisdom an appropriate substitute for knowledge when dealing with biomedical technologies? At best one can hope that individual states will not enact restrictive legislation, at least until national legislation has been considered. At this time (spring 1976), a national commission has been empowered to study psychosurgery and one hopes that it will develop an appropriate data base to help answer at least the following questions: (a) what have been the long-term consequences of various psychosurgical interventions? and (b) what have been the unexpected long-term side effects of these interventions? Psychosurgery is presently so vulnerable to regulation from outside the medical profession because the data base contained in the current psychosurgery literature is not adequate to support a rational procedure for deciding the justification issue. While having adequate data will not answer whether psychosurgery is justified in any given case, without such data *any* decision for or against is probably unjustifiable.

Question 4: If the relevant data base were available, how should the clinical use of psychosurgery be regulated? The answer would be very simple if there were never any good long-term consequences and all unexpected side effects were bad. This being the case for every possible psychosurgical intervention is so improbable that we are naturally led to consider the difficult final question: if some long-term consequences are good and some are not, and if some side effects, expected or unexpected, are good and some bad, when will physicians be justified in recommending or carrying out a psychosurgical procedure?

To illustrate this problem, let us consider the following model: international data base enables a national commission to make judgments about relevant variables on a scale from 0 (very bad) to 10 (very good). For example, after destruction of a tissue site in the right amygdala, which has been identified by depth EEG recordings as showing abnormal electrical discharge, the consequences are:

(a) short-term memory loss	2
(b) long-term memory loss	8
(c) short-term ward adjustment	4
(d) long-term ward adjustment	6
(e) postoperative I.Q.	No change
(f) long-term ability to function without hospitalization	7
(g) short-term ability to handle novelty	2
(h) long-term ability to handle novelty	4
(i) long-term employment record	6
(j) preoperative employment record	3

While this list could include other important and relevant variables, such an extension would only make it harder to develop a rational means for deciding when such a procedure is justified. The justifiability decision is not primarily a function of abstract data like those in the data base, but rather of general data about the surgical procedure and judgments about the potential patient. Only if the general data warrants the conclusion that inflicting the procedure would be tantamount to legally punishable mayhem (because the consequences are *always* bad), could we get an easy answer to the fourth question.

Because we cannot label psychosurgery unjustifiable mayhem, and also lack suitably complete data about the procedure, how could our present knowledge be the basis for legislation regulating the specific use of any psychosurgical procedure? Of course legislation could mandate that the physician be reasonable; but that is clearly no advance, since criteria for determining reasonableness—that is, for determining which patients are likely to benefit from the given procedure—would still be lacking. This latter question, "Is procedure X justified for patient P?," is always crucial in considering any intervention. In other words, as long as the condition of mayhem is absent, the question can never be is procedure X justified?. Indeed such a question, ignoring the variable of Patient P, is no more answerable than asking whether amputation of a limb is justified, unless the procedure is mayhem.

Although there are those who argue that psychosurgery is psychic mayhem, I think it unlikely that a full and critical evaluation of the available literature will lead any responsible national commission to condemn any and all psychosurgery as mayhem. Consequently, the final hard question, "For which patients is a given psychosurgical procedure justified?," is unavoidable. While I have no direct answer to give, I am convinced that this problem can be solved neither by legislation nor by the judicial system. The courts can, however, find liability in specific cases and thus develop what it means for a physician to act reasonably, an evolution that is precisely what medical malpractice cases and decisions should contribute to medical jurisprudence. While holding Doctor A liable for having amputated P's arm under a given set of conditions does not tell us whether amputation is ever justified, it does help us to decide if there are circumstances in which amputation is not justified. As with questions of justice generally, it is often possible to furnish standards for deciding what is unjust, even when establishing what is just in the given circumstances is not possible. So courts, administrative tribunals, or medical ethics boards in condemming specific uses of psychosurgery will at least develop operational standards for determining when certain psychosurgical procedures would not be justified. Comparable decisions are presently made for medical interventions generally even when "model" scientific justification is not available. This process would seem reasonable because unless all psychosurgical interventions are mayhem with adverse long-term consequences and consistently adverse side effects, one cannot understand why psychosurgery should not be governed by standard medical malpractice principles. Indeed, unless it can be shown that the consequences of a psychosurgical intervention are so bad that the patient's long-term prospects are worsened through the procedure, what rational basis is there for treating psychosurgery differently from other medical interventions?

Many readers will object that I rely too heavily on the free market mechanism to protect health and prevent medical frauds, and indeed the customary medical malpractice mechanism is far from perfect. However, such critics need to bear in mind at least two considerations. In the first place, criticisms of the current medical malpractice mechanism need not imply criticism or rejection of the underlying free market mechanism. If the attorney's contingent fee arrangement were replaced by an imposed fee scale, or if arbitration or an administrative remedy replaced the current conventional judicial relief, the free market mechanism would still not be affected. Its underlying principle would remain the physician's liability for doing something unreasonable in the given case. Even if there were a national insurance scheme to provide recovery for injuries or losses sustained in medical treatment, the basis of recovery could still be the reasonableness of what was done to the given patient by the specific physician. Only if there were a "no fault" insurance scheme might one be required to abandon the free market machanism as the means of determining whether a specific psychosurgical intervention was justified.

The second consideration touches on the much more general problem of the risk inherent in any search for improvement, a danger which might be called the risk of institutional anarchy. Surely anarchy is not an inevitable accompaniment of the search for improvement; however, I have deliberately exaggerated here to emphasize the need for great caution in changing deeply entrenched institutional arrangements which have been relatively successful in protecting important interests. Those who question my reliance upon the free market mechanism as the way to protect health and prevent medical frauds must tell me what is better, for it is rash to reject what is available, even for good reasons, unless there is a more plausible alternative. In my opinion, a "repaired" medical malpractice, free market mechanism is likely to be better than either national or state legislation (or any other currently plausible alternative) for the regulation of psychosurgery. A national or a local "no-fault" insurance scheme, which would cover injuries or losses occasioned by a medical intervention, will not be responsive to whether a particular psychosurgical intervention is justified in a given case.

Can the Meaning of "Justified" be Legislated?

Until reasonableness is produced by mandate, legislation will be unable to solve the psychosurgical problem unless the data base warrants concluding that certain psychosurgical procedures must be prohibited. As long as some psychosurgical procedures are justified for certain patients, legislation is unlikely to furnish criteria for identifying which patients should be given particular procedures. This legislative inability is almost certainly true for predominantly biomedical considerations, and surely the case for other relevant considerations. I shall illustrate what is involved by two hypothetical cases. Let us assume that the data base makes possible a statistical index for any possible psychosurgical procedure. For example, based on the kind of evaluation illustrated above in connection with a unilateral amygdalotomy, it might be possible to derive a rational rating mechanism by weighing and averaging the different relevant factors. Using some such technique, we learn that on a scale of 0 to 10, procedure X gets a 7. Do we now know whether X is justified for both Mr. A and Mr. B? Do we know this even if, as regards the relevant biomedical factors, A and B are undifferentiable? The disorder for which X might be justified is controllable if the patient regularly takes prescribed medication. While A has no family and there is no community institution which could insure that he would take the required medication regularly, B has a concerned and willing family. Is X then equally advisable for A and B? Could any legislation cover *all* essentially nonbiological factors so that, in addition to the rated procedure, there could be a similar scale for rating patients and their environments?

The answer here is obvious, and therefore I see only the following options:

(1) legislation will ban some or even all psychosurgery because available data demonstrates that such procedures constitute mayhem
(2) legislation will ban some procedures entirely and prohibit others until further authorized investigations furnish data which will justify the ban or use of these other procedures
(3) some procedures will be permitted

If some procedures are permitted, then further options arise:

(1) legislation will try to define the appropriate patient population by laying down general guidelines; e.g., no prisoners may choose X

(2) legislation will furnish criteria to identify those patients appropriate for X (I have tried to suggest why this will not get far.)
(3) legislation will mandate the mechanism which will be used to decide who is a proper candidate for procedure X

Because I believe this last option is the most viable, I shall conclude by suggesting a solution for deciding whether any specific patient is a suitable candidate for a specific psychosurgical procedure which has not been prohibited.

Although the methods of handling informed consent vary widely with different patient populations, my procedure initially presumes not only that a specific patient has been deemed a suitable candidate for X, but also that the appropriate procedure will be followed as regards consent. My suggested procedure further presumes that the proposed intervention is believed to be therapeutic for the specific patient. Only rarely does a potential psychosurgery patient first consult with a neurologist or a neurosurgeon, for these specialists are generally only seen upon the recommendation of the physician initially consulted by the patient. In such cases the referring physician is usually a general practitioner or a psychiatrist; therefore, in order to minimize the risk of improvident psychosurgery, the concurrence of the referring physician should be a necessary precedent condition. However, this procedure by itself is unlikely to provide much real protection since, even if the neurologist or surgeon is more convincing than the original referring doctor, and the patient then goes onh to consult a different general practitioner or psychiatrist, it is most likely that the recommendation of the convincing specialists will again be obtained. If the patient consults a physician recommended by his specialist he will almost certainly experience the self-fulfilling prophecy since a specialist will hardly recommend an antipsychosurgery physician. Consequently, the patient needs more assurance than the concurrence of the physicians he has employed.

While there are about 3,000 neurosurgeons in the United States, probably less than 150 do psychosurgery and they are probably all located in rather large urban areas where there are specialists whose professional judgments would aid in deciding whether a specific patient is an appropriate candidate for a proposed procedure. Therefore, a legitimate part of the cost of psychosurgery should cover having each case evaluated by a relevant specialist other than, and in addition to, the recommending neurologist or neurosurgeon and the concurring physician who referred the patient. Although one would think that before doing psychosurgery the neurologist or neurosurgeon would want the concurrence of at least a clinical psychologist, such has not always been the case. However, what I am suggesting goes considerably beyond this minimum "medical" concurrence, for I would require that the case be evaluated by qualified specialists who are not employed by the patient, even if they are paid by him or his insurance carrier. There are two reasons for such an unusual requirement. First, even though any medical intervention can generate significant costs for society at large, psychosurgery is often regarded as a measure of last resort and therefore likely to apply to those most nearly hopeless cases where society is already bearing significant costs. Second, the still controversial character of psychosurgery warrants greater public visibility and accountability in order to furnish important and appropriate protection to the patients and to the physician as well.

In addition to the biomedical and behavior specialists' evaluations, a prognosis by persons trained in determining the social and lifestyle consequences of permitting or denying the intervention would also be appropriate. Although evaluation by family, friends, or neighbors might be considered, I do not find much to recommend such a requirement. I am convinced that these groups are either too vulnerable or too distant, and that while their judgments should be sought by the evaluating trained social scientists, their opinions should not be a critical component in the decisional process.

A suitable procedure might then take the following form:

(1) The recommending physician(s) and specialists concur that the case should be laid before the evaluating specialists.
(2) Each of the evaluating specialists, after reviewing whatever records are pertinent and interviewing appropriate family, friends, neighbors, and employers, makes a written recommendation.
(3) Those physicians involved in (1) review all the recommendations made by those involved in (2).
(4) If the physicians decide not to proceed, that is the end of the matter.

(5) If, contrary to the recommendations of those involved in (2), the specialists wish to proceed, the matter could be laid before a suitable committee. Such a body might function under the auspices of the nearest university, and since almost all neurosurgery is done in urban centers, it should not be difficult to make necessary arrangements. The committee should function pursuant to the HEW rules which apply to committees that review biomedical or behavioral research proposals involving human subjects.

Clearly, alternative committee arrangements might be suitable or even more appropriate in some circumstances. However, the above plan seems to balance fairly most of the relevant competing social and medical interests so that patients, physicians, and society are reasonably protected in trying to determine whether psychosurgery procedure X is justified for patient A.

Chapter 5
LEGAL, MEDICAL, AND POLITICAL IMPLICATIONS OF PSYCHOSURGERY*

The Grounds for Debate

The current debate over psychosurgery is characterized by irrational extremist views, and this is perhaps why Dr. Bertram Brown, the director of the NIMH, when appearing as the first witness before Senator Edward Kennedy's congressional subcommittee, began by saying: "I welcome this opportunity to discuss with you, in what I hope is a balanced and rational manner, an issue which has served as a lightning rod for highly emotional responses on both sides of the issue: Should psychosurgery be encouraged or even permitted as a technique to bring about desired therapeutic changes in a patient's behavior."[1] Extremists have held their positions with little concern for compromise. For example, Breggin and his allies see all psychosurgical interventions as suspect, if not inherently wrong. Breggin, introducing his own testimony before the subcommittee, attacked the behavioral modifi-

*This chapter is based upon "The Emotional, Medical, and Legal Reasons for the Special Concern About Psychosurgery," in F. Ayd, ed., *Medical, Moral, and Legal Issues in Mental Health Care* (1974). With the permission of the editor and publisher, The Williams & Wilkins Company, Baltimore.

cation psychology of Dr. B. F. Skinner and his followers as "elitist" and "totalitarian," arguing:

> The theory and practice of behavioral modification is really at the root of psychosurgery, and whether or not Skinner himself supports psychosurgery, his mechanistic, anti-individual, antispiritual view, which I call totalitarian, is what gives justification to the mutilation of the brain and the mind, in the interest of controlling the individual. . . .
>
> The reliance on professional ethics and medical control over these issues leaves the physicians in charge of the situation. It creates for themselves an elitist power over human mind and spirit. If America ever falls to totalitarianism, the dictator will be a behavior scientist and the secret police will be armed with lobotomy and psychosurgery.[2]

On the other hand, many clinicians urge the extreme opposite view: the doctor, in his own unimpeded judgment, should decide what is best for each individual patient, regardless of the kind of intervention which is contemplated. In his testimony before the Kennedy subcommittee, Dr. O. J. Andy, a neurosurgeon from the University of Mississippi, urged:

> The ethics involved in the treatment of behavioral disorders is no different than the ethics involved in the treatment of all medical problems. The medical problem concerning behavior may have a more direct impact upon society than other medical problems such as cardiac or kidney dysfunction. . . . However, if treatment is desired, it is neither the moral or the legal responsibility of society to decide what type of treatment should be administered. The ethics for the diagnosis and treatment of behavioral illness should remain in the hands of the treating physicians. . . . [3]

It seems to me that both extremes lead to unattractive consequences, and if we are to avoid these consequences, it is necessary to understand that the problem is not simply legal or medical but political as well.

We are moving into a time when almost all medicine will be regarded as having political dimensions, and I refer not merely to the delivery of health care, but to the specific intervention which any doctor recommends, be it prescription of an aspirin or surgical intervention on the brain. Little imagination is required to appreciate that although psychosurgery is presently in the forefront of biomedical ethics, it will not be long before much of medicine is subjected to comparable consideration and attack. Surely this will be true for all forms of psychiatric intervention, for even if one does not entirely agree with Dr. Thomas Szasz,[4] it is easy to appreciate that psychotherapy will be a natural subject of bioethical concern. Psychotherapeutic interventions are at least as significant for personality modification and behavior control as are surgical interventions on the brain. One need read only a little of the literature of psychiatry to recognize the significance of psychopharmacological interventions and the present capacity for behavior modification and control through psychotropic drugs. A statement in *Psychosurgery: Perspective on a Current Issue,* emphasized this latter point by stating that "the ethical problems posed by the modification of behavior with drugs or psychotherapy are probably of greater import because these means of control are available to a much wider range of potential 'abusers' than are the techniques of psychosurgery."[5] Indeed, I am amazed that psychosurgery is the prime target of so many contemporary "reformers." If all neurosurgeons in the United States worked twenty-four hours a day, the number of surgical procedures which they could "inflict upon their victims" is minuscule when compared to the number of behavior modification victims who could be reached by drug-dispensing doctors.[6] Even if we leave aside behavior modification drugs dispensed by physicians untrained in psychiatry, prescribed for young children by so-called child psychiatrists, and prescribed by pediatricians, it is clear that the number reachable by drugs is enormously greater than the number reachable by surgery.

Thus the current attack upon psychosurgery is directed at the smallest tip of a large iceberg, since the infliction of a psychosurgical procedure is a rarity compared to the daily assault upon integrity and personality occurring in so many other ways.[7] Because of unavoidable exposure to blaring radios, newspapers, and television, we are constantly subjected to behavior modification techniques which are often more subtle, more insidious, more dangerous, more uncontrollable, and more obnoxious than a psychosurgical procedure carried out by an ethical doctor. Only a money-hungry surgeon inflicting a procedure on a brain merely for mercenary reasons might approximate the danger which already confronts us in compulsory public education, which is characteristically irresponsible in the sense relevant to the arguments about regulating psychosurgery. Radio, television, the press and communication media in general, including compulsory education, are "irresponsible" because they provide virtually no institutional mechanisms for any kind of public accountability. Nor is there any such accountability for medicine in general, let alone for such potentially serious psychologically invasive therapies as psychotherapy, chemotherapy, or electrical stimulation of the brain. In light of all these actually or potentially greater dangers, why does psychosurgery nonetheless generate so much more anxiety?

The Inviolability of the Brain Thesis

Although the metaphor seems to confuse proctology and neurology, at least part of the reason for the intense concern with psychosurgery is based upon the belief that "the seat of the soul is the brain." As is often the case in trying to translate feelings into words, it is difficult to be precise about just what is intended. Nonetheless feelings play an important role in the attack upon psychosurgery, especially with Breggin, who seems to find the essence of what is human existing in the brain. According to him, "What goes on in your mind is a very different thing from what goes on in your kidney or your heart. Blood passes through your heart and circulates in a rather limited fashion. I believe your eternal spirit passes through your brain and lives there for a while and then goes on. Tampering here in the brain is considerably different than tampering with the heart or the lungs. It must impair the expression of your spiritual self."[8] Just why one's "spiritual self" is more a function of brain tissue than say of heart, eye, or hand tissue, is hard to understand unless we recognize that "brain" in Breggin's context functions as an intellectual construct for character or personality rather than as a label for that two pounds of tissue inside the skull. Writing in the *Saturday Review/World* (September 1973), in an exceptionally well-balanced presentation, Dr. Richard Restak, a neurologist, made it clear that the brain is frequently regarded as "the essence of what we refer to as personality."[9] Understood in this special way, the "sanctity of the brain" theory begins to make better sense, and we may begin to understand those who defend such views.

In the course of a discussion about psychosurgery under its auspices, the director of the Hastings Institute, Dr. Willard Gaylin, a psychiatrist, suggested why psychosurgery is special. "To a psychiatrist at least, the fact that [psychosurgery] could produce this much passion, this much vitriol, suggests that it seems substantively different. We may come to the conclusion that there is indeed a substantive difference between entering the brain and manipulating it artificially as distinguished from manipulating it with ideas."[10] Dr. Perry London, a professor of psychology and psychiatry, added: "There is something about this new technology that is different from most of the issues of public versus private interests which have preoccupied men in the past. Unlike compulsory education, unlike vaccination, unlike the traditional domain of conflict between the state and the individual, the arena of discourse here is the executive apparatus of the individual."[11] Professor Robert Neville further added:

> The brain, I think, should be conceived as a special environment for the person. Behavior-control techniques, especially these, seem to me to be altering the environment to make possible certain personal actions or certain personal continuities, careers, certain highly prized human emotions and the like. By conceiving of the brain as an environment that inhibits or fosters these human activities, we can conceive the techniques relative to the freedom and values of the person. The question has been raised of the privacy of the brain in the wider environment. There are lots of ways of defining privacy but it seems to me that in the social context, privacy is something that people demand for certain spheres of their life, and that society grants. Individuals and society may not always agree. Sometimes we would not like to have our brain be private, if, in fact, we can be freer, better, or cured of disease by intrusion.
>
> I'm quite confused myself about the particular values used for defining what ought to be recognized as the private sphere. But it seems to me that the techniques we're discussing now raise two important practical questions. Modifying the brain, since it's the most intimate environment for our humanly prized emotions and thought, is likely to have more pervasive effects than modifying certain other kinds of environment.[12]

Dr. Herbert G. Vaughan, Jr., a professor of neurology, declared that he found "people do consider the brain to be one of the areas in which the possibility of a surgical or physical procedure is most feared. Is there, within each of us, perhaps inborn, some fear that requires us to protect ourselves against encroachment upon the brain?"[13] This less exalted view of why the brain is regarded as sacrosanct finally gives way to a complete dismissal of the brain's special character. In eleven terse words, Dr. Jose Delgado, professor of neurophysiology and author of *The Physical Control of the Mind* (1969), sternly urges: "The inviolability of the brain is only a social construct, like nudity."[14]

No matter how it is presented, and even if there is something intrinsically arresting about the "seat of the soul" theory, the problem of using language to state what the theory means clearly remains. Is there some advance in clarity or understanding when, instead of speaking about the sanctity of the mind, we talk about "the spiritual self" (Breggin), "a substantive difference" (Gaylin), "the executive apparatus" (London), "a special environment" (Neville), "the privacy of the brain" (Neville), or "inborn" fears of "encroachment upon the brain" (Vaughan)? Did Senator Kennedy learn anything special about the brain from Brown's answer? Referring to "thought control, a la '1984' or 'Clockwork Orange,' " the senator asked him, "Is there any validity to those fears?" Brown answered: "I think there is great validity in the sense that there is something special indeed about the brain. There is something very special about experimenting on the brain. And the anxiety of course is very deep in terms of the control of feelings, thought, and behavior. There is validity in the depth of concern with taking cognizance of the need of troubled people to receive help, of the need for us to develop more knowledge in order to treat these people, and in order to treat people with these difficulties, we must deal with that valid set of anxieties."[15]

In their recourse to metaphors we see brilliant men struggling to give a *feeling* they wish to share public life. I am not saying that such exercises in communication are somehow "wrong." On the contrary, I am suggesting that because of the need to deal publicly and not privately with psychosurgery, we should content ourselves with recognizing that even if there is some deeper layer of experience, incapable of expression by ordinary language, which supports the inviolability-of-the-brain thesis, this thesis is, as Delgado said, only a social construct. It may be that the inviolability thesis is an attitude which deserves recognition and even protection, despite its having no scientific basis and lacking any clear articulation in ordinary, nonpoetic, nonmetaphorical language.

My conclusion about the inviolability thesis is based upon the principle that even if unjustified, widely shared moral feelings deserve as much respect and protection as can be accorded them without compromising equally important feelings, whether or not the latter are more justified. Applying this principle to the psychosurgery issue means there should be at least sufficient public accountability to prevent abuses such as needless brain surgery, surgery performed on young or other incompetent persons unprotected by adequate legal institutions, and experimental human brain surgery initiated prematurely or otherwise scientifically unjustified. In addition, the principle suggests that institutional mechanisms should maximize public accountability wherever this can be done without compromising other important considerations. As regards psychosurgery, these other considerations would include some which are moral (e.g., trying to minimize human suffering), some which are scientific (e.g., trying to conquer the last great medical frontier—the functioning of the brain), and some which are both (e.g., trying not to discourage the search for new knowledge). In short, even if the inviolability thesis is incapable of scientific formulation or justification, it deserves at least as much recognition as is regularly accorded other "social constructs." To use Delgado's example, we do protect community attitudes about nudity—and it is surely not irrational to believe that widely shared community sentiments about the "seat of the soul" deserve nothing less. Just as there is no logical or scientific connection from tissue to body to nudity, so there is no such connection in the movement from brain tissue to mind to soul. But in neither case should the absence of logical or scientific connections imply that the "social construct," the attitude, therefore be regarded as unworthy of legal protection.

The Irreversibility Thesis

The second major reason for the intense moral and social concern about psychosurgery is based upon somewhat scientific grounds; however, here again serious difficulties arise in trying to formulate carefully just what is involved. The thesis is that psychosurgery is irreversible. In the course of the Hastings discussion, Dr. E. A. Bering, Jr., of NINDS, emphasized it, saying: "A very important point that has not been brought out is the difference between a surgical procedure on the brain and electrical stimulation of the brain. By stimulating the brain with electricity one can start and stop certain activities. The procedure is essentially reversible but a surgical lesion destroys part of the brain and is an irreversible, permanent anatomical change. If you don't like the result you're stuck with it and it can only be changed by making the lesion larger or another somewhere else."[16] In the Detroit psychosurgery case the plaintiff's primary "technical" witness, Dr. Ayub Ommaya from NINDS, also stressed that psychosurgery is irreversible, as did Breggin when he testified in that trial. In Restak's *Saturday Review* article, the argument is made that: "An important distinguishing feature of any psychosurgical procedure is irreversibility. Once the brain tissue is altered, it can never be the same again. Since the brain is the essence of what we refer to as personality, it follows that psychosurgery irrevocably alters personality."[17]

Although the irreversibility thesis may have better grounds than the inviolability thesis, it also lacks clear and careful formulation. The hypothesis upon which the irreversibility thesis rests may be referred to as the "integrated brain function theory." However, without exploring that theory, one can notice how loose, and therefore misleading, are the formulations of Bering and Restak, and I would emphasize that neither doctor was engaged in the emotional or extremist attack upon psychosurgery which has characterized much of the public literature. Bering suggests that unlike psychosurgery, ESB is reversible because electrical stimulation can be stopped, whereas a surgical lesion destroys "part of the brain" and is therefore a "permanent anatomical change." Similarly, Brown, testifying before the Kennedy subcommittee, noted that: "There are some who would also criticize, with some reason, the changing of behavior by stimulating the brain through implanted electrodes, even though this is a less drastic treatment because it does not cause irreversible damage to the brain."[18] While I shall not marshal the technical evidence here, I believe there are sound scientific reasons for questioning (1) whether electrical stimulation alone can cause "permanent anatomical change" and (2) whether destruction of brain tissue is necessarily either (a) a permanent or (b) an anatomical change. There is reason to believe that electrical stimulation of a certain intensity or of a certain duration, or of a lesser intensity, but with a certain frequency, may cause as much "permanent anatomical change" as a surgical lesion. There is also reason to question the concept of permanent anatomical change, since it may well be that in the above contexts it is either trivially true or false. It is trivially true in that by definition any tissue destruction is tissue destruction, and therefore if "permanent anatomical change" means only tissue destruction, then cutting one's fingernails is also a "permanent anatomical change." If this is all that is meant by the irreversibility thesis, then surely every surgical intervention, probably every chemical intervention, and possibly every psychotherapeutic intervention, is an equally permanent anatomical change.

While the irreversibility thesis need not be thus trivialized, I am suggesting that the usual formulation of the thesis, or rather its lack of formulation, provides little or no clarification. Restak writes that a psychosurgical procedure is irreversible because: (1) altered brain tissue can never be the same; and (2) since the brain is the essence of personality, (3) an altered brain necessarily produces an irrevocably altered personality. Although his argument has the appearance of a perfect syllogism, there are reasons for questioning both the minor premise and the conclusion, as well as the logic of it. As I said above, (1) is either trivially true or subject to considerable doubt. There is reason to believe that even if what is altered is altered irreversibly, altering some brain tissue does not necessarily imply that brain function is altered, altered irrevocably, or altered permanently. There is scientific evidence that the destruction of some brain tissue does not alter brain function, that some alterations in function which do occur are reversible, and that some alterations are not permanent. In addition, and indeed absolutely cardinal for the development of a rational analysis about the psychosurgery issue, it is necessary to recognize that even if step (1) in the irreversibility argument was correct, and even if we grant some plausibility to the major premise, step (2), step (3) would still *not* be the logically necessary conclusion. Again, using Restak's argument as the model, what I am urging is that even if his (1) were true, and even if we give some credibility and scientific meaning to (2), it would still not be the case (except in the trivial, definitional sense) that irrevocably altered brain tissue necessarily produces an irrevocably altered personality. It has yet to be demonstrated that:

(a) the loss of some brain tissue *necessarily* produces personality change; (b) that the brain is incapable of replacing lost tissue without change in personality; (c) that because for some functions we may have "two brains," unreplaced, irrevocably lost tissue necessarily produces an irrevocably altered personality.

It should be clearly noticed that in one important sense, the entire irreversibility argument is irrelevant to the core questions of whether psychosurgery should be regulated and, if so, how? Although there are surgical procedures which are reversible, and in some situations there may be a choice between a procedure which is reversible and one which is not (e.g., some kinds of sterilization), probably almost all surgical procedures are undertaken in the hope that the results will be irreversible. Indeed, the attractiveness of a surgical procedure may be due to the probability that its consequences will be permanent. In other words, the most important question about a surgical intervention, psychosurgical or otherwise, is not whether it is permanent, but rather what its consequences are. Even if a psychosurgical intervention always and necessarily resulted in a permanent alteration of personality, the real question would be missed. If a change is undesirable for social, political, moral, or anatomical reasons, it ought not be produced even if reversible, whereas if a change is desirable, irreversibility is a virtue. By itself, reversibility will not make an undesirable change desirable, and the core question concerns not the reversibility, but the desirability of a change. If personality changes resulting from psychosurgery are likely to be bad or undesirable, then such interventions are hardly rendered unobjectionable if reversible. Only when there is adequate scientific reason to believe that a change will probably be desirable, and at least permanent enough to warrant the discomfort and risk, should surgical intervention be considered as a potentially proper treatment.

Some "Medical" Reasons for Concern about Psychosurgery

There are at least ten major "medical" reasons why socially conscious and conscientious people are concerned about the clinical practice of psychosurgery:

(1) the integrated brain function theory
(2) the medical meaning of causal connection
(3) the evidence of organicity
(4) the accuracy of the lesion
(5) the identification of a syndrome which warrants a medical intervention
(6) the inadequacy of testing instruments for ascertaining the specific effects of a psychosurgical intervention
(7) the possibility that no intersubjectively communicable testing mechanism could be constructed to uncover all the important consequences of a psychosurgical intervention
(8) the possibilities for adverse side effects
(9) the possible unknowability of long-range effects, genetic or otherwise
(10) the meager scientifically acceptable literature about general human brain function and the virtual lack of any such literature dealing with the effects of a specific lesion in the brain.

To this list we could add even more subtle matters such as:

(11) the connection between epileptic and paraepileptic phenomena[19]
(12) the medical treatment of overt conduct even in the absence of medical evidence of abnormality
(13) the relevance of psychiatric evaluation in determining the appropriateness of a nonpsychotherapeutic intervention
(14) the relative efficacy of alternative treatment modalities in constructing a hierarchy of treatment choices

It is obvious that each of these issues must be carefully treated if a rational strategy is to be developed for dealing with the psychosurgery question. However, my immediate concerns are to show why the analyses of these seemingly medical questions generate important legal and philosophical concerns and to consider the argument raised by plaintiffs in the Detroit psychosurgery case as to whether depth EEG studies were justified. Plaintiffs, supported by their technical (medical) witnesses argued that such studies were not justified because: (1) depth EEG studies are, if not entirely worthless, of dubious evidentiary significance; (2) the high rate of morbidity, if not also mortality, connected with depth EEG work mitigated against such studies, especially if they would be inconclusive anyway; (3) even if the depth recordings supported or strongly suggested organicity in the tissue of the amygdala, that would not sustain a decision to proceed to a lesion; (4) since John Doe had no history of epileptic seizure sufficient to warrant a brain lesion, the lesion on the amygdala would be unwarranted even if there was evidence of organicity there, since it had not been proven that the patient suffered from any medical syndrome (uncontrollable aggressivity, it was argued, is not such a syndrome); (5) even if uncontrollable aggressivity were identified as a medical syndrome, it had not been proven that a lesion on the amygdala would be therapeutic; (6) even if such a lesion might be therapeutic, it had not been proven that the cure would not be worse than the disorder (the adverse side effects argument); and finally, (7) since surgery in general ought to be the treatment of desperation and not of choice, it had to be proven that less intrusive therapies had been tried and failed, or would fail if tried.

Can anyone not see that each of these arguments exudes philosophical, moral, legal, social, and political concerns? Clearly, questions are generated about the nature of causation, evidence, good evidence and good enough evidence, about brain function theory and the isolatability of function, and about the criteria for the identification of a medical disorder. In addition, questions arise as to whether every disorder is therefore a medical disorder, what it means to say that something is a medical disorder, how to ascertain whether electrochemical change is improvement, how to weigh electrochemical improvement against biological improvement, how to decide whether biological improvement is a socially or politically attractive gain, and how scarce resources are to be allocated.

In the Detroit psychosurgery case, the plaintiffs called no witness qualified in neurology or in EEG; indeed, their only witness with any kind of scientific background even remotely related to psychosurgery was a neurosurgeon from the NINDS whose specialty is cerebrovascular disease and head injuries. Yet Dr. Ommaya testified that there was no causal connection between a lesion in the amygdala and the control of aggressivity. He took this view because of his belief in the integrated brain theory and despite reports in the medical literature of about five hundred amygdalotomies or amygdalectomies. This literature had largely influenced the Lafayette Clinic investigator to undertake the project, since the reported cases suggested a connection between the amygdala and aggression. In my cross-examination of Ommaya, I wanted to discover what he meant, as a medical scientist, by causation.

Q. [I]s there some special sense of causal connection applicable in medical research?

A. No, it's exactly the same. It's the same as is used in physics, chemistry, science.

Q. . . . [I]f you place a depth electrode and you stimulate the electrode, and each time you do so the subject twitches in a certain place, would you say there's a causal connection?

A. There may be.

Q. What would be the evidence which would lead you to believe there is not a causal connection . . . ?

A. I think, as I described earlier, you'd have to show it in a significant number of observations, and you would have to show it in a significant set of observations, such that in a given group of patients, the same electrode in the same place, confirmed by pathological evidence, really did the same thing. Only then can you really accept a hypothesis as a fact, as a law, as a theory.

Q. In other words, a causal connection is not something which is determined by a litmus paper test, there's a body of evidence which has to be accumulated. Is that your view?

A. A syndrome is established at various levels.

Q. No, no, I'm not asking—I'm asking you about a causal connection.

A. A causal connection is established at various levels.

Q. Right. In other words, the level at which you establish it and how you establish it depends on the purpose for which you're going to use that causal connection?

A. Correct.

Q. And so . . . your theory, then, is that there is no connection between electrical abnormality and aggressive behavior for what purpose?

A. For defining a syndrome in patients. In other words, there is no data showing there are, say, 20 patients who invariably do this episodically violent behavior and who have this bad an EEG. This is not available. If you have that evidence, I'd like to know it.

Q. . . . [I]f, after a surgical procedure has been performed on the brain, the patient is better, does that show there is a causal connection between the surgical procedure and the condition which was sought to be alleviated by that procedure?
A. Not necessarily.[20]

At another time, in connection with his direct testimony, the witness was questioned by Judge Gilmore:

Q. You say no syndrome has been defined for neurosurgery to affect behavior. Now, are you speaking of the experiment in Michigan or are you speaking generally? Would you elaborate on that just a little bit?
A. Yes. It has been proposed that such a syndrome exists. In other words, the hypothesis has been advanced that there exists—and this is in all—I am talking generally now—that there exists a group of patients who are—have electrical abnormality in their brain and are subject to episodic bursts of violence. This is an idea that has been floating around for many, many years. There are patients in whom this association is found.

What has not been defined is that this is a causal relationship, that there is such a causal relationship between the electrical abnormality measured—or between the physical abnormality and the resulting aggression, the aggression being an episodic causal invariable consequence of that abnormality.

What has only been shown is an association, not a causal relationship. And until you show or have evidence for causal relationship, there is no syndrome in the clinical sense.
Q. How do you show causal relationship in a situation like that?
A. Well, it depends upon the category. . . . [21]

Here we have a competent medical scientist, who was conscientious, even if wrong, struggling to communicate to scientifically untrained judges conceptual material which is not scientific. Whether Ommaya did much worse than Aristotle, Kant, or Hume in trying to explain causation is arguable. Indeed, after this particular court session, the question was raised as to whether the intention had been to conduct a cross-examination or a seminar in philosophy! The conceptual constructions upon which the doctor relied in trying to deal with the questions included: (1) causal connection, (2) hypothesis, (3) law, (4) theory, (5) levels of causal connection, (6) purpose, (7) association, (8) syndrome, (9) relation between purpose and causation, and (10) relation between syndrome and association or causal connection. Would anyone argue that the elucidation of all, some or even any of these conceptual constructions was only or primarily a matter of medical science?

Judicial Management of Medicine and the Role of the Medical Expert

Not every court involvement with the practice of medicine amounts to management, and judicial management is not necessarily bad. But the Detroit psychosurgery case attracted so much international attention because it was a rare instance in which a court was asked to undertake the management of a whole field of medicine. This is in sharp contrast to the usual judicial intervention, where an individual patient seeks redress from an individual doctor or institution for an alleged, specific wrong. However, the important lesson in the Detroit case arises not from the unusual character of this particular judicial intervention, but rather from the general role of technical, scientific, medical witnesses when judges are asked to practice medicine. The potential abuses of expert medical witnesses are particularly discernible in the Detroit psychosurgery case because of the court's unusual role. From a limited legal perspective the court had as its primary concern the question of whether an involuntarily committed mental patient or his guardian could, under certain circumstances, consent to a psychosurgical intervention. However, in order to decide this limited question, it was deemed necessary to consider the much broader "status" of psychosurgery, and it is in this area, and not that of consent, that we perceive how a judicial proceeding can function as the institutional mechanism for evaluating the current status of a medical procedure.

To demonstrate the utility of depth EEG studies defendants called as their principal technical witness Dr. Richard Walker, the president of the American Electroencephalographic Society, and a physician of wide experience board-certified in the relevant specialties. They also offered testimony by one of the most distinguished living neurosurgeons, Dr. Earl Walker, a man with an international reputation who had recently retired from an important academic position. In addition, Dr. Ernst Rodin, one of the named defendants, also board-certified in EEG, testified on this subject; his expertise in this field was conceded and unquestioned. The plaintiff's single "technical" witness, Dr. Ommaya (who stated in court that he was not an expert in EEG and not board-qualified in EEG), testified that depth EEG was largely useless and had rather high mortality and morbidity rates. He conceded on cross-examination that the published literature did not support his estimates as to mortality or morbidity rates, and his statements were flatly contradicted by the medical experts who subsequently testified. He based his statements upon work done at NINDS, which, he stated, was as yet unpublished. Although while under oath he agreed to furnish the court with material to support his statements, to date none has been furnished. Interestingly, Dr. Breggin in testifying about the adverse effects of psychosurgery stated that his testimony was not supported by the published literature, and like Ommaya, also said he was relying upon unpublished "investigations." While under oath, Breggin also agreed to furnish the court with material in support of his views, but again none has yet been received.

What we see in the testimony of these two plaintiff witnesses is one of the most important lessons to emerge from the Detroit psychosurgery case. Lawyers interested in suppressing an experimental or innovative medical approach are not likely to have too much trouble in finding "experts" with a sufficient paper record to make their views admissible, regardless of how those views are supported or, indeed, contradicted by the primary criterion for determining what is scientifically acceptable as of a certain time—namely, the published scientific literature of the world. Indeed, the effectiveness of Breggin's advocacy is largely due to the fact that it is not scientific. Although in his testimony before the Kennedy subcommittee he referred to his "research papers in the Congressional Records,"[22] he did not characterize them that way on cross-examination in court. Rather, his "research papers" were there described as publications not designed to reach the scientific community. Instead, he said he was trying to present materials for a popular audience. Anyone familiar with Breggin's contributions in the *Congressional Record* or elsewhere will have little difficulty in seeing why his distorted, prejudicial review of the psychosurgical literature has not appeared, and is unlikely to appear, in any scientific journal. I am *not* criticizing Breggin for resorting to Madison Avenue techniques to attain a goal which he sees as political (as contrasted to medical), for in his testimony before the Kennedy subcommittee Breggin made it clear that he sees psychosurgery as a political, not a medical, problem. His closing statement urged: "It is time to give up study. I do not think [psychosurgery] is a medical issue. . . . "[23] But while I must concede the openness of Breggin's methods is admirably unhypocritical, I cannot praise him for eschewing science for propaganda nor be uncritical of the role he played in the Detroit case and with Congress. Whether the end ever justifies the means in politics, and if so, when, is a matter beyond my immediate concern, and so I leave aside questioning the propriety of a doctor using sales strategy to gain a political goal. However, I am deeply concerned about the medical expert's role and function qua medical expert, and hence I am highly critical of Breggin's role in court (and also critical, to a lesser extent, of his role before the Kennedy subcommittee).

Although Breggin's tactics are particularly egregious, the larger problem of separating the medical scientist role from other roles doctors play—for example, concerned and conscientious citizen—is more significant. While there are cases where it would be difficult or useless to make a distinction (e.g., a doctor sitting on a commission to decide whether a new hospital was warranted in a particular community), there are also instances where the failure to make and keep different roles separated can be destructive of important social, political, and scientific interests. The medical scientist who gains access as an expert to the institutionalized judicial decision-making process has a professional and political obligation to perform as a scientist and not as a political huckster. If a medical scientist comes into a decision-making institution and says that depth EEG work has a high degree of morbidity or that psychosurgery has very severe adverse side effects, the institutional decision maker should not be required to depend upon the wiles or guiles of opposing counsel to show that, in this instance, the scientist appears in politician's clothes. Psychiatrists have been particularly guilty of playing this double-agent role and have lent unnecessary additional support to Szasz's attack upon public-policy-oriented psychiatry. Of course, no profession has a monopoly on double-agent strategy and perhaps lawyers are even more frequent offenders than other professionals because of their willingness to characterize any problem as legal, thus creating the impression that political or social concerns are less relevant. One need not be a Marxist to appreciate that legal solutions to a problem either suppress or accommodate specific social and political values; a legal solution is probably never neutral.

There are instances when even if the medical solution to a problem is not value neutral, one still needs to distinguish between the medical scientist and the policial demagogue who also happens to be a medical scientist. The scientist, if he enters the political process as a scientist, will contribute only his expertise to the decision-making process; the demagogue will enter the process by creating reasonable expectations in the minds of the decision makers that he will perform as a scientist, but then he will perform as a demagogue. The scientist, especially when part of an institutional mechanism specifically structured as a court, will not perform as though his scientific and other roles were necessarily fungible. I am not suggesting that a scientist ceases to be a father or citizen while peering into his microscope; however, I am urging that it is still possible and sometimes necessary to recognize that a white laboratory coat is not an infallible guide to the role its wearer is playing.

Deliberately or accidentally packaging politics and social values as medical science is particularly objectionable because there is no effective way to protect the political decision maker from the deception. This is especially true of the institutionalized judicial decision process because its adversary character tends to polarize positions which are then tenaciously defended as if they were the private property of the witness. In addition, even where the relevant process is legislative and not judicial, the medical demagogue is particularly objectionable and difficult to deal with because those medical scientists who are his opposites characteristically refuse to come forward and participate *even as scientists* in the decisional process. As a result, the decision maker suffers from a double blindness. First, he receives the relevant scientific material deliberately filtered through a political screen, and second, he is left ignorant of that material as it exists in unfiltered form.

Although there were medical witnesses in the Detroit case who were deliberately evasive and willing, indeed anxious, to utilize their medical status for advancing political or social values, I do not imply that, for example, Breggin deliberately lied under oath. It is enough to say that he failed to perform as a medical expert ought to have performed, and that his failure came about because he did not see that the roles of medical scientist and citizen-politician are not fungible, even if they are never entirely separable.

None of the rich literature on the subject of the medical expert in a judicial proceeding and almost none of the concern about doctors in court have focused on a case like that in Detroit, in which the judges sat as a medical review committee passing on the scientific status of an entire field of medicine. The Detroit case should suggest what I hope is now the question in the reader's mind: if psychosurgery or some other entire field of medicine, or some field of new scientific technology, requires regulation, what should "regulation" mean, and is there some better way to achieve such regulation than through the judicial process?

Social Control of New Knowledge

According to an ancient tradition, social and political stability is valuable enough to justify the suppression of new knowledge, as well as to forbid its acquisition. Although Bruno and Galileo are not available, we can get a pretty good idea from Bertolt Brecht and Eric Bentley of what Galileo thought about the need to choose between stability and new knowledge. It is unlikely that one of my generation, or even a younger person, is unaware of the stability-versus-knowledge controversies that surrounded the development of atomic energy, genetic engineering, behavior control techniques, and new medical technologies. In view of the vast literature and general public familiarity with this matter, and since I have no formula by which to diminish the fears which many have about the 1984-like consequences of new scientific knowledge, it must suffice to call the reader's attention to a couple of points in these controversies which relate specifically to psychosurgery. Perhaps because I am a lawyer, when I am confronted with a problem in applied morality or politics I tend to ask what legally effective institutional models are available for constructing a mechanism which would prevent the worst consequences of whatever is creating the problem. Thus for me the issue is not whether new knowledge should be suppressed but how it can be controlled. This approach is both philosophically more defensible and, as regards psychosurgery, probably also inevitable.

If international espionage were not such a science, and had the relation between Roosevelt and Stalin been different at a certain crucial time in history (some say had Roosevelt not been so naive), it is conceivable that the American knowledge monopoly on atomic energy could have continued longer than it did. But could any similar monopoly of new knowledge survive in medical science? On the contrary, one of the features which distinguishes the development of medical knowledge is its international character. Van Rensselaer Potter wisely cautions that after we once have opened "Pandora's Box of Knowledge,"[24] it is impossible to return the contents. I would add, at least as regards medical knowledge, that a decision to keep the box closed can never be made effectively on a national level. Even if it were deemed better to suppress new medical knowledge because of its Orwellian potential, it probably could not be done internationally, and it surely could not be done on a national basis. Neither Narabayashi nor Sano in Japan, Hassler in West Germany, Balasubramaniam in India, Bailey in Australia, Crow in England, Baker in Canada, Chitanandh in Thailand, nor Delgado in Spain, to name only a few, will be deterred, let alone prevented, by the decision in the Detroit case nor even by congressional legislation from continuing their work on experimental brain surgery. Unless Congress also bans their publications from the United States and prohibits American doctors from attending conferences abroad or reading foreign medical journals, American doctors will acquire the "dangerous" new knowledge and be able to tell any sufficiently desperate patient that, in England or Japan, so-and-so has treated cases like his with some apparent success.

I have sketched this caricature of knowledge suppression in medicine to illustrate my belief that the real problem is not whether potentially dangerous new knowledge should be suppressed. On the contrary, especially as regards new knowledge in medicine, the task should always be at least twofold: first, to encourage the development of as much new knowledge as possible to insure that we will not make mistakes out of ignorance, and second, to institutionalize those restraints upon the use of the new knowledge as seem warranted by its potential for harm.[25]

Chapter 6

PSYCHOSURGERY AND FREEDOM OF THOUGHT

The Detroit Psychosurgery Case and the First Amendment Argument

In the preceding chapter I examined a number of the considerations which have influenced those who have been most critical of psychosurgery. In doing so, however, I did not confront directly the issue which is probably considered to be the heart of the matter by the critics of psychosurgery. It is the possibility of thought control as in George Orwell's *1984* and Anthony Burgess's *A Clockwork Orange*. I am therefore concerned here to place this general question within the political-legal context of the Constitution and to ask whether the First Amendment may prevent the use of psychosurgery.

I must stress initially that there was *no* relationship between the First Amendment argument and the "case or controversy" presented for decision in the Detroit psychosurgery case. Nonetheless, that court apparently was convinced that the First Amendment right to freedom of mentation constituted a barrier to coerced psychosurgery. That no coercion question was presented in the Detroit case can be inferred from the petitioner's devoting only one page in his posttrial brief to the question. In addition, neither the attorney general's brief on behalf of the state and all the named defendants, nor my brief on behalf of the named defendant doctors and Lafayette Clinic, contains a single sentence relating to the First Amendment argument. However, one need not rely on indirect evidence, for this case was unusual in that the precise questions on which the court was to rule were presented by agreement of all eight counsel, and subsequently accepted by the court as the basis for the exercise of its jurisdiction. Thus, ironically the court, in the very opinion in which it says there is a First Amendment barrier to coerced psychosurgery, also gives the questions agreed upon as the basis for its exercise of power. Since neither question in any way asks whether a state may impose psychosurgery upon an involuntarily committed person, how could the court nonetheless rule on the coercion question? Had the court stopped in its opinion when it held that no consent, whether from a patient or a guardian, was possible, it would have fully, finally, and emphatically decided the case or controversy before it.

In going on to consider a case which was neither argued nor about which it received a single word of testimony, the court either made a mistake in logic or simply wanted to deal with a constitutional question. I suspect that both motives operated. The error in logic was to infer that if institutionalized persons could not consent, the state could force the psychosurgery upon them anyway. "Anyway" is the crux of the matter, for it reflects the major premise that, with or without consent, involuntarily committed patients can be compelled to submit to certain therapies. However, the court's logical error resulted from confusing two entirely different questions: (1) may an involuntary patient or his agent consent to psychosurgery? and (2) may the state impose psychosurgery upon an involuntarily committed patient? An affirmative or negative answer to the first question logically implies neither an affirmative nor a negative answer to the second; and conversely, an affirmative or negative answer to the second question logically implies nothing about the first. It would be no logical contradiction to hold that whether or not an involuntarily committed patient could consent, the state could impose therapy. It would also be no contradiction to hold that whether or not a state could impose therapy, an involuntarily committed patient could not consent. In the Detroit case the court's mistake was in thinking that a negative answer to the first question somehow implied or required a negative answer to the second. Even if a state could impose therapy, it would be legally and logically possible to recognize a difference between imposed therapy and therapy furnished on consent; and conversely, even if the state could not impose therapy, it would be legally and logically possible to recognize that therapy could be furnished on consent, or withheld despite consent.

Thus, although there is surely a constitutional question about coerced therapy, the Detroit case did not present that "case or controversy" to the court. If there was any doubt on this issue, the statements of the principal defendant doctor, both in court and elsewhere, made it overwhelmingly clear that he did not consider himself involved in a situation where the state ordered the patient to have a given therapy. This doctor repeatedly insisted, "If the patient did not consent, I would not touch him. That would be the end of the matter."

This panel of unusually competent judges expanded its jurisdiction to decide an enormously important constitutional issue never argued to it in part because judges are regarded as "unusually competent" if they do not dodge difficult or important questions such as the constitutional coercion issue. What is regrettable is that the three judges thought themselves competent to decide the constitutional question without benefit of testimony or argument. It is to protect us from such overly aggressive judges that the legal principle that a court must decide only the case or controversy was established. It is unfortunate that in this first impression case, on such an important and complex matter, the judges exceeded their power.

The Structure of Shapiro's Constitutional Argument

The First Amendment argument has been best developed by Michael Shapiro in "Legislating the Control of Behavior Control," where he postulates that there is a fundamental right to freedom of mentation protected by the First Amendment. Shapiro formulates his argument in seven steps. The first five develop the argument that the First Amendment protects mentation; the final two seek to establish that it follows as a corollary that the First Amendment also protects against the coercive use of organic therapies.

(1) The first amendment protects communication of virtually all kinds, whether in written, verbal, pictorial or any symbolic form, and whether cognitive or emotive in nature.

(2) Communication entails the transmission and reception of whatever is communicated.

(3) Transmission and reception necessarily involve mentation on the part of both the person transmitting and the person receiving.

(4) It is in fact impossible to distinguish in advance mentation which will be involved in or necessary to transmission and reception from mentation which will not.

(5) If communication is to be protected, *all* mentation (regardless of its potential involvement in transmission or reception) must therefore be protected.

(6) Organic therapy intrusively alters or interferes with mentation.

(7) The first amendment therefore protects persons against enforced alteration or interference with their mentation by coerced organic therapy. (This last proposition would also be a valid inference if it read: "The first amendment therefore protects persons against certain kinds of *denial* of access to organic therapy, or psychoactive agents generally, which are used to alter mentation.")[1]

Coercive therapy affecting mentation, he argues, may neither be imposed nor denied by the state unless the state can meet the burden required to overcome a constitutionally protected fundamental right. Roughly, the state must show a compelling state interest which cannot be protected by some lesser invasion or compromise of the protected fundamental right. That is, the state must prove that the least intrusive alternative has been chosen.

While I have important reservations and questions about several aspects of the first five propositions in Shapiro's argument, I am primarily interested in his last two steps. The footnote to (6) makes it clear that virtually any organic therapy is sufficiently intrusive to fall within the scope of the protection, and that alteration or interference is value neutral. In other words, the effect (good, bad, or indifferent) of the therapy is irrelevant.[2] Ignoring whatever tiny escape hatch may be provided by "virtually all," it is apparent that (6), because its crucial terms are not defined, builds the conclusion into the premises so that "therefore" in (7) is not a logical deduction but a definitional consequence. There is nothing intrinsically wrong with defining virtue into existence, even when the crucial definitions are tucked into a footnote, but it is misleading to imply that there is some logical compulsion to recognize the "required" virtue. Even though state coercion for or against organic therapy may be morally objectionable on utilitarian or rule-utilitarian ground, to create by definition the impression of a legally compelling argument adds no strength to the case. In order to make "therefore" in (7) a conclusion to an argument, Shapiro should show (rather than positing by definitional fiat) that all (or virtually all) organic therapies are sufficiently intrusive to fall within the scope of the protection, that "intrusive" necessarily "connotes an interference with personal autonomy,"[3] and finally that "improvement" in mentation or behavior constitutes interference with personal autonomy. In other words, (6) looks like a plausible premise in the argument, but when its crucial terms are translated in accordance with the instruction in the accompanying footnote, the appearance of plausibility vanishes. Translated, (6) should read: "All organic therapy interferes with personal autonomy whether or not it effects an improvement in mentation or behavior."

Thus it becomes easier to question whether the first five steps in any way support "therefore" in (7). Do they establish that any interference with personal autonomy is an interference with mentation or behavior? Do they establish that all organic therapy is an interference with personal autonomy? I leave aside here the question of why any organic therapy, because it interferes with autonomy, falls within the scope of the protection while nonorganic therapies, which clearly interfere at least as much, are ignored. If there is a constitutional barrier to interference with personal autonomy, the organic/nonorganic distinction cannot effectively filter out objectionable from permissible coercion. Even granting the first four steps, and accepting (5) all mentation is protected, does it necessarily follow that coerced *improvement* of mentation is prohibited? I cannot see in the first five steps any basis for such an argument, and so despite its "therefore," (7) is not the logical conclusion to a legal argument.

At least part of the reason Shapiro thinks (7) is a deduction arises from his seeming confusion about the logical relation between mentation and communication. He maintains:

> It should be stressed that the connection between mentation and communication . . . is not simply an empirical connection which might put mentation in the same category as *tools* of communication (*e.g.*, printing presses, tympanic membrances, or auditoriums). It is by definition embraced in the term "communication," a term properly defined as involving the expression of ideas, thoughts, and feelings. To affect the nature of content of mentation is thus, as a matter of logical necessity, to affect communication involving or depending upon such mentation. Mentation is not simply a means of or aid for communication; it is a logically prior antecedent of *any* communication.[4]

This relation between mentation and communication is crucial to the First Amendment argument because mentation is protected only because, and to the extent that, it falls under the protected communication umbrella. A constitutional protection for thinking (mentation) per se is a very different matter from Shapiro's argument about protected communication. Yet, despite the relation between mentation and communication, pivotal for Shapiro's argument, the above quotation is the only place where it is mentioned. He does attempt to explain in a footnote why, within a formalized language system, some statements are logically true (that is, as a result of definitions, axioms or linguistic inference rules). Shapiro tenders this explanation to "elaborate" upon the idea "that mentation 'is a logically prior antecedent of . . . communication'. If X is a logically prior antecedent of Y, then the statement 'Y implies X' is necessarily or 'logically' true."[5]

By combining the quoted textual passage and the footnote, we see that Shapiro must either be correct by definition (his), or just confusing. If "Y implies X" it does not logically follow that X is a logically prior antecedent of Y. There are other reasons why "Y implies X" may be logically true; for example, "X is Y" or "X" exists if, and only if, Y exists. Since no axiom or linguistic inference rule posits that mentation is a necessary antecedent of communication, it is clear that their "logical" connection is created only by definitional fiat. Because the relevant language system (of the law) is a natural and not a formal language system, Shapiro cannot posit mentation as the "logically prior antecedent of *any* communication" and then pretend to have deduced the relation as a matter of logic. Whether the natural language system of law necessarily (by definition and not just empirically) presupposes mentation is quite another matter. To ascertain if this relationship obtains one must examine how the legal system deals with and protects communication, a process that clearly eschews putting mentation protection in by definition and then alleging to get it out by deduction.

There is a further difficulty with the "logical relationship" aspect of this First Amendment argument. If we assume that there cannot be communication without mentation, does it necessarily follow, as Shapiro and the Detroit court believe, that protection of the former necessarily implies protection of the latter? Even more importantly, does "protection" always necessarily denote the same kind or degree of insulation? Is a language system a logically prior antecedent of communication? Is such a language system constitutionally protected in the same way or to the same degree as constitutionally protected communication? I am not even sure what it means to say a language system is constitutionally protected because communication is. Many things, phenomena, and relations are logically prior antecedents to communication, but despite this "logical" relationship, no legal consequences follow either possibly or necessarily.

Thus, there seems to be no logical relationship between communication and mentation such as would support Shapiro's "logical" First Amendment argument. However, the reader should not infer that there is no basis for a First Amendment protection for mentation. I believe such an argument could be constructed along the lines of Shapiro's seven steps, but with this important difference: one must realize that the relation between communication and mentation is not a logical but an empirical phenomenon. This difference is particularly important in steps (4) and (5). Indeed, while (4) states that it is "in fact" (not in logic) impossible to make an advance determination of what mentation is necessary for communication, (5) seems to forget that the crucial relation in (4) is not logical but empirical. Once this latter relationship is recognized then (5) would more rationally become: because there is a present lack of knowledge about what mentation or what kind of mentation is necessary for communication, it is "therefore" preferable to err on the side of too expansive protection rather than risk compromising the fundamental right to freedom of communication. Stated in this way it becomes clear that constitutional questions about coercion and for or against therapy, organic or otherwise, are to be determined largely, if not exclusively, by the present state of medical knowledge and not by logic. Given such a formulation of (5), it becomes possible to consider the "evidence" about psychosurgery and its effects upon mentation; while if the "therefores" in (5) and (7) are regarded as logically warranted, empirical evidence about therapeutic practices and effects is irrelevant. To make this decision in advance seems strangely inconsistent with the basic philosophy of the First Amendment, which is that knowledge will make you free. While I am sympathetic to any attempt to find constitutional support for the argument that the state should not coerce to "health," I am perplexed because all organic therapies, including psychosurgery, are criticized more frequently and more intensely than nonorganic therapies. Consequently, even if Shapiro's steps (4) and (5) were interpreted as making empirical knowledge rather than logic the decisive factor, I would still regard these postulates as objectionable because they single out organic therapies.

Finally, it should be noted that Shapiro's "logical" argument and one based upon empirical evidence and relations differ not merely in matters of style but quite fundamentally as matters of context. If the alleged logical relation between mentation and communication existed, a First Amendment per se prohibition upon certain therapies might make sense and rigid statutory barriers protecting mentation might be warranted. When however the basis for protection is the relevant state of empirical knowledge, statutory barriers and per se prohibitions seem uniquely inappropriate because of the rapidity with which medical knowledge accumulates and/or becomes obsolete. This last point is well illustrated by the contemporary fiasco involving statutory schemes for dealing with phenylketonuria (PKU).[6] Well-intentioned, sincere people successfully lobbied for legislation in more than forty states on the basis of empirical knowledge about the disease; however, even before all these statutes were enacted, the relevant knowledge bank had been rendered obsolete. Where the knowledge accretion rate is high, and the basis for relevant legislation is a rapidly changing data bank, elasticity and not ridigity is required, and thus statutory per se tests are wrong. Given the difficulty of repealing legislation, such elasticity also mitigates against statutory "solutions" when the relevant base is in flux. Thus, the California legislation (and that elsewhere under consideration) which purports to solve "the psychosurgery problem" by imposing per se prohibitions or operationally nonfunctional criteria in order to discourage a particular set or class of procedures strikes me as paradigmatically wrong.[7] Given the three kinds of possible governmental intervention—executive, legislative, or judicial—legislative regulation of psychosurgery is probably the most impractical.

The Present State of Medical Knowledge about Psychosurgery

In order to cross-examine witnesses in the Detroit psychosurgery case, I read very extensively in the medical psychosurgery literature, which is on the whole comprehensible even to the nonspecialist. While I could read this literature with relative ease, its generally unscientific character is what most forcefully struck my philosophically disposed and legal eye. With the possible exception of some reports and analyses of the results of surgical treatment for temporal lobe epilepsy, the literature about psychosurgery and other surgical procedures designed to affect mentation or behavior was, almost without exception, anecdotal. Much of the material one would expect in a scientific evaluation of a new or controversial surgical procedure was missing or grossly inadequate; there was a striking lack of adequate pre- and postsurgical reports on the psychological, neurological, and general medical evaluations of the patient as well as nearly total absence of sociological data which might be relevant if not crucial. The literature also fails to provide any long-term follow-up histories without which the significance or value of any surgical intervention cannot be judged. While I am not certain that a comparable relevant literature exists for kidney or heart transplants, society regards the heart and kidneys as just organs and the brain as something generically different.

We must ponder what this data deficiency implies for the legal protection of mentation. Does such a deficiency require that legislators or judges must impose per se or functionally equivalent per se prohibitions on brain surgery? Since we are here considering only the regulation of certain surgical procedures on the brain, should certain procedures (e.g., "psychosurgery") be absolutely prohibited at this time, or for a certain class of potential patients? We have quickly reached a point that is far from Shapiro's First Amendment argument against coercion. Indeed, a major difficulty in Shapiro's coercion argument arises from the seeming gap between regulation of psychosurgery and regulation of the coercion it implies. His first five steps can be compressed as follows: (1) the First Amendment protects communication; (2) communication necessarily involves mentation; and (3) therefore, protection of communication requires protection of mentation. This is so (4) because the First Amendment guarantees the right to communicate about virtually anything, and it must therefore also guarantee the right to think (mentate) about almost anything. Indeed, Shapiro writes after step (5): "The argument thus far establishes that the first amendment protects mentation." My difficulty is in understanding what (6) and (7) add to the argument, since the footnote to (6) defines organic therapy as that which affects mentation and (7) merely repeats (4). If Shapiro's initial steps establish that mentation is protected as is communication, then we know that coerced mentation, like coerced speech, is prohibited. Since "intrusive" connotes interferences with "personal autonomy," Shapiro's declaration that all "organic therapies . . . probably fall within the scope of the first amendment" because "[all] organic therapies are considerably intrusive"[8] is tautological.

Shapiro has obviously defined into his premises everything he wants to get out of his conclusion. It is given that all organic therapy affects mentation by interfering with personal autonomy and that "interfere" is neutral; that is, the effect of the intervention, whether good, bad, or indifferent, is interference. My argument is that (7) can have legal significance only if it can be shown that the prohibition against coercively imposed thought control requires regulation of psychosurgery as well as of organic therapy because such procedures do in fact, and not just by definition: (A) affect mentation; and/or (B) affect it in a way which is not trivial; and/or (C) affect it so that there is some unwanted interference with personal autonomy. In other words, Shapiro's (6) is intrinsically defective because it ignores the possibility that even if we postulate that any brain surgery (or organic therapy) will satisfy (A) and (B), it does not therefore follow that such a procedure is objectionable. Consequently, accepting Shapiro's footnote interpretations of "intrusive" and "interference" does nothing to make (6) an argument which culminates in (7). Step (7) is well-entrenched without (6) because his first five steps already establish that coerced mentation is prohibited. Step (6) has relevance to the argument only if (C) is included, and it is precisely at this point that the relation between any proposed medical procedure and the First Amendment argument is most dependent upon empirical knowledge about the state of the art of psychosurgery. It is because of its ambiguity and vagueness that "unwanted" furnishes just the right adjectival modification for "interference." The plasticity of "unwanted" makes clear how necessary it is to work out the implications of (C) in order to develop principles to guide decisions.

Because Shapiro ignores the crucial "unwanted interference" dimension, current psychosurgery literature seemingly has no bearing on his argument. To me, on the contrary, the state of the art appears critically important, and a crucial question is, "What relation exists between the state of the art and the state of the literature?" Although I have not heretofore discriminated carefully between these two notions, they are by no means interchangeable. For purposes of legal prohibition or regulation of psychosurgery, the state of the art is almost irrelevant, while the state of the literature may be dispositive. The general comprehensibility but unscientific character of most psychosurgery literature becomes more meaningful once we acknowledge that significant legal consequences turn upon whether a proposed intrusion affects unwanted interference. This idea implies, as a minimum, that it is possible to know the inevitable (probable, likely, possible) effects of an intrusion, for without such knowledge there would be no way to determine whether effects are unwanted. Indeed, some psychosurgical procedures may have neither discernible effects, objectively ascertainable effects, nor subjectively perceivable effects. Yet the degree and kind of knowledge (information, data) communication between the doctor and the prospective surgical candidate, which is relevant in the legal context, can only be ascertained by the state of the literature. While an investigator could occasionally furnish more knowledge than would be warranted by the "state of the literature test," given the clinical practice of medicine it is the literature test which is likely to be dispositive on legal issues.

Psychosurgery and Personal Autonomy

Shapiro advances "three major propositions" which he believes lead to and warrant First Amendment protection. The second and third propositions are credible only if the first is, and so it is this first proposition which is the "basic norm" of Shapiro's construction.

> The first is a moral thesis: it is prima facie (presumptively) immoral for the state to effect substantial changes in a person's mentation against his will. That is, mind control is prima facie wrong and must be justified on moral grounds adequate to overcome the presumption of immorality. This proposition is simply an instance of the general moral principle of personal autonomy that forcing individuals to do what they do not wish to do, or preventing them from doing what they wish to do, is prima facie wrong.[9]

I strongly believe that mind control is immoral because contrary to the "general [and fundamental] moral principle of personal autonomy," and I also share Shapiro's belief that the moral principle of personal autonomy has constitutional status and therefore freedom of mentation is protected. Nevertheless, I still find Shapiro's First Amendment argument unconvincing. I find his attempt to substitute definitions for knowledge at crucial places in order to create the appearance of a logically deductive argument objectionable, and I would use knowledge tests rather than definitional fiats to develop a functional constitutional test for the requisite protection. This important difference is most discernible when we consider the relation between psychosurgery and autonomy, especially if intrusiveness is the test of whether and how far autonomy is comprised by a given medical procedure.

The three crucial terms here are "psychosurgery," "personal autonomy," and "intrusive." In chapter two I argued that Shapiro misuses the first of these terms because of his exaggerated belief that psychosurgery could be used solely to control aggression. In defending a statutory per se rule "which forecloses entirely both psychosurgery and ESB on patients lacking capacity for informed consent," Shapiro insists that it is "simply unjust to subject [such persons] to an intrusive, irreversible procedure whose therapeutic soundness is sharply in question."[10] His accompanying footnote adds that "it would seem that current psychosurgery is better described as representing efforts directed toward control of aggressive, violent, or 'emotional' outbursts rather than as efforts toward restoration of decision-making competence."[11] The significance of his last observation for understanding what personal autonomy means is seen when "restoration of decision-making competence" is contrasted with Shapiro's statement about personal autonomy in the first of the "three major propositions" which underpin his First Amendment argument. There he indicates that personal autonomy is defined by whether individuals are forced "to do what they do not wish to do, or [prevented] from doing what they wish to do."[12] Much if not all of the difficulty with Shapiro's analysis results from a confusion between autonomy as self-competence and autonomy as insulation from coercion. The two concepts are dramatically different, even if the latter is a necessary condition for the former. The crucial point is that insulation from coercion can never be a sufficient condition for decision-making competence, and so knowledge about what a psychosurgical procedure may do is absolutely essential for developing any functional constitutional test for the protection of mentation. The per se rule prohibiting psychosurgery or ESB for someone lacking competence to give informed consent suggests an inconsistency, in that important consequences (the denial of access to a particular therapy) turn upon the absence of the very criterion which is supposedly necessary before important consequences can attach. This rule implies that the subject is protected against coercion because he is competent, but he is coercively denied access to a particular therapy if incompetent.

The difference between the noncoercion and competence tests of personal autonomy becomes even more important if prevention of coercion means only prevention of unwanted interference, as urged above. If the relevant standard for the constitutional barrier is prevention of unwanted interference, then the noncoercion element of autonomy merges into the competence element and the basis of decision becomes whether the intervention increases, diminishes, or leaves unaffected decision-making competence. Shapiro appears to deny that psychosurgery can ever increase competence autonomy; although in one place he recognizes that even if psychosurgery has a "dampening" effect on mental functioning, "this very dampening may also involve the elimination of dysfunctional responses to certain stimuli, and thus enlarge the set of opportunities for rational action."[13]

If one appreciates this competence-enlarging possibility of psychosurgery, how can he favor per se prohibition, or a First Amendment barrier which operationally forbids such procedures? Shapiro favors prohibitions because of his belief that "current psychosurgery'' is concerned primarily, or even only, with the control of aggression rather than with the "restoration of decision-making competence," and because of his related belief that psychosurgery's " 'therapeutic' value is seriously in doubt."[14] In other words, Shapiro favors some per se prohibition upon psychosurgery because he prejudges such procedures to be therapeutically valueless and directed toward control of violence rather than restoration of competence. Although there is absolutely no hard evidence to support the latter belief, it is not difficult to understand why a competent scholar might have adopted such a position. The kind of psychosurgical procedure which has received the greatest attention in the popular media has been that which is directed toward control of violence. In addition, probably the most widely read "scientific" book about psychosurgery is Mark and Ervin's *Violence and the Brain.* This book is "scientific" rather than scientific, because although its authors are prominent medical scientists who purport to describe and evaluate their research on the title subject, they blatantly manipulate a scientific, biomedical "style" in order to encourage a belief in hard-core relationships between medical interventions and "disorders," even though scientific data does not support the existence of such relationships.[15] Such bad "science" lends credibility to the fictional persuasiveness of *A Clockwork Orange,* and with the aid of newspaper stories about prison wardens who favor psychosurgery to control their violent inmates, makes it easy to believe that psychosurgery *is* violence control!

In reality the range of procedures covered by "psychosurgery"—whether defined by Shapiro, the NIMH, or me—is very broad and includes many which do not involve violence control. It is therefore unwarranted to emphasize the correlation between phychosurgery and violence control while ignoring psychosurgery's usefulness in competence restoration. Indeed, the information I have acquired from those neurologists, neurosurgeons, and phychiatrists willing to discuss the matter, clearly shows that the overwhelming majority of private clinical cases in which a psychosurgical intervention was recommended or carried out had competence restoration, and not violence control, as its aim. While it may be that competence restoration is not the target, so far as institutionalized patients are concerned, I wonder whether competence restoration, making patients manageable, is not at least as important as violence control for "selfishly" motivated institutional managers.

Shapiro's second reason for advocating per se prohibitions upon psychosurgery is the single glaring departure from a generally high level of scholarship in the article. It is disconcering to find him insisting that the " 'therapeutic' value of [psychosurgery] is seriously in doubt." While his text moves on to a different subject, there is a footnote which refers the reader to a later footnote. However, neither in the text nor in the accompanying footnotes is there any plausible defense for Shapiro's sweeping condemnation of all psychosurgical procedures. Shapiro's reliance upon the writings of Breggin is particularly objectionable because anyone even vaguely familiar with the literature about psychosurgery knows that in addition to lacking any special professional competence about it, Breggin has neither done any original work nor published any scientific papers in any scientific journal on psychosurgery.[16] Breggin's nonscientific writings about psychosurgery are probably the least reliable source of data or analysis on the subject, and it is dismaying that a scholar like Shapiro depends so much upon them.

Shapiro's readiness to support his sweeping condemnation of psychosurgery without carefully reviewing more of the relevant literature is a further result of his fixation upon psychosurgery for the control of aggression. Because he ignores the range of procedures which are covered by "psychosurgery" he can write: "Consider the contemporary practice of psychosurgery, which has come under heavy attack from many quarters. Psychosurgery, whether successful in inhibiting aggressive urges or not. . . . "[17] Notice the jump from psychosurgery in the first sentence to psychosurgery for controlling aggression in the second, an identification Shapiro repeatedly seems to make. Shapiro would have been more consistent had he said: "Consider the contemporary use of psychosurgery to control aggression, which has come under attack. . . . "

I have mentioned Shapiro's mistaken identification of psychosurgery and aggression control so often because the point he is trying to make about the valuelessness of some, or even all, psychosurgery is entirely irrelevant to his own First Amendment argument. His logical First Amendment argument, directed as it is primarily toward insulation from coercion, cuts both ways as regards psychosurgery: the state may no more impose than deny such procedures. Shapiro is perfectly aware of this consequence although it receives only modest attention in his article. At the very beginning, where he outlines the seven steps of his argument, his concluding seventh step reads:

> The first amendment therefore protects persons against enforced alteration or interference with their mentation by coerced organic therapy. (This last proposition would also be a valid inference if it read: "The first amendment therefore protects persons against certain kinds of *denial* of access to organic therapy, or psychoactive agents generally, which are used to alter mentation.")[18]

Near the end of the article, commenting upon this alternative formulation of (7), Shapiro writes:

> The first amendment argument presented earlier in a seven step derivation reaches the conclusion that if "communication is to be protected, *all* mentation (regardless of its potential involvement in transmission or reception) must . . . be protected." It was then observed that since organic therapy intrusively alters or interferes with mentation, the first amendment protects against coerced alteration or interference with mentation by organic therapy. Another valid inference is that (7') "the first amendment therefore protects persons against certain kinds of *denial* of access to organic therapy, or psychoactive agents generally, which are used to alter mentation."
>
> State denial of access to organic therapies should, on this theory, oblige the state to establish a compelling interest to justify such denial. . . . The state, then, should have to explain why the constitutionally mandated presumption against substitution of judgment is overcome in any given case of denial of access to an organic therapy, or in banning certain organic therapies outright because they are "inherently unsound."[19]

As I have already suggested, disproportionate amounts of attention have been paid to the First Amendent ban against imposing therapy and its ban on denying access to therapy. Shapiro is not insensitive to this imbalance, and in a footnote which points out that the Constitution cuts both ways on the coercion issue, he argues:

> We should review briefly the problem of possible inconsistency between requiring full deference to competent refusal of therapy while not doing so with respect to competent consent for available therapy. The issue of access involves an assessment of the costs and benefits of a desired therapy. Such an assessment contemplates preventing a therapy's use when it is so dangerous that gravely impaired autonomy is very likely. The denial of access might thus be charac-

> terized as a prevention of active self-destruction. Deference to competent refusal, however, allows stasis of a condition of impaired autonomy. The moral preference is thus for inertia—for omissions over acts. This latter per se practice may generate less adverse macro-moral effects than permitting dangerous therapies, because of this generally felt preference for inertia. One who omits to secure medical help for himself is regarded with somewhat less disdain than one who affirmatively acts to inflict injury upon himself. . . . On these views, then, there is no inconsistency between requiring complete deference to informed refusal but not to informed consent. On the other hand, if there were little difference, between autonomy foregone and destruction of autonomy, the macro-effects of the practices might be the same.[20]

Shapiro's thesis here is not very convincing. As the last sentence makes clear, a good deal of specific data about the effects of various procedures is essential to making the necessary judgments. However, as urged above, the same consideration erodes Shapiro's well-developed argument against imposed therapy. Thus the constitutional protection for autonomy as insulation from coercion (let alone as decision-making competence) is ultimately dependent upon empirical knowledge rather than logic.

The futility of substituting definitions for knowledge in order to create an apparently logical argument becomes even more noticeable when one considers state coercion to deny access to "therapy" requested by one competent to do so. Shapiro's analysis of this aspect of the coercion problem rests upon: (A) an argument about paternalistic coercion which I believe sound and convincing; (B) an assumption about organic therapy which I believe clearly wrong; and (C) a further clearly inaccurate assumption about psychosurgery. He develops (A) by using utilitarian and rule-utilitarian arguments to build upon J.S. Mill's famous defense of individual liberty, which declares that the state power cannot force a competent individual to act solely for his own benefit. I think Shapiro convincingly shows that good motives neither dissolve nor even weaken the constitutional barriers against coercion. Consequently, it would seem that requested organic therapy, even psychosurgery, ought not to be barred if the request is made by one who is competent. Yet Shapiro hedges on this logical corollary because of mistaken beliefs underlying assumptions (B) and (C).

The error in (B) arises from his belief that "involuntary intrusive organic therapy is in general a far greater destruction of personal autonomy than physical confinement, but this is a value judgment not shared universally."[21]

His mistake here is in arguing that *any* organic therapy is worse (more destructive of autonomy) than *any* confinement. It is entirely possible that I am misreading Shapiro, for his emphasis may be upon the coercion and not the remedy: he may be urging, for example, not that psychosurgery is worse than jail, but that coerced psychosurgery is worse than coerced jail. However, if that is his purpose, he advances no reasons in its defense, and one must surely wonder why psychosurgery is more destructive of autonomy than jail—unless psychosurgery "recycles"[22] the subject-prisoner more than does prison. If that is Shapiro's argument, then we are back to (B) as I have interpreted it. Neither of us then can muster any evidence from controlled studies to support or defeat either theory. However, (B) strains my credulity by suggesting that lifelong imprisonment on a Devil's Island or a nineteenth-century southern prison farm would leave the subject more autonomous than some nonaversive conditioning. Indeed, I would suggest that such imprisonment is more destructive of what is left of autonomy than either an aversive organic therapy or some psychosurgery procedures.

Assumption (C), which further disposes Shapiro to avoid the hard-line consequences of the First Amendment protection against paternalistic coercion, is that psychosurgery is more destructive of autonomy than other organic therapies and more destructive than any nonorganic therapy. He comes to this conclusion because he finds psychosurgery more intrusive upon mentation than any other therapy. While I shall examine this notion of "intrusiveness" below, the relevant point to the argument against paternalistic coercion is that psychosurgery is thought to be more destructive than other therapies. What is troublesome about (C), as about (B), is that there is simply no data either to support or to refute the belief. I again find it hard to imagine that every psychosurgical procedure (not just those directed toward control of aggression) is more destructive of mentation (and therefore of autonomy) than any other organic or nonorganic therapy.

Because of the premises which underlie (B) and (C), Shapiro is more amenable to restrictions upon First Amendment prohibitions against denial of a requested therapy than he is to restrictions upon protection against imposed therapy. His fear of psychosurgery ultimately leads to this imbalance in the interpretation of the constitutional protection against coercion. My own fear of psychosurgery is so considerably less than my fear of state coercion that I would not shift the balance in favor of the latter unless there were very strong reasons and clearly manageable principles and standards for doing so. (We must remember that the balance here is between coercion to deny therapy and a request for such therapy by one admittedly competent.) Shapiro's principle for deciding when the state may deny requested therapy is that such a demand can be denied only if it is inherently unsound.[23] He recommends allowing psychosurgery to proceed if certain conditions are met.

> To the extent that (1) deliberate self-mental-mutilation is not the patient's object, (2) there is reasonable medical opinion supporting the therapeutic value of psychosurgery and (3) little likelihood exists that the patient's condition will create substantial social costs after the therapy, then the case for allowing the patient to take his chances in accordance with his own preferences seems rather commanding.[24]

Interestingly enough, the current state of the art is specifically made the relevant decisional base here; why this should be so when the question is imposition of therapy is never made clear. In addition, there is nothing about the "inherent unsoundness" principle which suggests it is more appropriate for coercive denial than for imposition. In short, I find no convincing reasons either in the logic of the First Amendment argument or in the evidence provided by the state of the medical art to justify this asymmetry between protection against imposition and denial of therapy.

The Relative Intrusiveness of Psychosurgery

Most of what has been discussed in this chapter, and in Shapiro's article, culminates in the analysis and application of the notion of intrusiveness, particularly as it applies to psychosurgery. Shapiro urges:

> "Intrusiveness" is a standard invoked *both* to establish whether certain practices create a threshold first amendment claim *and* to

> determine whether it is constitutionally permissible to use a given organic therapy, rather than a less intrusive one, upon someone lacking the capacity for informed consent. The distinction drawn between certain organic therapies which are effective in a *relatively* nonintrusive way and those which are effective in a highly intrusive way is thus perfectly consistent with premise (6). . . . All organic therapies are considerably intrusive and thus probably fall within the scope of the first amendment. . . . As used in this Article, the term "intrusive" by definition connotes an interference with personal autonomy: the greater the degree of intrusiveness, the greater the assault on autonomy.[25]

I have previously considered some consequences of defining "intrusive" as connoting any interference with personal autonomy regardless of whether or not the intrusion's effects were wanted. There are some further consequences which arise from this strange definition.

Shapiro recognizes that:

> Since therapies vary in the degree to which we are inclined to view them as intrusive, or nonintrusive, we must address some obvious questions. . . . How do we identify among the infinitude of stimuli or conditions which have *some* effect on mentation those which should be deemed so assaultive . . . that the state should be heavily burdened with justifying their use in altering mentation? . . . In short, not every effort to change behavior by changing attitudes, emotions, or mentation generally constitutes coercive mind control.[26]

The principle used to distinguish objectionable from permissible mind control is "intrusiveness," and the criteria which measure the intrusiveness of an intervention include: (1) the reversibility of its effects; (2) the extent to which its effects create an "unnatural" state rather than restore the person to his prior state; (3) the rapidity of the change; (4) the scope of the change; (5) the extent to which the change can be resisted; and (6) the duration of the change. More interesting than these specific criteria is that "it is immaterial whether the change effects a constriction or amplification of a person's mental functioning, or whether the effects are 'good' or 'bad'."[27] Apparently dichotomies of amplification versus constriction and good versus bad cover the same range of variables as the dichotomy of improvement versus deterioration which Shapiro previously excluded as relevant in determining interference with mentation. It is very tempting to consider separately each positive and negative criterion for intrusiveness and to see if every amplification of mentation is an improvement (let alone good) or whether every constriction is a deterioration (and therefore bad). I believe the answer to both questions is no, but I will eschew considering these criteria individually in order to concentrate upon the larger issue—the principle of intrusiveness.

The problem with the interpretation of this principle, and the application of those criteria Shapiro uses to support it, is the same difficulty we encountered in his analysis of personal autonomy. While the bifurcation in that analysis was between autonomy from coercion and autonomy as decision-making competence, the bifurcation of intrusiveness is between intrusiveness as a function of involuntariness and intrusiveness as a function of the goal of the intrusion. After briefly analyzing his six criteria, Shapiro suggests:

> These criteria of intrusiveness may be roughly captured in part by some notion of voluntariness or self-help in altering thought and behavior patterns. If such alterations seem to be more the joint product of the therapy and the person's voluntary efforts in changing himself rather than the product mainly of mentational effects over which the person has no control, then a conclusion that the regimen (forcibly imposed though it may be) is beyond the first amendment's protection seems justified. Something was done *for* the person with his help, and not to him, or to his mind or personality.[28]

This formulation clearly puts forward the dominant meaning of intrusiveness as the principle by which objectionable is distinguished from tolerable mind control. However when he later analyzes those bases by which the state might overcome First Amendment protection against coercion affecting mentation, Shapiro seemingly develops a different test of intrusiveness. If mentation is protected by the First Amendment as a fundamental right, then to overcome this barrier the state would have to prove both that there is a "compelling state interest" and that the coercively imposed or denied therapy is the "less onerous alternative." That is, even if society's interest is sufficiently great to warrant some state action against the individual subject, is the action taken only as intrusive as is necessary to protect those legitimate state interests? Shapiro goes on:

> Let it be assumed that [the] goal [''rehabilitation,'' ''cure,'' or ''control'' of mental dysfunction causing aberrant behavior] is indeed a compelling state interest. The task is to relate this interest to the process used for effecting conforming behavior. . . . [29]

He then talks about the goals of rehabilitation and mental health, and in a footnote asks:

> To what goal is there, or is there not, a less onerous, equally effective alternative? Without appropriate limitations on the characterization of such goals, the notion of 'less onerous alternative' becomes vacuous, and perforce so does the fundamental right at stake.[30]

While there is no intrinsic inconsistency between intrusiveness tested by voluntariness and intrusiveness as a function of the goal of the intrusion, there are surely some important differences which could be relevant. There is a third test of intrusiveness which permeates much of Shapiro's analysis, and again, this test is not intrinsically inconsistent with either of the others. This third ''meaning'' of intrusiveness is linked to the idea of individual integrity. ''The more gradual the change, the more likely we are to regard it as voluntary and consistent with the maintenance of the integrity of individuality.''[31]

What I find revealing about Shapiro's various tests for intrusiveness, which is *the* crucial principle for determining the scope of First Amendment protection, is that they reflect the two quite different senses of autonomy previously considered. The voluntariness test of intrusion fits autonomy as freedom from coercion, and the goal test of intrusion fits autonomy as decision-making competence. The integrity test, as Shapiro presents it, would come closer to the freedom from coercion sense of autonomy. He apparently intends this test to safeguard the subject's right to remain as he was before the intrusion—be he passion killer or compulsive pyromaniac. I find this use of ''integrity'' in no sense ungrammatical, but when considered in Wittgenstein's sense of language as a shared form of life, rather contrary to the prevailing ''forms of life.''[32] Perhaps this is why Shapiro speaks about the ''integrity of individuality'' rather than the ''integrity of the person,'' since ''person,'' in the sense of human being, gives a flavor to the idea of integrity which does not suggest that integrity is maintained or achieved by retaining whatever may be at least human. Thus "integrity," "autonomy," and "intrusion" all function in two quite different ways: as insulations from change or coercion, or as efforts to attain the *goal* of decision-making *competence* which is necessary for the integrity of a *person*. It is clearly the latter, goal-competence-person sense of "autonomy," "intrusive," and "integrity" which I find most useful in trying to develop the right questions about the regulation of psychosurgery and other organic therapies. Shapiro, on the other hand, seems primarily interested in the no-change, no-coercion sense of these crucial terms. As a result, his questions and answers are less relevant than those which should be considered. It is too easy to lay down per se prohibitions and functionally equivalent rules which serve to bury, rather than solve, real problems. Shapiro's rather mechanical logical approach—if mentation, then no change, no coercion—offers a neat litmus paper test. However, while a mechanical test may be adequate for questions whose answers are only "base" or "acid," "yes" or "no," it is clear that no important questions about psychosurgery are of that order. The distortions generated by Shapiro's simplistic identification of psychosurgery and aggression control thus finally vitiate his analysis and illustrate Wittgenstein's admonition: "A main cause of philosophical disease—one-sided diet: one nourishes one's thinking with only one kind of example."[33]

Chapter 7

INSTITUTIONALIZATION AND INFORMED CONSENT FOR AN EXPERIMENTAL PROCEDURE*

The Detroit Case Opinion

The most troublesome feature about informed consent is the requirement that there be "competence" or "capacity" to give such consent. Except for the Detroit psychosurgery case, there is little relevant case law or legal literature on the criteria for competence or capacity, particularly as regards informed consent for an unconventional procedure. This paucity of explicit case law accounts for the HEW statement preceding its recently proposed regulations on biomedical or behavioral research involving human subjects requiring special protection. In response to the suggestion that its proposed regulations on informed consent be expanded to include "language concerning . . . assurance that the subject comprehends the disclosure," HEW stated that this "suggestion . . . goes beyond requirements for informed consent as they have generally been articulated by the courts."[1]

The already decided cases indicate that competence is pre-

*I have presented the major arguments of this chapter in "Patients, Subjects, and Voluntariness," in J. Schoolar and C. Gaitz, eds., *Research and the Psychiatric Patient* 50 (Brunner/Mazel, 1975).

sumed and that the doctor's judgment on competence should stand. In other words, if the doctor obtains consent, it is presumed that the patient was competent because otherwise the doctor would not have solicited the consent. This "rule" means that the plaintiff will have the burden of proof if it is alleged that his consent was not informed because of incompetence. It requires little imagination to appreciate why, in an age of "consumer protection," it is time to reexamine the legal consequences of the doctor's self-serving statement: "I would not have solicited the consent if I did not think the patient was competent."

One reason why courts have not been more critical about this aspect of the informed consent requirements is that any operationally effective, alternative procedure is likely to be expensive, burdensome for both the patient-subject and the doctor, and unwarranted in more than 90 percent of the cases. Given these disadvantages, and the enormous difficulty in developing criteria to identify cases where more should be required than one doctor's judgment, it is understandable that this aspect of the law on informed consent is underdeveloped. The problem is further exacerbated because cases may need to be distinguished on the basis of what kind or how much competence is required in terms of who is the patient or subject, what is the proposed procedure, and how rational are available alternatives? The last item is particularly subtle because existing law suggests that the irrationality of the patient's decision does not defeat the claim to competence; however, what law there is has not been developed in connection with investigative medicine.

In the Detroit psychosurgery case, the court decided that "involuntarily detained mental patients cannot give informed and adequate consent to experimental psychosurgical procedures on the brain." In other words, regardless of the empirical realities surrounding each individual and his case, being involuntarily detained automatically makes any consent legally inadequate. It is hardly surprising that even a sympathetic commentator has written that "the internal logic of [the court's] holding is difficult to comprehend. If no one can presently give valid consent to any amygdalotomy 'knowledgeably,' as parts of the opinion suggest, it is unnecessary to create a special per se rule for involuntarily committed mental patients. And if the court's holding is limited to such mental patients, 'voluntariness' alone would be a criterion of consent which could not be met in any case. Thus, there is no need to cumulate doubts to reach the opinion's result."[2]

While institutionalization surely complicates the entire informed consent problem, both as to doctor-patient and doctor-subject relations, should it be dispositive on competence, as suggested by the Detroit case? Although the court's statement that institutionalization merely diminishes rather than defeats capacity was applied only to diminished capacity for consent to psychosurgery, the implications of its position are potentially more far-reaching. There is no reason to restrict this argument to psychosurgery if it can be shown that other procedures are comparably complex and subject to unspecifiable uncertainties. In addition, there is no reason to limit this analysis to experimental procedures because the degree and kind of damage to capacity allegedly attributable to institutionalization is independent of any proposed procedure, whether experimental or conventional.

The principal reason that the court's opinion in the Detroit case is an unsatisfactory treatment of the capacity element is because of the mechanical way it dealt with the phenomenon of institutionalization. Being institutionalized is regarded as determinative for the questions of capacity and voluntariness when the basis for determining answers to those questions should be empirical. It may well be, as the Detroit psychosurgery decision suggests, that in an experimental context, the subject's choice of available options (options as to his total life style and not merely ones of health) may be relevant in assessing competence. However, at this point the distinction between competence and voluntariness becomes even more obscure than in the "ordinary" case. In the Detroit case the court declared:

> Although an involuntarily detained mental patient may have a sufficient I.Q. to intellectually comprehend his circumstances . . . the very nature of his incarceration diminishes the capacity to consent to psychosurgery. He is particularly vulnerable as a result of his mental condition, the deprivation stemming from involuntary confinement, and the effects of the phenomenon of "institutionalization."

Commenting upon this argument, a law review writer concludes that the "court's position, then, is that involuntary commitment which removes the patient's normal psychological defenses and offers him no chance to make autonomous choices can only work to erode the competency required to give adequate consent to experimental psychosurgery."[3]

HEW Proposals for Regulating Consent

It is encouraging that proposed HEW regulations on biomedical or behavioral research which involve institutionalized mentally disabled as subjects do not adopt the approach of the Detroit court. While HEW's proposed regulations may significantly restrict research in which such persons may be involved as subjects, they also provide for "the individual's legally effective informed consent to participation in the activity or, where the individual is legally incompetent, the informed consent of a representative with legal authority so to consent on behalf of the individual. . . . "[4] This regulation can be contrasted with the mechanical, exclusionary rule adopted by the Detroit court, which on the question of proxy consent held:

> Equally great problems are found when the involuntarily detained mental patient is incompetent, and consent is sought from a guardian or parent. Although guardian or parental consent may be legally adequate when arising out of traditional circumstances, it is legally ineffective in the psychosurgical situation. The guardian or parent cannot do that which the patient, absent a guardian, would be legally unable to do.

Pursuant to the July 1974 HEW regulations on the protection of human subjects, institutions which receive substantial National Institutes of Health (NIH) research funds will probably review and revise their institutional policies and procedures on research involving human subjects, and past institutional practices on informed consent will also undoubtedly require reappraisals. Such reconsiderations are likely to lead to procedures which maximize the probability that the research subject and/or his proxy comprehends, understands, and appreciates the subject's role in the proposed research. In other words, the new HEW requirement, although not explicitly demanding that the subject or proxy be "competent" to give consent, in effect imposes a competence requirement. This requirement means that the investigator will be faulted when only "mechanical" consent is obtained, even if it is "informed."

Potentially the most influential feature of the HEW regulations on informed consent for research with the mentally disabled is in the provision following that which provides for proxy consent:

> (c) The individual's assent to . . . participation has also been secured when in the judgment of the consent committee he or she has sufficient mental capacity to understand what is proposed and to express an opinion as to his or her participation.

The significance of this provision lies in its distinction between "assent" and "informed consent." Obviously, both are terms of art requiring elaboration and development. But no matter how these terms are defined, the added requirement of subject assent, when the subject is incompetent, creates an enormous new set of complications. No one can foretell whether this new requirement will incline courts to interpret informed consent more or less expansively than they would if proxy consent were alone legally adequate. While there are good reasons for being less demanding about informed proxy consent if the subject also assents, the intrinsic difficulty is that such "secondary" assent requires that the subject have "sufficient mental capacity to understand," a condition that leads one to ask why anything less than the subject's own informed consent should be accepted.

It is impossible not to be sympathetic to the problem which confronted the drafters of the proposed HEW regulations. There is the real possibility that an individual will be declared incompetent for some civil purposes, such as disposition of property, and thus declared incompetent to give informed consent to an experimental medical procedure. In such a situation, if a procedure is therapeutic but places the individual at risk, he might be cut off from his only remaining therapeutic hope unless proxy informed consent were possible. On the other hand, given all the real dangers about inadequately sensitive proxies who might unthinkingly consent, how could potential subjects be protected? The proposed assent requirement may be a workable alternative to the unattractive extremes of no incompetent ever being able to be a subject and any incompetent being made a subject by proxy. If it were necessary to choose one of these almost equally grotesque alternatives, a court might well favor the position adopted in the Detroit case. However, that decision is objectionable because it is not necessary to choose between such extremes. Whether the HEW assent mechanism is the best way to avoid either extreme is not immediately apparent, but that it is better than what the Detroit court did is obvious.

In dealing with the proxy consent problem there are clearly alternative models, some of which are: (a) judicial approval of the proxy consent; (b) an independent "committee of protectors" (rather than an individual family member or friend); and (c) technically competent independent consultants furnished to the family member or friend. While each mechanism presents difficulties, just as the assent technique does, any of these mechanisms is preferable to the Detroit court's blanket ban. A necessary but nonetheless regrettable rule under the proposed HEW regulations is that all regulated research activities must adopt the same mechanism for dealing with the proxy informed consent question. I should have preferred that HEW encourage experimentation on this matter, indicating by regulation only the permissible scope of the alternatives and reserving to the secretary of HEW the power to refuse approval.

Proxy informed consent is potentially important because it may easily be extended beyond institutionalized subjects. Not only is proxy consent important for the mentally disabled and for minors, but the idea of proxy consent may come to play a cardinal role in all unconventional procedures. Indeed, the institutional review committee mechanism now required by HEW regulations and the consent committee mechanism required by its proposed regulations are both proxy mechanisms for determining whether a subject may consent at all. Thus, HEW regulations consistently provide a layer of paternalistic insulation around the consent process in the form of a proxy mechanism.

Another more vexing facet of proxy informed consent arises from the realization that there may be good reasons for doubting whether patients or subjects themselves are *ever* sufficiently competent to give legally adequate consent. The HEW regulations make it clear that in an experimental context individuals cannot give adequate consent by themselves, since such consent becomes adequate only if accepted by the relevant committees and, in effect, by the secretary of HEW. The obviously well-intended paternalism of these HEW regulations on the protection of human subjects raises all the usual problems about state paternalism, and also leaves these questions unanswered. There are good reasons to be suspicious whenever the state bestows an unwanted "advantage," such as protecting patients or subjects from a "wanted" advantage. Unlike the paternalism of motorcycle helmets, warnings about smoking, prohibitions upon marijuana, or high tax rates on alcohol, all of which aim at protecting the individual from his own follies, the paternalism in the judicial or HEW informed consent requirements tries to protect the individual from the follies of others. This latter kind of paternalism is potentially more justifiable because of the enormous disparity between the authority, competence, experience, and other relevant variables possessed by the patient-subject and by the treating or investigating doctor. As Rousseau argued so powerfully, nothing comes close to inequality as a cause of corruption and hypocrisy. Since informed consent requirements cannot aim to remove all inequality, they should try to provide protection against the worse abuses of such inequality. Unhappily, the legalistic tendencies of HEW and the courts discourage the kind of personal and professional morality which frequently provides more real protection than externally imposed and enforced restraints. The familiar tendency to accept compliance with imposed standards in order to avoid seeing that such standards achieve their intended purpose will, I fear, become all too real in this situation. While HEW regulations may protect subjects from those relatively few mass producers of biomedical research who never remember that their subjects are also people, these rules will probably diminish the protection already accorded subjects by that larger group of research doctors who will now no longer feel any personal responsibility for the rights and welfare of their subjects because that obligation has devolved upon various review committees.

Despite my fears that the new HEW regulations may dull an investigator's sense of involvement and personal responsibility, it should be recognized that these rules are a reaction to the accumulated evidence of moral and social insensitivity, if not impropriety, in biomedical and behavioral research. While this insensitivity represents a failure by the relevant professions properly to educate their members about the morality of responsible research, it is debatable whether the new regulations, which represent an exaggerated attempt to adjust the pendulum away from laissez faire research, will create a greater individual concern about morality among researchers. Although many investigators would not agree with legally oriented civil rights enthusiasts who regard the new regulations as long overdue and barely adequate, most of my colleagues in biomedical research are considerably more sympathetic to the general objectives of those regulations than they would have been five or ten years ago. I am inclined to believe that the new regulations may be the required antidote for perceived, even if exaggerated, abuses; however, I also recognize that these new regulations will significantly deter and encumber legitimate research and add to the financial cost of all biomedical research. Whether the new regulations are justified on a cost-benefit analysis basis will probably never be known, yet it is to be hoped that the relevant professions will not require any further federal or judicial prodding about their long-ignored responsibility to teach not only technical expertise but also moral and social competence. The tokenism of medical schools offering one or two elective hours on medical ethics will no longer do.

"Patients," "Subjects," and Informed Consent

Among the many unexamined premises in currently fashionable formulations of the informed consent doctrine is one which distinguishes between patients and subjects. This distinction supports the view that while the usual "commercial" standard of informed consent is appropriate when dealing with patients, something more is required when dealing with subjects. The very influential Declaration of Helsinki, promulgated by the World Medical Association, and officially endorsed by the American Medical Association (AMA), while requiring informed consent for all nontherapeutic experimentation (dealing with subjects), also provides that when the experimentation is intended to be therapeutic (dealing with patients), informed consent may not be required if "consistent with patient psychology." Perhaps the justification for this distinction is the expectation that a doctor treating a patient will heed the ancient Hippocratic admonition, "first of all, do no harm." Thus the treating physician will not even consider an experimental procedure which might harm the patient and so rigorous informed consent is not necessary.

Clearly, apart from the dubious assumption that treating physicians respect the Hippocratic admonition more than do investigating physicians, this justification for requiring less informed consent for patients suffers from many infirmities. Even if treating physicians adhered to the Hippocratic admonition, a further problem would still remain. Does this greater respect in fact *improperly* deter treating physicians from being experimental when they should? Moreover, since almost every treatment as applied to a particular patient is in varying degrees experimental, why should one believe that treating physicians are less likely to do harm than investigating physicians, who if they take risks with subjects are more likely to be deliberate about those risks? We also must note that in medicine doing nothing is doing something; that is, deliberately pursuing no treatment is a deliberate treatment. Consequently, when the treating physician goes no further than nonexperimental procedures, he *is* experimenting because he "does nothing."

I hope I have suggested why permitting a different quality of informed consent for subjects or patients is of dubious propriety. One might be tempted to conclude that if patients and subjects are to be beneficiaries of the same informed consent requirements, there would be some lessening of those requirements when dealing with subjects. However, the long overdue legal concern for the protection of consumers has recently resulted in an elevation of the informed consent required for patients rather than in a lowering of the consent required for subjects. The higher disclosure standard required by recent cases reflects not only the new consumerism but also the changing character of the doctor-patient relationship. While there are probably still some doctor-neighbor relations, it is now less likely than before that a doctor knows enough about his patient's psyche, life style, and his life prospects to indulge in that medical paternalism which protects the doctor who makes less than full disclosure because he is acting in the patient's "best interests."

In the most important recent informed consent cases where a patient (not a subject) sues the treating physician for damages, the federal circuit court for the District of Columbia, and state courts in California, Pennsylvania, Rhode Island, New York, and Wisconsin have refused to hold that informed consent requires only that a doctor disclose those risks which are generally disclosed by other doctors practicing in the community.[5] This objective medical community standard, for which expert testimony was essential, has been replaced by a disclosure requirement virtually identical to that which obtains, pursuant to HEW, FDA, or Veterans' Administration (VA) rules, for research subjects. In *Canterbury*, the leading case, the court concludes that the jury decides: "(1) whether a reasonable patient would have deemed undisclosed information 'significant' in deciding whether to submit to a course of treatment (materiality); and (2) whether a reasonable patient would have foregone that treatment had the information been disclosed (proximate case);" the commentator on the case then suggests that the "courts could provide a welcome simplification of the law if they were to recognize this overlap and focus upon the one relevant question—whether, had all undisclosed information been made known to him, the average prudent patient would have withheld his consent to treatment."[6] In replacing the objective medical community standard by the subjective reasonable man test, the *Canterbury* court found that a risk is material and therefore to be disclosed "when a reasonable person, in what the physician knows or should know to be the patient's position, would be likely to attach significance to the risk or cluster of risks in deciding. . . ."[7]

The Problem of Therapeutic Privilege and Informed Consent

It is worth recalling that feature of the Helsinki Declaration which compromises the requirements for informed consent for *patients* who are "subjected" to therapeutic experimentation. The declaration permits the requirement for informed consent to be waived when "consistent with patient psychology." This is currently known as the "therapeutic privilege," and constitutes one of several rather well-entrenched exceptions to the usual requirements for informed consent. The best known exception is in cases of emergency treatment, and there are also less clear exceptions tolerated by some courts. For example, some require no disclosure if the patient will suffer no serious consequences, or if the risks are such that any reasonable person would have known of them.

It is difficult to develop an impressive justification for the therapeutic privilege even for patients in a nonexperimental situation. Such justification is probably based upon vague notions about "first of all, do no harm," the theory being that if a patient's medical condition would be worsened by full disclosure, then disclosure is not required. The unstated presumption is either that "patient condition" is the same as "medical condition of the patient" or that the patient has no right to regard any other condition as more important than his medical condition. The first is patently false and the second is simply a reflection of one of the dangerous, but deeply entrenched, prejudices of our time—that if you have good health, you have everything. Although the privilege is easily abused even as applied to patients receiving conventional therapies, it ought to have no relevance when applied to subjects for biomedical research. Further, it ought to have no relevance when a "patient" is to be the "subject" for innovative or experimental therapy.

The therapeutic privilege is easily abused because treating physicians can so readily manipulate patients and situations to create an environment in which fuller disclosure plausibly would have "worsened the patient's 'condition'." The therapeutic privilege thus becomes a mechanism by which a sincere but authoritarian physician, convinced that the patient's medical condition cannot be improved except by a proposed therapy, can insure the receipt of informed consent by defending the nondisclosure of relevant risks. He will do so by arguing that the patient's psychological state would have rendered the latter incompetent either to consent or deny consent. However, it is perfectly clear that one principal aim of informed consent is to prevent the physician from saying the patient is "better off" because of the procedure, and that therefore the doctor's having induced the consent ought never to be actionable (or wrong). Because paternalistic coercion is not any less coercive than self-serving coercion, and an imposed "benefit" is not any the less imposed, coercively induced benefits are as incompatible with the right of self-determination as are coercively induced disadvantages. Incidentally, the usual physician defense of nondisclosure maintains that fuller disclosure of relevant risks would scare the patient into denying consent and thus deprive him of what he needs. However, the empirical evidence to support this widely held belief is simply not available.

It is also worth questioning whether the therapeutic privilege, even as to patients, is not somewhat inconsistent with the competency required if consent is to be regarded as informed. The competency required for informed consent is such that the patient can evaluate, understand, and appreciate the relevant material information. Yet if he is incompetent to handle such information because it would be too upsetting, how can the consent be regarded as informed? The courts have not explored this apparent inconsistency, probably because a doctor might be liable for causing psychological stress by disclosing too much, and since a patient may have a right to waive disclosure entirely, he may partially waive it by implication. However, neither reason for tolerating the apparently inconsistent therapeutic privilege seems very convincing; the preservation of a rigorous competence standard seems so essential to informed consent that a continued physician reliance upon therapeutic privilege to justify nondisclosure would hardly be well advised.

In at least one notorious informed consent case, admittedly involving research subjects and not patients, the therapeutic privilege line of thinking was relied upon as a defense. The case is notorious because of the newspaper coverage and the prominence of the persons involved, and because it dealt with the injection of cancer cells into already hospitalized persons suffering from disabilities other than cancer.[8] The experiment was financed by the United States Public Health Service (for which the principal investigator was a consultant) and the American Cancer Society. The principal investigator was also a consultant for the National Cancer Institute which recommended recipients for American Cancer Society research grants, a full member of the Sloan-Kettering Institute for Cancer Research, an associate professor at Cornell College of Medicine, and on the staff of at least two distinguished hospitals in New York City. Thus this case, which occurred only ten years ago and hence two decades after Nuremberg, did not involve a young, inexperienced investigator at the county hospital in Podunk who hoped to make his reputation by finding a cancer cure. Nonetheless, this experienced distinguished investigator defended his failure to obtain informed consent because "within any reasonable definition of the words 'no risk' there was no risk"[9]—and, therefore, why risk upsetting the "patients?"

There are four aspects of the cancer cell case which are germane to our present inquiry: (1) the experiment was successful; (2) the investigator was correct that there were no risks for the subjects; (3) the investigator knew that informed consent was required; and (4) the improprieties of the experiments were exposed by a doctor on the hospital staff and not by the subjects, their families, friends, or attorneys.

(1) The experiment provided confirmation for the very important hypothesis that persons seriously debilitated by diseases other than cancer would reject live cancer cells as quickly and completely as healthy persons. (Interestingly but not surprisingly, prison volunteers were used to establish the rejection rate for healthy persons.) Thus we see that research "success' is no more relevant than failure in determining the need for, or propriety of, informed consent.

(2) Even the investigative committee failed to challenge the investigator's claim that research subjects were not exposed to risk. Two of the subjects died soon after the cancer cells were injected, but they were already seriously ill and it was never maintained that the injections caused or hastened their deaths. Thus we see that the investigator's correct perception of the risk also does not immunize him from liability for failure to obtain appropriate informed consent. This fact is particularly important in light of the 1974 HEW regulations for biomedical research on human subjects. These regulations are clearly directed at research in which subjects are at risk, and thus one might be tempted to conclude that under these most recent federal standards, the doctors were improperly condemned in the cancer cell case where the subjects were not at risk. However, the definition of "subjects at risk" in the new regulations suggests a quite different conclusion.

> "Subject at risk" means any individual who may be exposed to the possibility of injury, including physical, psychological, or social injury, as a consequence of participation as a subject in any research, development, or related activity which departs from the application of those established and accepted methods necessary to meet his needs, or which increases the ordinary risks of daily life, including the recognized risks inherent in a chosen occupation or field of service.[10]

Since healthy persons, let alone those already nearly terminal, suffer the possibility of psychological injury if injected with live cancer cells, it would be necessary to comply with the HEW regulations if they were otherwise applicable. Indeed, the cancer cell case illustrates why HEW may have been correct in using such seemingly broad language for the definition of "at risk."

(3) It is the consent aspect of the cancer cell case which makes it so appalling, even if there were no possibility of psychological injury. It is perfectly clear that the investigators knew consent was required, and they did obtain oral consent from their subjects. However, the Board of Regents of the University of New York found these investigators guilty of fraud and deceit. The doctors did not merely deem themselves as sufficiently right so as to justify less than full disclosure of all material facts, but used their superior knowledge to justify disclosing none of these facts. Yet although the investigators had a deep confidence about their hypothesis, nonetheless they could not be entirely certain. When asked why he did not use himself as a subject, the principal investigator reportedly said, "Let's face it, there are relatively few skilled cancer researchers, and it seemed stupid to take even the little risk."[11]

(4) Perhaps the most interesting feature of the cancer cell case is that the medical profession itself brought the matter into the open. This was accomplished largely through the persistence of Dr. William Hyman who, although having been a director of the hospital since its inception of 1926, was not re-elected to this position after he sued the hospital to force disclosure of the medical records of those patients used as research subjects. In addition, some hospital personnel resigned to protest the experiment. This aspect of the matter is important because it supports my belief that despite external restraints imposed by law, it is perhaps even more important to cultivate and encourage internal restraints.

The Definition of Patient and Subject

The basis for the distinction between patients and subjects is often only dimly perceived except for cases at the polar extremes. It is evident that the same human being may be both clearly a patient and clearly a subject, even as to the same doctor. The cancer cell case illustrates the more usual situation: to the hospital staff not knowingly involved in the experiment those twenty-two people were patients, while to the investigators and the hospital staff who collaborated they were subjects. It is of course possible that at different times the same person is both patient and subject to the same doctor. Usually in such cases the time differences will be sequential, and normally the patient will become the subject, although there are numerous cases where this normal pattern does not obtain.

Let us consider these two situations:

Case A: Mr. A has been seeing Dr. P, a psychiatrist, for two years. He was referred to P by his family doctor because of a hand-washing compulsion. A has not benefited from his psychotherapy and faces severe poverty as he is about to lose his job because he is so frequently washing his hands. P recommends that A see Dr. N, a prominent neurologist, who after appropriate evaluation recommends a surgical procedure on A's brain. In consultation with Dr. S, a prominent neurosurgeon, it is agreed between S and N that A should have a __________. A is confronted by S and N and his consent solicited.

Case B: B has been imprisoned for many years. Even before entering prison, but more so now, he has suffered from a hand-washing compulsion. Dr. N, Mr. A's neurologist, is seeking persons who have such a compulsion in order to test the controversial hypothesis that __________ does favorably affect such a compulsion. In consultation with Dr. S, the same neurosurgeon as in Case A, B is identified as someone who has the appropriate symptomology and his consent is solicited.

Although anyone's initial reaction would be that A is a patient and B a subject, I have considerable difficulty in finding rationally attractive and operationally manageable criteria for distinguishing these cases. Of course there are differences, but the question is whether these differences justify dissimilarities in the character or extent of the relationship between A or B and the doctors. N and S owe the same obligation to A and B, as to both diagnosis and performance, and their malpractice liability is measured by the same standards in both cases, since the right of recovery, the burden of proof, and the measure of any damages are the same. Under the recent consent cases, the kind and degree of disclosure required for effective informed consent is also the same. Why then would we nonetheless probably say A is the patient of N and S, but B is their subject? The principle which emerges is that if a person can mount a legal assault upon a doctor who recommended or carried out some procedure because the procured consent was defective, then the legal efficacy of the consent will not be any more or less realistic because of the plaintiff's status as patient or subject. But this is not much of a "rule," since we still face trying to formulate functional, realistic principles for identifying cases in which informed consent is required and for determining competence, proxy competence, materiality of risk, and voluntariness, as well as the scope and depth of required disclosure.

Consent and the Involuntarily Committed

The post-*Canterbury* trend in informed consent cases suggests that each situation must be considered on its own merits. Furthermore, these recent cases imply that the same considerations should determine if a consent was informed and legally effective whether the case involves patients, subjects, involuntarily restrained persons, or volunteers. This emerging individualizing but egalitarian development in the law of informed consent is attractive because it recognizes each human being's personality and right to be treated as something more than the general labels he embodies. "Prisoners," "the mentally disabled," "involuntary" or "voluntary hospital patients," "ordinary patients," "subjects," or "volunteers" are all attributions made by socially sanctioned and institutionalized mechanisms. One is not an individual human being because of such an attribution; clearly more respect should go to a unique, complex personality than to any reductive labels imposed by society's role-manufacturing agents. Treating informed consent as a matter peculiar to each individual case respects our basic individual humanity, while decisions based upon class or category do not. The post-*Canterbury* cases affirm that individual personhood is worthy of greater respect than category or status. The Detroit psychosurgery decision, alas, does precisely the contrary.

In the Detroit case the court concluded that although a "patient, institutionalized or not" could give "truly informed consent" for "a regular surgical procedure. . . . Informed consent cannot be given by an involuntarily detained mental patient for experimental psychosurgery. . . . " The court so concluded because it found: "Involuntarily confined mental patients live in an inherently coercive institutional environment. Indirect and subtle psychological coercion has profound effect upon the patient population. Involuntarily confined patients cannot reason as equals with the doctors and administrators over whether they should undergo psychosurgery. They are not able to voluntarily give informed consent because of the inherent inequality in their position." The court further found: "Although an involuntarily detained mental patient may have a sufficient I.Q. to intellectually comprehend his circumstances . . . the very nature of his incarceration diminishes the capacity to consent to psychosurgery. . . . Institutionalization tends to strip the individual of the support which permits him to maintain his sense of self-worth and the value of his own physical and mental integrity. An involuntarily confined mental patient clearly has diminished capacity for making a decision about irreversible experimental psychosurgery."

What reason is there to believe that a committed patient who enjoys sufficient competence and equality of "bargaining power" to give "truly" informed consent for such complex but nonexperimental surgery as a portal-caval shunt for cirrhosis, an internal mammary artery myocardial implant, or even an ilestomy for ulcerative colitis, suddenly loses that competence and equality because the procedure is experimental psychosurgery? Is there *necessarily,* that is, logically by definition or empirically, some greater intrinsic complexity or subtlety about any and every experimental psychosurgical procedure than any "regular" surgical procedure? The court's answer to this key question is a clear non sequitur. What it appears to say is that because as a matter of law the involuntarily committed patient cannot consent to experimental psychosurgery, he lacks the requisite capacity. But the patient only lacks this capacity *after* such a decision. Therefore, translated into plain English, what the court has said is that these patients lack capacity as a matter of law because the court holds, as a matter of law, that they lack capacity. The court is forgetting that it was not only to decide questions but to do so in a particular way, namely by the use of rules, principles, and reasons. If all we wanted were a "decision," we could save much effort and money by rolling dice. Unfortunately, in this important case the court did not furnish any reasons for its conclusion. To have done so would have required that the court show why, not as a matter of law but as a matter of fact, any procedures denominated experimental psychosurgery are necessarily so much more complex or obscure that a patient sufficiently competent and endowed with equality of bargaining power to understand "regular" surgical procedures suddenly loses both capacities. To tell us that the nature of the contemplated procedure affects the equality of bargaining power or the patient's competence is only to demonstrate that if the conclusion is built into the premise, it can be no surprise if it appears in the conclusion.

The court's method of decision by definition or non sequitur is illustrated by two further aspects of its opinion. Some thirteen involuntarily committed patients from the institution where John Doe had been kept, after reading newspaper accounts of the pending trial, wrote a letter on their own initiative stating that they did not want to be considered for the research project. I have suggested that their action mitigated against the argument that institutionalized patients are necessarily so overwhelmed by their environment that they will readily consent to any medical procedure. The court apparently thought it was responding to this argument in declaring: "The fact that thirteen patients unilaterally wrote a letter saying they did not want to be subjects of psychosurgery is irrelevant to the question of whether they can consent to that which they are legally precluded from doing." One need not be a Ph.D. in mathematical logic to wince at this substitute for an argument. The court is quite right in saying the letter is irrelevant if the patients could not consent as a matter of law. However, the question which the court was supposed to be deciding is precisely whether, as a matter of law, there could be consent. Presuming the answer to the question in putting the question hardly seems a rational principle for decision making.

The same technique for evading the question is used by the court when it discusses whether and how a legal guardian could give informed consent for an involuntarily committed patient. Since this was a specific question put to the court, one hoped that the court would at least analyze the matter. Instead, the entire subject is disposed of by finding that "a guardian or parent cannot do that which the patient, absent a guardian, would be legally unable to do." Although the finding is probably wrong as a matter of law (couldn't a guardian effectively execute a contract or dispose of a patient's assets, even though the patient "would be legally unable to do so"?), the statement is even more objectionable because the court is again "deciding" by definition or non sequitur. To say that we will hold, as a matter of law, and the patient cannot consent, and to argue therefore that the patient cannot consent is bad enough, but to say that because we so hold, the guardian cannot consent either, is clearly to have left the substantive question untouched.

The court's entire analysis of whether a guardian can consent if the patient cannot consists of urging: "Equally great problems are found when the involuntarily detained mental patient is incompetent, and consent is sought from a guardian or parent. Although guardian or parental consent may be legally adequate when arising out of traditional circumstances, it is legally ineffective in the psychosurgery situation." "Equally great" arises from the belief that: "Institutionalization tends to strip the individual of the support which permits him to maintain his sense of self-worth and the value of his own physical and mental integrity. An involuntarily confined mental patient clearly has diminished capacity for making a decision about irreversible experimental psychosurgery." As I already pointed out, the conclusion of the court vis-à-vis guardians is logically irrelevant and it should now be clear that it is empirically irrelevant as well. Granting the truth of all that is said in the opinion about institutionalization, what is the significance of those factors as regards consent by a guardian? Is it presumed that the guardian has also been institutionalized? Or on the contrary, doesn't the question about guardians presume that a guardian will be chosen who does not suffer the disadvantages of the ward? Couldn't a guardian be chosen who would not only be of equal bargaining power to the doctors, but even superior to them? Or couldn't it be required that independent scientific experts be furnished to the guardian so that any gap in bargaining power between him and the doctors is diminished, if not eliminated? Obviously, there are many crucial questions which the court never even considered; yet it did decide that a guardian may not do what the patient cannot do!

In addition to the court's decision being logically defective and failing to take account of important empirical realities, the court's conclusion about informed consent is further objectionable because it gave no consistent weight to the realities it did consider. Had it done so, we might now have a useful opinion about how to proceed when, for any surgical or medical procedure, a doctor wants to comply with the legal standards established for obtaining consent from an involuntarily committed patient.

Although my analysis of the consent issue has been primarily legalistic, it is easy to see that large social and political problems lurk just below the legal veneer which so often disguises troublesome matters. In terms of the real social problems which surround experimental psychosurgery, experimental surgery, or experimental medicine, have we been helped at all by the informed consent analysis of the Detroit court? It is clear that we have not been aided largely because this court was unwilling to confront the difficult real social problems. Among these are concerns about what to do with those committed patients for whom society is willing to furnish only enough resources to ensure continued confinement, but not enough to do what may make them well. There is also the related sociopolitical problem about institutional management when scarce resources are by legislative decision deliberately withheld from an organization which must nonetheless function. Finally, there is the political problem of the so-called basic civil rights of committed mental patients. Does the court's decision about informed consent suppress or protect those rights?

The Civil Rights of the Involuntarily Committed

Although the court's analysis of the civil rights issue was undertaken to support its conclusion about informed consent, the thrust of the argument is largely toward the question of who will be a suitable candidate for some special surgical intervention. Will anyone qualify for any procedure if he can afford it? Should no one qualify regardless of ability to pay? Should entire classes of persons be declared unqualified as either a matter of law (e.g., those involuntarily committed) or as a matter of social policy which is not primarily legal (e.g., those who are poor, or poor and black)? One of the "scare" pieces in the popular media dealing with psychosurgery is an article in *Ebony* (1973) suggesting that psychosurgery is a new white man's tool for "taming" black people.[12] Here again, even if no evidence exists to support such a view, there may nonetheless be good policy reasons for disqualifying all black people from psychosurgery. Of course, the question as to whether disqualifying black people or those involuntarily committed best serves even their sociopolitical or medical interests still remains. Even if we assume that political or social interests are better protected by such wholesale group disqualifications, further questions of how they are to be decided, by whom, and whether the protected sociopolitical interest is worth the possible loss in biological or psychological health are still to be faced.

I am troubled even more by a fear that in declaring entire classes of persons ineligible for any experimental psychosurgery out of a concern for their civil liberties, we may be asking already unfortunate people to suffer further so that the civil liberties of those who are allegedly protecting them can be advanced. I can illustrate this possibility by slightly rearranging the facts of the John Doe case. Supposing that John Doe was not committed under an unconsitutional statute, what then would be his present social-political-legal-biological-psychological position? Instead of being free in the community because he had been detained pursuant to an unconstitutional statute, John Doe would be back in a facility for the criminally insane where each day he would be free to tell himself and the world, "See, the ever vigilant courts in this great land have guaranteed that I can continue spending my natural life in confinement consoled by the knowledge that no one took advantage of my legally manufactured incompetence to consent."[13] I cannot help feeling that the already long-suffering John Does of our society are not getting much in exchange for their civil rights which would supposedly be compromised were they or their guardians permitted to give legally adequate consent for experimental psychosurgery. Indeed, when I see a case even worse than those of the lost John Does, in which the person is perhaps also self-mutilating or otherwise tormented, I wonder which of his conceivable social or civil rights would not be worth compromising to ameliorate his biological or psychological condition. Even the quite properly cautious NIMH recognizes the need to consider a lobotomy permissible, and when the Detroit court condemned all psychosurgery it was not talking about anything as serious as a lobotomy. The NIMH said: "Faced with the choice of leaving a patient raving in the back ward of a mental hospital, soiling himself with his own feces, and attacking other patients and staff, or performing a lobotomy with a reasonably good chance of improving his condition so he can be moved to a ward with better conditions, many reasonable people would make the latter choice. Although in many cases lobotomized patients who were able to be discharged from the hospital functioned at a lower intellectual level than prior to the onset of their illness, this was better than the realistic and grim prospect of spending the rest of their lives in the hospital."[14]

Who then are the real beneficiaries, if any, of the decision that neither involuntarily committed persons nor their guardians can consent to experimental psychosurgery? Can it be maintained that those who remain in confinement or torment somehow have their lots improved, or is this another instance where the class of persons least able legally to protect themselves are used to advance the interests of those much better off? Even if there are legitimate fears about the possibilities of behavior control by surgery, whose fears are assuaged and allayed by the "no consent" doctrine—those people who have access to law and lawyers or those who lack such advantages? We surely have reason enough to be anxious about protecting our civil rights, but I wonder what has happened to our sense of justice if we permit those who already are surviving on crumbs to pay for our "right" to sit at the banquet tables of life.

It would be naive to suppose that those who support the no consent doctrine are unaware of its consequences for the John Does. What these no consent proponents would argue is that the entire area of involuntary commitment must be reexamined and perhaps even abolished. I share the belief that, with very narrow exceptions, incarceration because of social deviance should be abolished.[15] However, those who favor the no consent doctrine also strongly believe that a committed person has a right to treatment which is reasonably calculated to improve or cure. In addition, many who favor these positions, as I do, would also argue, as I would, that even if the committed patient has a right to treatment, it does not follow that the state has a right to impose treatment. Yet it is precisely because I believe a committed person has the right (1) to treatment, (2) to effective treatment, and if competent (3) to refuse some or any treatment, that I find the no consent doctrine morally, socially, and legally objectionable. We may refer to these three rights as the basic civil rights of the committed mentally ill.

Because I believe that committed people deserve to have every opportunity for improvement, I find it wrong to shut them off from that which scientifically untrained judges believe is medically unimpressive. I share the court's belief that we should maximize the conditions under which a person, voluntarily committed or not, may consent to any surgical or even any nonroutine medical intervention. In my view this requires more stringent conditions than those which now govern such consent; however, from these convictions it follows only that scrupulously careful concern should be exercised by doctors and equally careful vigilance by courts to ensure that in each case the proper consent procedures are followed. The no consent doctrine is inherently contrary to the intellectual and moral bases of the civil rights package of the mentally ill because it disenfranchises and further dehumanizes them. By holding, as a matter of law, that they can consent under no circumstances, the court in effect has further separated involuntarily committed persons from society. The philosophy behind the basic civil rights package ensures that the committed are not further alienated, forgotten, or removed from the community by treating them differently when their legitimate interests can be protected without so treating them. Holding that the involuntarily committed, as a matter of law, are so different from the rest of society that they cannot consent, or even have a guardian do so, is absolutely antithetical to their best interests and inconsistent with the moral and political foundations of their basic civil rights.

Chapter 8

SCIENTIFIC MANIPULATION OF BEHAVIOR*

Evolution and Man's Unique Position

About 100,000 years ago, probably in East Africa, as a result of natural selection, some apes acquired that gene pool from which *Homo sapiens* evolved. For nearly 95 percent of the time since, figuratively as well as almost literally, the jungle law of survival has determined the fate of those 100,000 genes. Largely due to errors in the reproduction of deoxynucleic acid (DNA) molecules, that gene pool has had at least half of its components changed since, some more than once. This differential reproduction of genotypes, which is the jungle law of evolution or natural selection, has perpetuated adaptive mutational changes and the process has been "natural." What distinguishes the latest 5 percent of elapsed time is man's escalating ability deliberately to affect his evolutionary "progress" by manipulating his environment. Unlike any of the 2,000,000 other species, man, as the most self-conscious form of life, has been able to create his own biofeedback loop through manipulating the environment to accommodate his given gene pool. Despite their larger and heavier brains, neither whales nor porpoises seem able to alter

*This chapter is based upon a paper prepared for the International Association of Legal and Social Philosophy world congress, 1975 (in press).

their gene pool, even though they face extinction because of the "light-brained" environmental manipulations of lighter brained man.

We can disregard Bernhard Rensch's hundred "rules" of evolution, but we cannot ignore current knowledge about the genetic code which makes it statistically impossible for man to have been a chance accident of evolution.[1] Contemporary man is not the result of natural selection in the sense in which that term is usually understood. The common understanding of natural selection, that species-beneficial traits will be perpetuated because members of the species carrying less desirable traits fail to reproduce successfully, is too simplistic to explain the development of a species that has the capacity to reform its environment to suit its preexistent traits, rather than adapting its traits to its environment. In the case of the lower animals, natural selection, like mathematical logic, is deaf, dumb, blind, and temporally neutral; the adaptivity value of any trait is a function neither of the future nor of the perceived present, but only of the immediately given.[2] Man's species-unique language and culture, however, enable him not only to manipulate the environment to accommodate his natural gene pool, but also to do so with a sense of the future consequences. In other words, the adaptivity value, to man, of a man-made, man-dominated, and man-manipulated environment inevitably reflects how he perceives the past, the immediately given, and the future. As Theodosius Dobzhansky writes:

> Mankind's unique position in the biological world is due to its biological evolution having developed the genetic basis of culture. Man is the creator and the creature of culture, a body of traditions and skills transmitted from person to person and from generation to generation not by genes in the sex cells but by instruction and learning, chiefly through the medium of symbolic thought and symbolic language. . . . Simpson . . . has compiled a list of 22 characteristics of the human species. . . . In Simpson's words: . . . "language is . . . the most diagnostic single trait of man. All normal men have language; no other now living organisms do."[3]

Although the connection between language and culture is possibly deeply relevant to the question of behavior control, the cardinal point here is that our species's specific genotypes enable us to anticipate the future, learn from experience, and acquire and transmit culture. Because of his genetic disposition to acquire culture and use experience, man, unlike other animals, can consider how to protect society from itself by discussing "The Scientific Manipulation of Behavior." There is no reason to believe that animals with larger brains or with better biological mechanisms (for example, some species of fish, flies, or mice which have biological self-regulatory mechanisms to control population density) convene to collectively worry about why or how they are manipulated by one another.[4] It is only man, and especially that subspecies *Homo sapiens philosophus,* who convenes for such purposes because, as Dobzhansky puts it:

> In having given rise to man, biological evolution has transcended itself. Mankind is the only species engaged in two evolutions at the same time—the biological and the cultural. The two evolutions are distinct in principle. Biological inheritance is transmitted by genes in the sex cells, cultural inheritance by instruction and learning. . . .
>
> The contrasting properties of the cultural and biological domains are evident. Probably a majority of social scientists believe these domains to be wholly disconnected. It has even been asserted that in having acquired culture, mankind has escaped biology. This is certainly an illusion. Culture and biology are connected by feedback relationships. Cultural changes have genetic consequences. . . . [5]

Recognizing that man is genetically species-specific in having language culture, does it follow that his species is also unusually intelligent and capable of using intelligence to maximize his capacity for culture? Anthropological evidence as to the correlation between culture and intelligence is hardly conclusive and, for quite some time, largely due to Alfred L. Kroeber, it was believed that man's capacity for culture developed very suddenly.[6] This theory about human culture is the anthropological equivalent of the big bang theory for explaining the origins of our solar system. However:

> The belief that the capacity for culture emerged very suddenly in the history of man received a cruel blow with the discovery of the australopithecine fossils. These man-apes lived between 5,000,000 and 750,000 years ago. . . . As more and more of these fossils have been discovered, palaeontologists have begun cautiously to accept the

> view that they represent the oldest known forms in the evolutionary process leading to modern man. . . .
>
> The evidence indicates that these semi-erect, small-brained proto-men were apparently capable of acquiring some of the elements of culture. They manufactured simple tools; the oldest tools found so far date back 2,600,000 years. Apparently they hunted small animals, and they may have had some system of communication more advanced than modern apes but considerably short of true speech. It seems highly unlikely that they could have had a culture comparable to even the most primitive cultures that have survived today, but they represent the start of what must have been a continuous, rather than a sudden, evolution of the capacity for culture.
>
> In short, the australopithecines, with a brain one-third the size of modern man's, possessed an elementary form of culture. The obvious conclusion, therefore, is that the rapid evolutionary increase in cranial volume did not precede the evolution of culture, but followed it.[7]

If then there is a connection between culture and intelligence, does it necessarily follow that intelligence maximizes the individual's capacity for culture? Even though there may be times and places where stupidity can be an evolutionary advantage (e.g., as when there is an oxygen shortage),[8] the selective advantage of intelligence must have been enormous, judging from the rapidity with which brain capacity increased.[9] Given that selectively adaptive traits normally develop over millions of years, that our present brain capacity was probably acquired not more than 100,000 years ago, and that even the enormously quick development of our present brain capacity prior to that time required at least several hundred thousand years, are we perhaps demanding too much of our intelligence in expecting that it will maximize the advantage of having a capacity for acquiring culture? Or should we ask instead whether intelligence can minimize the disadvantage of the capacity for culture? Jean Rostand, the French biologist, points out that since man emerged 100,000 years ago he has not evolved at all physically, particularly his brain—except that it contains knowledge about the five millennia of civilization.[10]

Unfortunately man's cultural knowledge has not diminished his capacity for intraspecific aggression—a trait not common to most other animals. In view of the apparent evolutionary failure to select genetically transmissible altruism rather than aggression,[11] Rostand and others now ask: Does man have the language-culture-intelligence to develop technology for either (1) accelerating evolution by positive eugenics which will eradicate intraspecific aggression from our gene pool, or (2) manipulating the environment to prevent or diminish the adverse consequences of uneliminable, objectionable genetic aggression? Moreover, if such technology can be developed, should it be? Because of the rapidly emerging technologies for genetic surgery, psychosurgery, ESB psychotherapy, drug therapy, and behavior therapy, the answer to the first question is, or may soon be, yes. Therefore, man must collectively worry about the far more difficult second question—should we do whatever we can do? The idea that we should is what one biochemist, Erwin Chargaff, has called "the Devil's Doctrine."[12]

Technology and the Evolution of Man

Stephen Toulmin reminds us: "A century ago, people still looked to science, first and foremost, for *enlightenment*. It was a source, not of physical comforts and conveniences, but of fresh ideas and insights. It challenged men's views about the world they lived in, its history and destiny, and about the significance of human beings in that world. It helped them, in Thomas Henry Huxley's admirable phrase, to understand, not just Nature but *Man's Place in Nature*. In a word, its interest to the lay public was not technological but cosmological, or even theological."[13] But in the mid-twentieth century, what the public seeks as a by-product of scientific research is less likely to be enlightenment than physical comfort. In any case, the intrinsic complexity of scientific knowledge increasingly makes enlightenment inaccessible to nonspecialists. The result is a mounting alienation between science and society. Even professional scientists are confused and uncertain about the relations between general scientific theory and the practical objectives of derivative technologies. Nevertheless, "scientism is still the headiest drink served in the barroom at the intellectuals' saloon,"[14] because of various reasons. First, only scientists seem currently plausible successors to the "priests, witchdoctors, shamans, wizards, soothsayers, oracles, clerical castes, and priestly orders" who previously, with varying success, furnished "enlightenment."[15] Second, scientism is enervating because of the popular transformation of the scientist into the technologist by a society which believes that only technology can solve the problems created by science-technology. The latter thesis urges that since the social problems precipitated by technology are inevitable, only technology can control what ought be done; and this argument is then used to justify going *Beyond Freedom and Dignity* (B. F. Skinner, 1971) to develop the *Technological Man* (V. C. Ferkiss, 1969). A slightly different reason for a continuing faith in technology is advanced by Sir Peter Medawar, who argues that since we are still only at the beginning of our cultural development, and since science has yet to find a definitive solution to any grand social problem, we may still develop the requisite technology for managing our technological accomplishments.[16]

Even though one feels that the basic thesis reflected in Skinner, Ferkiss, and Medawar is essentially incestuous (technology keeping technology honest), it is also compulsively attractive.[17] Its appeal arises from the fact that man is the result of natural selection functioning within his self-made and transmitted culture. Thus, man is "necessarily" a technological animal whose technological disposition is just as innate (and in the same sense) as his disposition to suffer death. Man cannot choose to be antitechnological because to become such an animal he would still have to use technology to remake himself. It is logically conceivable, and perhaps with psychosurgery even technologically possible, that the human gene pool could be manipulated to eradicate the uniqueness of *Homo sapiens* so as to let the species try to start again from where it was five million years ago. But this extreme "nature-knows-best" thesis, trusting only to natural selection, suffers from two overwhelming inconsistencies. First, even if man could deliberately revert to the apes of five million years ago, he might not again evolve to *Homo sapiens*, and second, deliberately going back entails having and using the requisite technology. Thus, we really do not have any choice about being technological animals. Even if it is incestuous to argue that we must develop technology in order to develop technology, we can only choose among alternative technologies. The choice is so illusory in contemporary society because of general acceptance of the Devil's Doctrine—because we can do it, we should—and because of the "most noxious combination . . . joining . . . technological possibility with demands for survival."[18] Even more seriously, man lacks any genetic or technological mechanism for lowering "the base-line of expectation and demand, neutralizing the sense of restlessness, unrequited desire, and obsessive attempts to achieve still more happiness through technology," all of which precisely characterize "advanced industrial society."[19]

Individual scientists do resist the Devil's Doctrine; indeed, many workers in the biological sciences have refused to participate in weapons development programs, thus continuing a great scientific tradition with which Leonardo da Vinci was associated.[20] Chargaff quotes from da Vinci's diary, where after sketching a submarine design, Leonardo wrote: "How and why I do not describe my method of remaining under water for so long a time as I can remain without food; and this I do not publish or divulge on account of the evil nature of men who would practice assassinations at the bottom of the seas by breaking the ships in their lowest parts and sinking them together with the crews who are in them."[21] The problem about the Devil's Doctrine, however, is not that individual scientists are unable to resist it, though that is too often true, but that the strength and persuasiveness of the popular belief that new technologies expand human freedom by generating otherwise unavailable alternatives is overwhelming. After all, we *can* go to the moon and President Nixon probably expressed the sentiment of much of the world when, after the first moon landing, he said that it had been the "greatest week since the Creation." But if going to the moon is somehow equal to the act of creation, then ought not going to the moon be just as imperative as the creation of the universe? The opportunity to choose creates an obligation to make a choice, even though having the choice by no means expands the freedom of those who now must choose. Daniel Callahan makes the point this way:

> The history of technology shows that specific developments are almost always justified on the ground that they will increase freedom of choice and maximize voluntary options. . . . Specified choices—usually in the name of a "responsible" use of freedom—quickly make the new options mandatory, either by law, economic force or social custom. . . . Genetic counseling was originally hailed as a means of giving people the freedom to choose the avoidance of a defective child, if they wanted to avail themselves of that option.

But signs are already present that they will in the future be considered socially irresponsible if they do not make use of their "free" choice to choose against bearing defective children.[22]

Scientific "Neutrality" and Scientific Role Fascism

Increasingly man's ability to manipulate the environment threatens the social stability achieved by sentiment and religion, and it is probably no accident that the rise of the great oriental religions accompanied the decline of science. The second great wave of science began with Copernicus and almost ended when Galileo was sacrificed for social stability; yet, for a multiplicity of reasons science has survived, flourished, and become the most powerful surrogate for religion. Talcott Parsons has shown why science has replaced religion as the primary source for current conceptions of social order.[23] Like religion, science is charismatic in that it purports to provide enlightenment about reality and man's place within the universe. From science we expect "information in terms of which human life can be patterned [and which organizes] extrapersonal mechanisms for the perception, understanding, judgment, and manipulation of the world."[24]

Although knowledge is still power, and science is still the dominant source of knowledge, the post-World War II years, and especially the last decade, have witnessed a deepening distrust of and even antipathy to science. This has been largely due to the realization that the reason for science's success in replacing religion—its seeming objectivity and universality—is a chimera.[25] There are three major reasons for this increasing disillusionment. First, because all human activity involves decision making it therefore reflects subjective values, and it follows that since science is a uniquely human activity, it not only causes environmental changes but reflects them as well.[26] Second, because of mistaken beliefs about its value neutrality, science lends itself to overt and covert political and economic manipulation. Third, because of mistaken beliefs about science's value neutrality, scientists can exploit their alleged objectivity to advance particular values. These three problems arise from three myths about science identified by the British

Society for Social Responsibility in Science. The first "myth states that the activities of science are morally and socially value free. Science is seen in the pursuit of natural laws which are valid irrespective of the nation, race, politics, religion or class position of the discoverer. . . . The second myth is that of the technological imperative. This states that whatever it is possible to conceive of being done by science and technology must be and will be done. . . . The third myth . . . is the accidentalist myth . . . [which] implies that the developments of science are not only unforeseeable but unexplained."[27]

Although both difficulties are dependent on its neutral image, the witting or unwitting exploitation of science must be distinguished from another aspect of exploitation in which earlier work is used for purposes unintended and even unimagined by the researchers. An almost classic illustration is the Ph.D. thesis of Arthur W. Galston which showed how a chemical substance (TIBA) could increase soybean production. In 1971, after defoliants had been used extensively in Vietnam, Galston wrote in an article entitled, "The Education of a Scientific Innocent,": "I have some reason to believe that my early investigation on TIBA helped several researchers at the chemical warfare laboratories . . . in their design and understanding of the defoliating action of chemicals. . . ."[28] Similarly, some of the most potent nerve poisons were developed from studies of plant physiology and nerve-muscle transmission, while conversely, the infamous mustard gas of World War I has been used for research in molecular genetics and to treat cancer. The point about such "exploitation" is that any control of science or technology based upon unforeseen, let alone unforeseeable or unimaginable future uses, is practically if not also logically impossible. There is only one way to prevent undesirable future uses if no controls over technology can be effective—stop all research.

The exploitation problem is related to the matter of scientific manipulation of behavior because it raises the issues of the political and industrial use of science and scientists. Current antiscience sentiments run deeper than the romantic idealism which seemingly motivated Goethe and others during the eighteenth-century wave of distrust toward science. This deeper contemporary feeling arises in part because the halo of neutrality has been taken from science, and in the process, science has become too closely connected to technology.[29] Even "pure" science is sometimes big business, and as such subject to the characteristic machinations for survival in a competitive economy.[30] Thus, lifting the veil of neutrality has raised the veil of innocence as well. The popular image of a value-free innocent working in a garret before a picture of Galileo could hardly have survived the post-World War II pattern of research funding dominated by military needs.[31]

While we are fortunate that Hitler's fanaticism blinded him to the scientific and technological resources available in Germany,[32] the politicizing of science arises not merely because funding is guided by military considerations. Instead, "scientists' influence in policy making . . . is shaped significantly by political forces and interests. Legislators, special interests, political executives, and the public all set forth the objectives and courses of public policies. Scientists may tempt these people with possibilities and knowledge, but the decision to forge and pursue a policy remains with these people alone. Scientists have rarely foisted anything on society that its policy-makers, citizens, or politically significant groups did not feel they wanted or did not encourage."[33] A potentially far-reaching contemporary illustration of this thesis was President Nixon's deliberate plan to make the NIH more responsive to political considerations. An assistant secretary for HEW even went so far as to urge that the NIH suffered from a "misguided sense of the place of research in the nation's efforts to solve its health problems." An overwhelming majority of senior NIH research scientists responded (in a letter to the *Washington Post*) that the worldwide eminence of the NIH was achieved "by operating on the principle that scientific and medical criteria, rather than political considerations, must be the basis for policy decisions related to bio-medical research."[34]

That part of the neutrality problem which I call "role fascism" is most crucial to how science is used to manipulate behavior, even though all three aspects of the neutrality problem are closely interconnected. Role fascism is the belief that scientists intrinsically possess special knowledge about areas other than their scientific specialties, and it is dramatically illustrated by the NIH case. The NIH scientists argued that *policy* decisions about research must be guided by scientific criteria, rather than by political considerations, but it should be apparent that science itself is anything but value free. Why, for example, would knowledge about their scientific specialties endow the 514 NIH signers of that letter with any special knowledge about allocating research funds? I do not wish to imply that either President Nixon or the assistant secretary had a better basis for deciding the future research functions of the NIH; indeed, if I had to choose, I would prefer that the 514 senior scientists make such a decision, but that is not because they are scientists!

The role fascist often crudely minimizes or destroys the effectiveness of his "scientific" input. We need to see role fascism at its most obvious levels in order to appreciate the more complex forms in which it often appears in debates about psychosurgery or other organic therapies and behavior control. Testifying that the motion picture "Deep Throat" had redeeming social value, a psychiatrist "told the court that oral-genital contact is 'healthy and legitimate' when it is enjoyed *and* 'practiced out of love and devotion and not coercion' *and* 'provided [it is] no more than a part of the foreplay that builds up erotic tension to climax in coitus.' "[35] Presuming that there is a scientific basis for believing the questioned conduct is "healthy," what possible psychiatric basis is there for believing that such conduct was "legitimate" (rather than deviant), when legitimacy and deviance are in the context of an obscenity trial not matters of mental good health? That is, no one can pretend that the political and legal criteria for obscenity are determined by criteria about good health. It is regrettable, but true, that almost all psychiatric testimony in criminal proceedings tends to illustrate, in varying degrees, rather crude role fascism.

An even more extreme and recurrent form of unsophisticated role fascism is what Robert Veatch has aptly called "the as-a syndrome." He illustrates this syndrome by the following hypothetical statements: " 'As-a neurosurgeon, I am concerned about the increasing use of psychosurgical ablation to control behavioral deviation. . . . ' 'As-a psychiatrist, I cannot condone involuntary psychiatric commitment. . . . ' "[36] Because it is a classic illustration of "as-a," egregiously crude role fascism, I quote at some length a 1971 lecture before the Royal Institution of Great Britain by a distinguished biologist.

> In choosing the subject matter of this discourse . . . I . . . had in mind the exhortation, frequently voiced these days, that it is the responsibility of research scientists, not only to bring to light new knowledge but also to draw attention to the implications of any new knowledge for society. So I propose to discuss the bearing of some general biological knowledge upon problems now facing society.

What are the problems facing society? They are the weaknesses, if not sicknesses, summarized under such headings as ever-increasing criminality, increased senseless vandalism and hooliganism, increased drug addiction, student unrest, industrial unrest in the form of reckless unofficial strikes, excessive absenteeism (i.e., absence from work without good reason) the precarious position of the national economy, the irresponsible exploitation of natural resources causing pollution and destruction of amenities. . . .

Although the branches of study concerned with the working of society—the social sciences—have grealy expanded in recent decades, this has not led to a cure for the ills of society. Thus, to judge from this failure and the deterioration of many aspects of society, the causes of the troubles have not been established, and therefore new diagnoses and new remedies ought to be looked for. These considerations have prompted me to search for possible causes of the "diseases." My approach is based on my training as a physician and a biologist, and the thesis which I shall put forward argues that one of the roots of many troubles is an inadequate appreciation of basic biological priniciples—of the facts of life—which govern the conduct and wellbeing of *Homo sapiens*. . . . What I propose to discuss, then, is the question whether, and to what extent, the current sicknesses of society have to do with a failure by policy makers to understand human nature, especially the animal in man; in other words has there been a neglect of what biology can teach us? . . .

I mentioned the neglect of a number of basic biological principles—facts of life. . . .

Fact No. 1: Unless life is constantly renewed by hard effort, it runs down. . . . [T]o earn means that [the individual] must render some service for which somebody is willing to pay. He who does not render such service to society fails to contribute to life and has to be carried by others. . . .

Number 2 is the fact that the lives of societies, such as nations, are, in principle, subject to the same laws as the lives of individuals. A nation, like an individual, has to earn its living in the face of tough competition. . . .

Number 3 is the fact that *Homo sapiens*, like all other species, does not by nature work unless he has an incentive. . . .

If producing work is one of the bases on which the well-being and strength of society rests, the laws and social organisation should do

> everything to encourage work. Amazingly a situation has developed during this century in this country where laws all too often do exactly the opposite. . . . By far the most amazing inefficiency of management is that of successive governments which, through tax laws, deters [sic] people from making their optimal contribution towards the welfare of the country. Let me emphasise that this is a mistake of successive governments, irrespective of party. I am not concerned with party politics but with biology; the need for incentives is a biological phenomenon. . . . [37]

In other words, biological expertise somehow also generated sufficient competence to make the biologist an expert in economics, labor relations, crime—indeed an expert about anything first labelled (by the biologist) as "disease."

Because role fascism has deeply colored the public and scientific debate about behavior control techniques, I will illustrate three further forms of the phenomenon. One manifestation of the "as-a" syndrome currently very popular is illustrated by the regularity with which, for example, biologists and geneticists meet to develop population policies. In environmental policies, Paul Ehrlich illustrates role fascism, especially in his best seller, *The Population Bomb* (1968), which one commentator characterized as "more reminiscent of a fundamentalist tract than of a contribution to a debate."[38] In the field of psychosurgery, the work of Breggin is, as I have pointed out, even more susceptible to such criticism. However, Ehrlich and Breggin differ because the former has an impressive history of scientific achievement in his own field and an important academic position, while Breggin has neither. Thus Ehrlich clearly qualifies as a "scientian" as that species is identified in a 1972 article in *Harper's*. "There are three distinguishing marks of a scientian. First, he must be a scientist. He must have an impressive base in his own specialized field. And this field must be some recognized branch of science that strikes an immediate and general cord of understanding. . . . [Second, he must] get the 'call' [and] use his background to extrapolate the currently known data of his field . . . to discourse on the *whole* of man. . . . [T]he third mark of the scientian [is that] his extrapolation lead him to proclaim the existence of a force, an evil reality, in man's world. . . . [This force is] the unidentified fly in the cosmic ointment, the worm in Eden's apple."[39] For Krebs the "fly" is the failure to appreciate the "biological" facts of life, while for Ehrlich it is overpopulation.

The "as-a" role fascism of the scientian is particularly objectionable and even dangerous when he becomes a government consultant. It should be noticed that current controversies about behavior control techniques have arisen because the subject has reached governmental concern through would be scientian consultants. Breggin's attack upon psychosurgery, for example, began in collaboration with a congressman who had the material printed in the *Congressional Record.* The government's use of consultants on behavior control, however, has been less frightening than it might be because there has not been an executive monoply on scientific consultants. A gross imbalance between Congress and the executive branch, particularly when the executive branch has a nearly exclusive access to scientific consultants, easily leads to exploitation and manipulation of the public, as with the supersonic transport (SST).[40] In the field of behavior control neither branch has yet gained a monopoly of advisory talent and that is why the deliberate effort to politicize the NIH is potentially so important. The scientific role fascists who serve government do not do so under duress. On the contrary, it is very easy to find scientists who believe science solves rather than exacerbates political problems. Yet the characteristic rationality of science is almost antithetical to whatever rationality is in politics, and efforts to treat the two as fungible (or even closely connected) have produced, among other things, Lysenkoism and the thirty-year blight in Soviet science.[41]

Before dealing with the behavior control kind of subtle role fascism, it may be helpful to illustrate this phenomenon further. Scientists in the health field are particularly susceptible to the temptations of role fascism—in part because of the World Health Organization (WHO) definition of health as "a state of complete physical, mental, and social well-being and not merely the absence of disease or infirmity."[42] Thus encouraged by WHO and by the "natural" expansionist tendency found in almost any professional field, it is not surprising that increasing numbers of medical doctors utilize their special knowledge to justify social activism, efforts which nearly always result in rather easily spotted cases of the "as-a" syndrome. While I would not even imply that doctors or other scientists who become overt political activists (Ernesto Guevara and Salvadore Allende, for example) are merely engaged in the "as-a" game, it is still necessary to distinguish between those easily identified cases where an individual scientist plays the "as-a" game and the harder instances when the whole profession or its official organization engages in the role fascism maneuver. Even this latter form of the game can sometimes be easily perceived, as in the AMA fight against national health insurance. Cases where self-serving economic or other motives are not so discernible are obviously more difficult.[43]

The problems of role fascism are particularly severe in connection with psychosurgery. If important questions about psychosurgery were rated from zero to ten, and if zero represented matters purely legal and ten those purely medical, then there would probably be no tens. The following items fall on the six and above side of the scale:

(1) the nature of organic brain damage—about nine
(2) the existence of organic brain damage—about eight
(3) the relationship between organic brain damage and overt aggressive violence—about seven
(4) the relationship between the brain's biochemistry and overt aggressive violence—about six
(5) the relationship between a specific lesion in that part of the brain where organicity is found and postoperative overt aggressive violence—about seven
(6) the relationship between a specific lesion in the brain, even though no organicity is found there, and postoperative overt aggressive violence—perhaps six
(7) the relationship between electrical brain waves and overt aggressive violence—eight or nine
(8) the relationship between a specific lesion in the brain and the subsequent five to twenty-year side effects—about six
(9) the relationship between a specific brain lesion and the long-term or genetic side effects—about six

In the Detroit psychosurgery trial there were varying amounts of "expert" testimony on all these matters; however, as quickly became apparent, it was virtually impossible to keep the several different questions separated as the experts testified. This complexity inevitably generates confusion as to what questions the expert has supposedly answered and the proper weight to be given to expert testimony. When parts of an expert's testimony are closely juxtaposed, both temporally (in the court) and as to content, and the witness's expertise is vastly different for the several parts of the given testimony, it is virtually impossible for a judge to have the skill or perspective to evaluate such testimony properly. For example, an "expert" witness testifies about (1) and then about (5), and in the course of his testimony makes additional comments about (6) and (9). Later, when writing his opinion, the judge uses this witness's testimony about (6) or (9). Now, although an expert has testified about a matter where his expertise is crucial, if not dispositive (1), the court relies upon him where his acknowledged expertise is clearly not dispositive and possibly not even crucial (6) and (9).

Let me illustrate this process with an example not taken from a trial situation. One of the participants at a symposium on war and peace was a physician, a professor of neurology at a distinguished Ivy League university, and chairman of the neurology department at a major eastern hospital. In his comments which follow the numbers placed inside parentheses indicate my opinion of how significant (zero to ten) his acknowledged neurological expertise is to the matter he is discussing.

> There is no suggestion that the brain today is greatly different from what it was 40 years ago (8), but it is conceivable that we are starting to use it better (1). . . . But I mean to talk briefly about a bit of gray matter that, unhappily (1), we *do* use. It is called the limbic system. The brain is like an orange, if you like, and the skin of the orange is the cerebral cortex. . . . This is what you use when you take part in a symposium (5), or cook a dinner (3), or write a sonnet (2)—or plan a war (2). This is the intellectual part of the brain, and normally, in balanced men (4) it controls the rest (3). . . .
>
> The general conclusion from what we know physiologically is that man is naturally aggressive (3) but can learn self-control (2). . . . Many people mature, their cortex taking over the control of these primitive centers (5) and thus you get a human being who is civilized (2). . . . In planning any world order, in planning any society, we have to remember this fundamental fact: that man's brain contains a physical entity called the limbic system (9) which is concerned, among other things, with aggression and violence (8). We have to remember that normally (4) it is kept under control (5) as the result of education, example, and a process of social conditioning (4) which employs both penalties and rewards (3). We sometimes forget the penalties these days.

> I do not mean to say that all aggression is limbic in origin (5)—on the contrary. War is only too often planned by the human cortex (2). This is cold aggression, or aggression for profit—national, social, personal, or racial. However, the limbic variety of aggression can also precipitate nations into war (1), as in the case of Hitler (1). He used his limbic rages as a weapon to overcome opposition and those who have listened to him on the radio and have seen him on the screen will know what I mean. He exhibited a dualism in that he planned his aggression at the cortical level, but coupled it with personal limbic aggression. This is what can happen when unstable individuals come to power. It has been so in history, and may be so again unless we look to it.

I have probably been generous in my ratings, especially in omitting ratings from the last few sentences. I have purposely not identified the speaker, however, because I do not want to imply that this distinguished scientist was "wrong" to talk about war and peace. My point is, rather, that his errors arise from his doing so as a neurologist rather than as an intelligent, humane, concerned person. This example suggests the kind of intellectual game judges would have to play to evaluate properly the complex "scientific" testimony which took up the nine problems of psychosurgery I rated earlier.

Medical Role Fascism and the Identification of Deviance

If, as I have argued, science is never value free, if even well-intentioned scientists are prone to role fascism, and if the public (including medically unsophisticated courts) are willing to accept "as-a" arguments without questioning their bases, then clearly there is another important issue that must be considered in relation to psychosurgery or indeed any other procedure which might be used to control or modify behavior. As I shall use the term, "behavior control" means control of *deviant* behavior. The most serious questions about behavior control are not how to do it or about the clearly political judgments which are made when it is done. Rather, the most difficult questions about these techniques relate to the initial triggering attribution—the decision that S is deviant.

It is hardly surprising that in deviance labeling one encounters the most insidious role fascism. The pernicious belief that disease and illness are the same, when coupled with the pervasive belief that the only models for identifying either are morphological or anatomical, generates a nearly incontrovertible justification for doctors, psychiatrists, and other health field specialists to regard themselves as appropriate and exclusive labelers of deviance.[44] Although a mushrooming contemporary literature demonstrates that health specialists function as role fascists when they regard themselves as the *only* appropriate labelers of deviance,[45] it was Thomas Szasz who, long before his contemporary peers, sounded the alarm.[46] Even though he has not avoided the exuberant exaggeration characteristic of someone who first recognizes an important truth, Szasz's fundamental thesis about role fascism, particularly in psychiatry, has made him influential and widely read. Szasz, R. D. Laing, Erving Goffman, Ronald Leifer, and others consistently stress the difference between structural-morphological diseases and socially affected judgments about mental disorders.[47] It is quite right to characterize this dichotomy as "unsophisticated,"[48] since it overestimates the biological component of nonmental diseases and underestimates that component in mental disease. However, in addition to this double exaggeration, Szasz and his cohorts reject the idea that psychiatric health scientists deal only with facts about the brain-nervous system's structures and processes.[49] Much recent literature applies the argument of Szasz and his followers to the rest of medicine to show that health specialists (like other scientists) never engage in purely objective, value-free work—even when engaged in professional scientific activities.

By way of illustration, let us assume that six doctors examine S, and the following reports are made:

(1) S has fever and is vomiting.
(2) (1) and S has a disease.
(3) (1) and S is sick.
(4) (1) and S has a mental disorder.
(5) (1) and S has a mental illness.
(6) (1) and S is faking. (Emerging literature about the ability to control the homostatic system suggests that "fever" levels may be manipulated by S.)

Let us ignore the theory that all understanding presupposes sociocultural constructs and the question whether description, like understanding, is a function of a system of sociocultural constructs. Even so, if the first doctor had merely said, "The red line on the measuring instrument is at 101" (instead of saying "S has fever"), we could still not avoid the question of whether description (unlike evaluation or prescription) is value free. If we ignore questions about the essential subjectivity and relativity of all knowledge, would we be able to make a judgment about the relative objectivity of the six reports, and if so, what criterion distinguishes more from less objective reports? The general view is that where there is discernible organic-structural destruction, deterioration, or mal- or misfunctioning not subject to voluntary reversal by S, then the report describing that condition is more objective than one reporting a condition where there is no discernible organic defect.[50] This principle for identifying objectivity is suspect because, from among the whole range of possible organic defects, each doctor chooses only certain ones to establish or suggest that a particular condition exists. S not only had fever and vomited, he was also shortsighted, flat-footed, bald, and overweight. In addition to choosing from among the available involuntary organic defects, (2) reflects a further deliberate premise that only certain involuntary organic defects will be regarded as disease or disorder. Is aging a disease?[51] If high blood pressure is a disease, why not low blood pressure? "The standard textbooks reject 'ideopathic hypotension' as a disease. Harrison's textbook . . . states: 'Chronic hypotension is not a disease. . . . Thus, persistent low blood pressure should never be treated as such'."[52] In some parts of North Africa hookworm was not regarded as a disease—it was "normal" to have it. In one place in South America the *absence* of dyschronic spirochetosis is pathological.[53]

In addition to the cumulative choices of (1) and (2), which affect the diagnosis, (3) makes an important further choice in characterizing an involuntary organic defect as sickness. Neither old people nor those who uses eyeglasses or arch supports are regarded are sick. Report (4) and the subsequent reports escalate difficulties about the voluntariness of the defect and the absences of organicity. However, enough has been shown to suggest that even (1), let alone (2) or any subsequent report, is not a description of S but rather an *attribution* to S. Among these attributions the most important as concerns the scientific manipulation of behavior is that which labels S as sick. Thus delineated, S becomes the beneficiary (or victim) of the primary feature of the medical sick role—exculpation from personal responsibility. If an alcoholic cannot control his body chemistry's interaction with alcohol, then he is not to blame for being an alcoholic; he suffers from a disease.[54] The AMA so concluded in 1956 and the courts followed suit. There is, of course, some difficulty with this argument since there is no way to prove that the alcoholic's peculiar body chemistry requires him to drink. On the other hand, heart disease is a paradigm of involuntary organic defect, yet S could voluntarily have eaten less, exercised, and thus prevented the disease. The blood chemistry of the heart disease victim does not require that he overeat, and if the alcoholic is not to blame for his condition, why is the heart patient not equally innocent?

If the psychological components of the precipitating conduct in alcoholism and heart disease are rightly ignored in order to immunize patients from blame, why does this same distinction not also obtain where no disease state intervenes between the psychological cause and the unwanted, objectionable consequences? Apparently, in alcoholism or heart diesease, S is the victim of that affliction and therefore his having the condition because he drinks or overeats is ignored. Yet if this were a persuasive argument, it would require concluding that when S is the victim of his own crime, and for victimless crime in general, S should be just as blameless (criminally and otherwise) as the alcoholic or heart victim. On the other hand, it could be argued that, if others besides S are victimized by S's condition, we should take account of the psychological components of the condition (that is, label it deviance and even criminal or blameworthy). However, we could not then regard heart trouble or alcoholism as sickness (and thus blameless) since clearly S is not the only victim of his overeating or drinking.

Talcott Parsons, while clearly recognizing that disease is both a physical condition and the most prevalent type of deviance, makes the most sustained sociological effort to differentiate medical from other kinds of deviance, especially criminal deviance.[55] One of the most salient features of his analysis is that, unlike sickness which involves the whole man, crime is deviance from relatively well-particularized norms. What has been suggested by the examples of heart disease and alcoholism is the artificiality of such a distinction. Modern "whole man" theories of medicine and psychiatry also make it increasingly difficult to accept Parsons's distinction. The definition or standard usage of "medical disease" is thus likely to function as a litmus paper test for determining which S's shall be the beneficiaries or victims of scientific manipulation. This political use of "disease" is by no means an exclusively modern exploitation of medicine, and it is hardly surprising that "medicine's position today is akin to that of the state religions of yesterday" in which "medicine is really a moral enterprise."[56] The ever-accelerating expansion of the concept of health, typified by the WHO definition, when coupled with the realization that health is a social concept,[57] foreshadows that the legitimation of political authority will increasingly come from health field specialists. As a result, a new, legitimate tyranny will rise from the duty to be healthy;[58] and what healthy-minded person could possibly object? From television we learn that using almost anything from Preparation H to Geritol is justified if it bestows some advantage upon health, because "If you have your health, you have everything." However, even the tyranny of good health is still tyranny.

Scientific Manipulation and the Freedom of the Subject

Dissenting in *Olmstead,* Justice Brandeis argued:

> The makers of our Constitution . . . sought to protect Americans in their beliefs, their thoughs, their emotions and their sensations. They conferred, as against the Government, the right to be let alone—the more comprehensive of rights and the right most valued by civilized man.[59]

Thirty-six years later, in a case involving the question of whether an adult Jehovah's Witness could refuse a blood transfusion, now Chief Justice Burger, then on the Court of Appeals, added:

> Nothing in this utterance suggests that Justice Brandeis thought an individual possessed these rights only as to *sensible* beliefs, *valid* thought, *reasonable* emotion, or *well-founded* sensations. I suggest he intended to include a great many foolish, unreasonable and even

absurd ideas which do not conform, such as refusing medical treatment even at great risk.[60]

If the "right to be let alone" was important in 1928 and more important in 1964, the technology and knowledge which has emerged in the last decade make it even more important now. With the available and emerging techniques for genetic surgery, psychosurgery, drug therapy, and other forms of medical manipulation, it is even more realistic to fear that freedom—the right to be let alone—will be eroded by the imposition of health, better health, or good health. The suppression of freedom through an appeal to society's supposed right to require healthy citizens is especially threatening because of a growing tendency to regard the diagnosis and treatment of political or social deviance as properly within medicine's province. If it were possible to reverse this trend toward the medicalization of social deviance, it would be well to concentrate all our efforts on achieving that goal. However, energy spent fighting that movement is not likely to succeed, and therefore, rather than trying to stop inevitable scientific tinkering with man, it would be better to develop institutions and technology to control whatever tinkering takes place.

Whether it is "manipulation" for someone other than S deliberately to cause S to behave in a predictable way is a subtle social, psychological, and political question. It would rob "manipulate" of its potential communicative utility if every instance of someone deliberately causing S to behave in a predictable way were characterized as manipulation. Rather, the essential elements for the core meaning in paradigm cases of manipulation would seem to be: (1) that there be deliberateness on the part of the manipulator; (2) that the manipulation involve some skill; (3) that there be some lack of fairness in regard to S; and (4) that there be some service to the manipulator. The third edition of the *Shorter Oxford Dictionary* (1933) gives three standard usages of "manipulate," as do the *American College* (1947) and the *Webster's Third New International* (1967) dictionaries. The first usage in all three emphasizes the skill element identified above. The third standard usage given in the *Oxford* is: "To manage by dexterous (esp. unfair) contrivance or influence." The third usage in the *American College* is: "To adopt or change . . . to suit one's purpose or advantage." In *Webster's*, the third usage is: "To change by artful or unfair means so as to serve one's purpose." *Webster's* 2b(2) is even closer to what is suggested as paradigm usage in the present context: "To control, manage, or play upon artful, unfair, or insidious means especially to one's own advantage." In such a light, and in view of what "manipulate" means, several important questions arise about freedom and scientific manipulation.

Question 1: Can science as technology or science as knowledge expand the domain within which someone can deliberately cause S to behave in a predictable way or enhance the skills with which someone can cause S to behave?

Question 2: Is there some inevitable connection between scientific technology or knowledge which "advances" the managing or controlling of S and the capacity or opportunity for doing so deliberately, unfairly, and to the manipulator's advantage? Does progress in skill imply or even entail, as a matter of historical truth, erosion of individual autonomy?

Question 3: Can there be "unfair" ways of causing S to behave, if doing so maximizes S's autonomy? What if the manipulator acts on the motive that his own advantage is served best by maximizing S's autonomy?

Question 4: Is there some standard for determining biomedical unfairness as to how (not for what purpose) S is caused to behave, perhaps analogous to procedural due process in law, which would distinguish between scientific manipulation and scientific propriety? Are there scientifically and socially plausible, as well as rationally and emotionally attractive, criteria which could decide whether certain techniques or knowledge may not be employed to cause S to behave predictably, regardless of whether they benefit him or society? Thus for example, in a given area A nearly everyone eligible to vote does so, and in a referendum X percent supports the proposition that Z (a biochemical agent) shall be regularly added to the water supply because the drug is not known to have disastrous side effects and is the most efficacious technique for preventing (or enhancing) condition C. In this case are there attractive criteria for deciding such issues? Are there such criteria regardless of the content of A, X, Z or C? What if, instead of Z to prevent tooth decay, the issue is genetic surgery before birth, or psychosurgery at birth, to prevent war?

Question 5: Are there moral, social, or political virtues or goals which could reliably be used to measure the trade-off between permissible manipulation (which thus perhaps ceases to be "manipulation") and the incremental attainment of these virtues or goals? For example, why do so many of the same psychiatrists, pediatricians, general practitioners, and parents who willingly, even eagerly, rely upon drugs to control children said to be hyperkinetic, overactive, and uncontrollable, recoil in horror at the prospect of controlling them by operant conditioning or surgery? Why is drug manipulation an acceptable trade-off for "manageable children" while other manipulative strategies are not? No more is known about the relevant chemotherapy than about the relevant operant conditioning or surgery, even though the contrary position is often argued by those who manage to avoid feeling guilty when they bribe Johnny to "just take the little pill." These guilt feelings are repressable because the little pill looks so innocuous, lends itself to easy, almost secret administration, and does not disrupt daily routines. These practical advantages rather than any scientific knowledge about the drugs make the trade-off of manipulation for manageable children acceptable, whereas with surgery, for example, the scalpel is not innocuous and hospitalizing a child can hardly be kept secret because it is so disruptive of routine. Is there, finally, a sufficiently greater scientific knowledge about manipulative drug therapy, or even psychotherapy, to make them worth the trade-off, as compared to similar manipulative behavior therapy, psychosurgery, or ESB? Even though there is no difference in degree or kind of knowledge to warrant treating drug therapy or psychotherapy differently from psychosurgery, there may still be reasons other than knowledge for our differing feelings about the alternative techniques.

Question 6: How do we identify the S who is manipulated? For example, if a fetus is manipulated by genetic surgery at a time when the mother could legally choose abortion, is S the mother, the fetus, or both? If S is the fetus, then serious questions arise as to who could, should, or does "represent" S, even if there is some institutional protection of subjects.

The Regulation of Scientific Manipulation

All of the general questions that I have raised above about the scientific manipulation of behavior demand thoughtful answers. But in the minds of many, the most important questions concern the courts' role. Because courts have traditionally developed and protected civil and social rights, and because we customarily give over to the courts those controversies which do not lend themselves to other institutional dispositions, there is a widespread belief that the courts should balance the legitimate demands for deviance control by scientific manipulation and the right to be let alone. However, my own experience as counsel in the Detroit psychosurgery case has only reinforced my belief that it is unrealistic to expect even competent judges to comprehend and appreciate the subtleties of relevant scientific materials. In addition, judicial "regulations" inevitably tend to operate on an ad hoc, unsystematic, case-by-case basis, and so there is no effectual way to prevent judges from treating scientific and sociopolitical concerns as fungible.[61] These reservations do not imply that courts have no place in developing rational doctrines about science and behavior control. Even if it is reasonable to expect that courts will understand how science (especially medical science) legitimates political authority, it is grossly unrealistic to expect courts alone to make decisions about: (a) the state of the art in any given developing scientific field; (b) the comparative efficacy (i.e. cost-benefit) of alternative intervention possibilities (e.g., psychotherapy versus drug therapy); and (c) the scientific (as contrasted to the political) advisability of any intervention as opposed to doing nothing. Doing nothing in the control of deviant behavior is another kind of intervention, since deliberately doing nothing is doing something. These facts raise another set of important questions.

Question 1: If the courts cannot perform this balancing miracle, can legislation do so, or at least do better? After the Detroit psychosurgery case legislation was introduced and considered (but fortunately never taken seriously enough to be passed in Michigan) which would have required that a jury decide on a case-by-case basis whether psychosurgery could be used.[62] While better but hardly remedial legislation has been introduced in Congress,[63] the general history of legislation as a mechanism for controlling medical science is highly distressing.[64] The rapidity with which medical knowledge increases, the character of the legislative process, militating against the rationality characteristic of scientific decisions, and the ease with which role fascists can lobby for a particular position are all reasons for such a dismaying record. This last matter significantly exacerbates the situation, because most scientists, unlike eager role fascists, shy away from involving their specialties with politics. The combination of overeager role fascists and excessively shy scientists virtually ensures that any "knowledge" upon which the legislator acts will be incomplete and distorted. Breggin's effort to arouse congressional ire over psychosurgery fully illustrates how incomplete and distorted information can successfully achieve the eager role fascist's goal.

Question 2: If neither courts nor legislation are likely to solve the problems, can something better be expected from executive action? Various federal agencies (VA, HEW, and FDA) have made important contributions to developing guidelines for resolving many difficult problems about science and behavior control; if it were necessary to choose from among judicial, legislative, or executive mechanisms to control science, history would favor the last. The executive branch has not only had the greatest access to the widest spectrum of relevant scientific talent but through power over the purse strings has been able to govern effectively most scientific developments relative to behavior control. However, as I indicated above, the executive monopoly of relevant talent is not without serious disadvantages. In 1974 Congress enacted the National Service Award Act, P.L. 93.348, and created pursuant to Section 201(a) of that act the National Commission for the Protection of Human Subjects. Section 202(a)(3)(c) provides:

> The Commission shall conduct an investigation and study of the use of psychosurgery in the United States during the five-year period ending December 31, 1972. The Commission shall determine the appropriateness of its use, evaluate the need for it, and recommend to the Secretary policies defining the circumstances (if any) under which its use may be appropriate.

The development of such a national data bank may help prevent excessive local discretion in regulating psychosurgery, a much needed development since the newest techniques for making a sterotoxic lesion may make "office" psychosurgery a real possibility.[65]

Question 3: Apart from judicial, legislative, or executive institutional mechanisms, are there other procedures which have been or could be important in this area? Scientific review, peer review, human rights, and subject protection committees have all been used with varying success. While much can be done to strengthen these institutions (for example, giving greater attention to committee memberships, written records, and the importance of full disclosure),[66] their procedures are also unlikely to balance adequately legitimate scientific behavior control against unnecessary or improper losses of freedom. Such committees, unlike courts, are unlikely to appreciate the political significance of medically controlling deviance or to deal effectively with those issues that I have identified which courts cannot adequately handle.

Although new institutions may emerge for regulating the scientific technologies of behavior control, there is an immediate need to consider what can be done while we await this panacea. It seems to me that a number of "affirmative action" possibilities should be considered. Even at their best, external institutional controls for science are not nearly as important or effective as the right kinds of science and scientists, and so the primary focus of affirmative action should be on attaining the latter. I would therefore suggest the following goals for the professional associations of scientific specialities:

(1) They should emphasize the social and political character of their work by recognizing and publicly dealing with its value consequences and its potential use in controlling behavior. They should, in effect, deliberately shed the neutrality pretense.
(2) They and their members should ensure that a handful of eager role fascists does not monopolize political decision makers.
(3) They and their members should deliberately ensure that an adequate and representative sample of relevant talent is available to *both* executive and legislative decision makers. When either branch begins to monopolize relevant talent, these associations should have a mechanism by which to take deliberate remedial action and should do so because they are better able to do so than any group of nonscientific citizens.
(4) Because they have such great influence in shaping the educational requirements of their future members, they should make certain that future medical, psychological, biological, and other specialists learn, and if possible understand, that these sciences are *human* sciences. They cannot just offer an elective course on "medical ethics,"

but must make a real effort to eradicate the neutrality mentality by which health and other scientific specialists insulate themselves from social reality.

I recognize that these four suggestions rely heavily upon the scientific specialists regulating themselves and thus avoidance is a real possibility. However, there are now an increasing number of medical scientists willing openly to confront and consider the value consequences of medical decisions. Furthermore, there is evidence that even among the inner core of recognized specialists who deal with psychosurgery there are some who are fully capable of careful and unbiased evaluation of the scientific data base. The single best analysis on the scientific status of psychosurgery is by one such specialist, Elliot Valenstein, in *Brain Control: A Critical Examination of Brain Stimulation and Psychosurgery* (1973). Furthermore, if the specialists, who at least begin with knowledge of the relevant data base, do not effectively deal with the problems of their profession, there are always judges with varying degrees of competence, harried legislators, eager and over eager role fascists, and executive decision makers willing to do so. In short, I would encourage those with the most technical competence to deal with their specialty's problems, and seek redress elsewhere only if they fail. Perhaps the National Commission for the Protection of Human Subjects will encourage just such a development, but in any event I hope the commission will discourage further piecemeal, state-by-state judicial or legislative actions.

While I believe we are most likely to avoid serious problems by "internalizing" controls, it is essential to recognize that some problems will not be amenable to internal solution or capable of being solved at that level. It is therefore necessary to encourage the "institutional pluralization of power" which avoids concentrating the decision-making mechanism in the judicial, legislative, or executive branch.[67] This pluralization is necessary if there is to be a rational and deliberate policy which weighs the individual's right to be deviant against society's rights, if any, to use science to socialize, resocialize, or reconstruct the individual, by suppressing, preventing, or diminishing his deviance.[68] My final point though is that before any further exercise of such pluralized power takes place, it would be helpful if some national standards about the practice of psychosurgery were articulated.

Chapter 9

THE RIGHT TO BE UNHEALTHY*

The Threat of Medical Imperialism

The right to be unhealthy has always been in jeopardy.[1] What makes this jeopardy even greater now is medicine's institutional tendency toward territorial expansion and the medical imperialism implied by the WHO definition of health as "a state of complete physical, mental, and social well-being and not merely the absence of disease or infirmity." Medical expansionism and imperialism are abetted by the rise of the welfare, service, facility conception of the state, characterized by the demand that the state furnish and insure "complete physical, mental and social well-being." The welfare service state's increasing reliance upon medicine to legitimate what the state should do leads to its ready accession to medicine's imperialistic demands. As the state legitimates the expansionist claims of medicine, it assures itself of the subsequent ability to legitimate state action within new medical provinces. In helping to legitimate medical approaches to new areas such as sex, drugs, alcohol, education, and crime, the state lays down a basis for the later legitimation of its own intervention in such areas. As the legally enforceable obligation to be healthy (and not merely a moral or religious obligation to be good) expands, the area within which the individual may choose to be unhealthy necessarily diminishes.

*With permission of the editors, reprinted with changes from 22 *Wayne Law Review* 61 (1975).

It is in this sense that medical imperialism is antithetical to moral autonomy and contrary to that individual personal freedom which characterizes the modern democratic state.

While the legitimating reciprocity between medicine and the state (to the detriment of individual freedom) is alone sufficiently awesome, there is another factor which enables medicine further to compromise autonomy for reasons of "good" health. One of the essential qualities of the doctor-patient relationship is that the patient must put faith in his doctor. How often does a patient tell "his" doctor, "I'm in your hands," or "Doctor knows best"? If we recognize that in this relationship the patient is always an individual human being while the doctor is often the state's surrogate, the significance of the faith relation becomes obvious. Since moral autonomy depends upon faith in internalized moral principles which determine action in individual cases, it is easy to see how such faith can be compromised by the doctor (state)-patient relationship. While the state versus the individual may result in a power versus faith confrontation, the state *as doctor* precipitates a faith versus faith confrontation. Once the doctor-patient relationship has been initiated, the good health about which doctor knows best is insulated from moral scrutiny because the relationship *itself* dictates that the "prescription" be taken on faith. While it is hardly surprising that many ancient cultures had doctors as religious functionaries and treated disease as a symptom of sin, it is curious that in modern society we are still so reluctant to "defrock the medical priesthood!"[2] Thomas Szasz has gone so far as to urge that "most people, on both sides of the Iron Curtain, now believe in health rather than salvation; in pills rather than prayer; in physicians rather than priests; in medicine and science rather than in theology and God."[3]

In addition to the faith underlying the usual doctor-patient relation, there are further features of the doctoring role which bestow an aura of moral, not just medical, authority upon the physician. This moral quality of the medical role is dramatically illustrated by cases where the doctor can, and often alone does, decide who shall be kept alive. When a doctor decides to refrain from heroic means which would sustain the life of a terminally ill patient, he can expect to be asked: "Aren't you playing God?"[4] Yet even without resorting to such extreme cases, it is readily apparent that doctors constantly make moral as well as technical decisions and, what is more, are expected to do so even by the very patients who may be the victims of such decisions. Indeed, every time a doctor labels a patient as "sick" there are clear moral and social consequences which attach; for example, the patient is exculpated from responsibility for his condition. It is important to appreciate that doctoring has a heavy overlay of morality because we then better understand why medical decisions about good health can be morally lethal. The individual, at most armed with a right to choose what "health" shall mean for him, must do battle against the medical scientist who comes armed with technical knowledge, the charisma which attaches to those who officiate at the most critical moments in life—birth and death[5]—and, most importantly, moral authority. In this almost grotesquely uneven struggle between individual moral autonomy and the technically overwhelming, charismatic, and morally authoritarian doctor whose role and cure have been legitimated by the state, is it any wonder that the right to be unhealthy has never been, and is not now, very healthy?

The obligation to be healthy has probably always been a major source of social pressure, but that pressure in now greater and more threatening. Much more territory is now included within the domain of good health, technically sophisticated mechanisms such as genetic surgery, psychosurgery, and operant conditioning are available for imposing good health and preventing or suppressing bad health, and we have witnessed the rise and spread of the welfare-oriented therapeutic state, which is expected to prevent crime by insuring that its citizens are normal and healthy. The primitive belief which underlies this expectation is that crime is a function of abnormality because healthy people do not commit crimes; yet, to the contrary, certainly one lesson we should have learned in the twentieth century is that it is entirely possible that only the "healthiest" will commit what at a certain time and place is defined as a statutory crime.[6]

The Problem of Medical Relativism

There are two basic assumptions underlying any justification of medical imperialism: (1) diseases are biophysical realities not invented by doctors but found "out there" waiting to be discovered;[7]

(2) the definition of "normalcy" is a medical problem. A subthesis of (2) is that psychiatric normalcy may be biologically determined, but even if it is not, the elaboration of the relevant criteria is nonetheless still a medical matter. Actually, what is behind both assumptions is a particularly tenacious, but pernicious, form of the myth about the value neutrality of science. Even though the significance of the Kuhn-Popper[8] controversy about scientific autonomy versus scientific relativism is well-recognized in the theoretical hard sciences, the medical sciences continue to function as though immunized again the relativism virus. It has been nearly fifteen years since Popper showed that there is not a category difference between theories and statements of fact, and that observations do not "prove" factual statements. "[E]very description uses universal names . . .; every statement has the character of a theory, of a hypothesis."[9] In other words, even before Kuhn, Popper attacked scientific autonomy on grounds very similar to those which Hume relied upon in his analysis of induction. Hume argued that no concatenation of singular statements "warrants" a universal law; Popper urges that no combination of singular sensations warrants a singular statement and, consequently, basic statements are agreed-upon conventions. To this Kuhn adds that such conventions reflect the social and political perspectives of those who participate in the decision as to which singular statements are "warranted" by experience. In other words, the hard core facts of science are a function not of sensation, but of community. Science, even hard science, is not autonomous, but rather a part of sociology and psychology.

Given the vulnerability of the physical sciences to these arguments, one would think that the life sciences, and particularly medicine, would aim at the constriction of their territories, yet the very contrary has been the case. There are probably many reasons for acknowledging the expanded applicability of the medical model, if one accepts medicine's exaggerated claims to objectivity. In addition, as the lack of objectivity in the hard sciences has become more obvious, and as it becomes clearer that man's place in the cosmos is largely a function not of the universe but of man, the vacuum created by the accompanying loss of objective certainty can be filled by almost anything. Compared to the "reality" experienceable by psychedelically zapping out into space, ignoring the subjectivity in much of modern medicine may not be such a bad alternative. Of course, we are helped to ignore the subjective quality in the medical "description" of normalcy because of medicine's reliance, wherever possible, upon a morphological model of disease, as well as upon biological structures and functions as the initial criteria for identifying abnormality.

In view of the fact that scientific relativism is due to the absence of some lawlike connection between sense experiences and singular observation (reporting) statements, the medical reliance upon biological structures and functions can only be seen as an effort to escape the inevitable relativism. That there is no escape, even though there may be a diminution in the degree of the relativism which would otherwise obtain is quite clearly seen in much of the current work directed toward ascertaining criteria for what constitutes genetic good health. It would appear that one of the few really firm lessons of genetics is that "health"—even when regarded as only the absence of disease, let alone as defined by WHO—is necessarily contextual. "Health" must be a function of a given environment, and this is so even as to biological structure and function.

> [In] genetic counseling, "genetic health" usually means being free of genes or chromosomes capable of causing clinically significant disease or disability if passed on to one's progeny. As straightforward as this definition appears at first glance, it has proven strangely unserviceable. A gene which has been transmitted with seeming impunity for one or two generations may cause terrible suffering years later—when the environment changes, or when the gene is finally transmitted in conjunction with a like gene (as with carriers of Tay-Sachs disease). . . . But does a minimal definition of "health" apply as well to "genetic health"? Take, for example, a definition of "health" as the *absence of disease*. Would a person who carried the gene for Huntington's chorea prior to the clinical manifestations of that condition properly be considered healthy?
>
> As long as this diversity exists, there will be genetic disease and disability due to the chance coming together of the same deleterious recessive genes and from the random assortment of genes which are adaptive in combination with one genotype and maladaptive with another. Thus, the greatest paradox of the concept of genetic health is that while from a population point of view, the "healthiest" individuals are probably those who carry the greatest number of genes in the heterozygous state, they are also the ones at greatest risk for transmitting genetic disease.[10]

In addition to these several problems and paradoxes which Lappé connects to any attempt at establishing a medical base for determining biological-genetic good health, it is worth noticing that such proposed criteria presume what is clearly not, or at least not exclusively, a function or structure of biology—the desirability of species survival. In a way, all theories about what is normal or healthy are essentially circular in that they presume that what is normal or healthy is therefore desirable, and that what is desirable is therefore normal or healthy. Yet the relationship between normal-healthy and desirable is clearly not symmetrical.

An interesting illustration of the belief that straight biological criteria for what is medically normal avoid, or at least significantly diminish, otherwise inevitable relativism may be seen in a letter by James Burtchaell, the provost of Notre Dame, written in response to an attempt by Dr. Joseph Fletcher, a distinguished teacher of medical ethics, to outline what it means to be human. In his paper presented to the National Conference on the Teaching of Medical Ethics, Fletcher suggested that, treacherous as the enterprise may be, "if we mean business" about developing some rational principles for biomedical ethics, then an effort must be made to develop a " 'profile of man' in concrete and discrete terms."[11] He then listed and briefly discussed fifteen "positive human criteria" and five negative ones. Burtchaell found these criteria "much too abstract and remote from *empirical observation*. . . . Dr. Fletcher is not exactly speaking in the language of the hospital or the lab. . . . In matters of life and death, I would much rather trust a *straight bio-medical* profile of humanhood. . . . "[12] Two questions inevitably arise. First, why would one prefer to trust empirical observations reported in "the language of the lab" rather than unempirical observations reported in whatever is contrary to the language of the lab? Second, what distinguishes a "straight bio-medical" profile from one which is not? There are at least three, and perhaps four, presumptions behind the provost's argument: (1) observation reports are not relative to the observer, or at least less so than other ways of relating to the external world; (2) knowledge about the external world is the only, and therefore the necessary, way to minimize relativistic generalizations about that world; (3) warranted specific statements about the world are constructed from observation reports; and (4) warranted generalizations can be constructed from specific statements about the world.

The Kuhn-Popper theories, however, show how dubious these several assumptions are, and we are therefore confronted by the "real" question—are there good reasons, or any reasons, for trusting straight biological criteria for normalcy in preference to criteria which are frankly sociological or psychological? In addition, we need to understand what it means to trust in this context. If normalcy criteria will be crucial or even relevant for determining who will be eligible to receive benefits beyond and above those generally regarded as necessary for a decent existence (e.g., advanced schooling), then perhaps we may be more relaxed—more trusting—about the criteria no matter how derived. However, what quite rightly bothered Burtchaell was that the primary use of these criteria would not be for bestowing benefits, but rather for determining who may live and who shall die. Since the ascription of deviance almost certainly implies that disadvantages and not benefits would attach, his objections would be equally well taken in this case. Ultimately, the right to be unhealthy may not deserve the protection accorded, for example, First Amendment rights, so long as choosing to be unhealthy carries no greater penalty than exclusion from benefits and privileges not necessary for a decent existence. However, the increased availability of scientific techniques for attaining an identified standard of "health" and the prevalence of the belief that the coerced production of health standardization is therapy and not punishment make it clear that the right to be unhealthy may need and deserve at least as much protection as First Amendment rights. Liberty and freedom, as well as the very right to life itself, are more and more frequently made contingent upon the prevailing criteria of health. In addition, access to the escalating benefits and privileges of an expanding, service-oriented welfare state is increasingly contingent upon compliance with government approved standards of health (that is, access depends upon failure to exercise the right to be unhealthy). Thus, Burtchaell's "straight biological" standard for health upon analysis may turn out to be significantly unattractive (even for him) because it is less relative than an overtly sociological or psychological standard. It may be fun to move from straight sociology to straight biology, but it is a sideways move which only substitutes one set of obscurities for another.

Although they are not essential to the argument I have been developing, Fletcher's twenty specific criteria are worth some attention because they purport to be "operational terms" which enable us to "get down to cases—to normative decisions." Apparently he believes that the development of such criteria will somehow furnish a more rational basis for solving bioethical problems. He suggests that there "are always some people who prefer to be visceral and affective in their moral choices, with no desire to have any rationale for what they do. But *ethics* is precisely the business of rational, critical reflection. . . . To that end, then, for the purposes of biomedical ethics, I am suggesting a 'profile of man' in concrete and discrete terms."[13] His fifteen positive criteria are: (1) minimal intelligence, (2) self-awareness, (3) self-control, (4) sense of time, (5) sense of futurity, (6) sense of the past, (7) capability to relate to others, (8) concern for others, (9) communication, (10) control of existence, (11) curiosity, (12) change and changeability, (13) balance of rationality and feeling, (14) idiosyncrasy, and (15) neocortical function. His five negative criteria are that man is not: (1) non- or antiartificial, (2) essentially parental, (3) essentially sexual, (4) a bundle of rights, or (5) a worshipper.

It is interesting to compare Fletcher's list with the distinguished biologist Robert L. Sinsheimer's effort to develop criteria for health. In presenting his criteria at a conference on genetic counseling and on the use of genetic knowledge, Sinsheimer asks, and then answers: "What, in an evolutionary sense, are the distinctive characteristics of humanity which—as we seize our destiny—we may wish to enhance? . . . 1. Our self-awareness; 2. Our perception of past, present, and future; 3. Our capacities for hope, faith, charity and love; 4. Our enlarged ability to communicate and thereby to create a collective consciousness; 5. Our ability to achieve a rational understanding of Nature; 6. Our drive to reduce the role of Fate in human affairs; 7. Our vision of man as unfinished."[14]

There is nothing on Sinsheimer's list to which biological expertise is uniquely relevant, and virtually nothing on Fletcher's list for which biomedical knowledge would be crucial, let alone dispositive. Because none of the criteria on either list is "straight biology," these lists suggest that even straight biological criteria would probably be of little value for dealing with the problems of bioethics. Moreover, the intrinsic reliance of both writers upon sociological and psychological criteria supports my point that there is not likely to be a significantly more autonomous, more scientific, or less relativistic mechanism for deciding major questions about the right to be unhealthy even when medicine furnishes the criteria. If scientifically autonomous or less relativistic criteria were available, they would surely have surfaced in these lists. I draw three conclusions from the inevitble relativism inherent in any effort to develop generalizations about good health, be they allegedly biological, sociological or psychological: (1) there is no difference in kind, but at best only of degree among the alternative general classificatory devices for distinguishing good from bad health; (2) the reasons for "trusting" one classificatory scheme in preference to others are not determined by our knowledge of biological structures or functions; and (3) the right to be unhealthy is accorded a degree of protection inversely proportional to the need for such protection.

Arguments Against the Right to be Unhealthy

The third conclusion is worthy of further development because it relates to an important aspect of almost everyone's life. There is relatively little institutional pressure exerted when an individual chooses to reject available therapy to correct what the community perceives to be a biological mis- or malfunctioning structure or process, so long as the consequence of being unhealthy in this way is either quickly terminal or relatively inconspicuous and unlikely to impose significant financial burdens upon the community. It is relatively easy for an individual to reject a cure for cancer or even to refuse repairs for a broken bone. In such cases, society is generally content with relying upon moral persuasion to encourage the right attitude about health. These are cases in which the individual can be most easily convinced to opt for what the community regards as good health because these "illnesses" are characterized by a shared perception that what requires therapy is a biological structure or process. Thus, if we begin with the *shared* belief that the disorder *is* biological, it is easier to procure consent for any therapy which allegedly restores good health, and this is why so much of the debate about psychosurgery centers upon the identification of brain organicity. The underlying presumption is that if there is a "damaged" brain, why would anyone resist the repair?

Of course, cases where the right to be unhealthy is most likely to be troublesome are ones where exercise of the right carries with it considerable social cost. It is quite probable that cost savings, at least as much as concern about human suffering, explain the escalating concern about procedures such as genetic surgery, psychosurgery, drug therapy, and operant conditioning. In these cases there is a double pressure. First, there is increasing evidence establishing a causal connection between anatomical function and socially expensive deviance, such as uncontrollable aggressive violence. Second, the alleged increase in objectionable violence makes it easier both to find a "causal" connection and to compromise the right to be unhealthy when the social cost is thought to be high. It should perhaps be added that currently acceptable mechanisms for controlling and preventing violence suffer an inverse relationship between program costs and payoff, so that by comparison the cost-benefit ratio for procedures like psychosurgery, which while still regarded as experimental, is potentially very attractive. In combination, these several factors discourage protection for a right to be unhealthy and make an impressive argument in favor of being normal—even if you don't want to be.

The most impressive argument for rejecting or severely limiting the right to be unhealthy can be summarized as follows: (1) disabling anatomical or physiochemical dysfunctions are regularly accompanied by biological symptoms and therefore organic (objective) criteria identify the dysfunction; (2) since "dysfunction" means "not functioning properly," proper function should be restored or created, if possible; (3) no intellectually or emotionally competent (normal) living person would deliberately choose to be disabled by repairable biological dysfunction; (4) therefore anyone who chooses to be unhealthy vis-à-vis repairably dysfunction is abnormal and lacking even the minimum qualifications for exercising the right to be unhealthy. In short, the argument is real life *Catch 22!* A comparable argument is made about persons whom doctors or psychologists believe require drug therapy or behavior conditioning. If informed consent is the prerequisite to initiating therapy, how can the subject consent since, if he had the capacity, he would probably not require the therapy! Sometimes it is suggested that the subject's consent should retroactively validate the initiation of therapy so that his consent is sought only after the therapy has progressed far enough to enable the subject to meet the minimum qualifications of intellectual or emotional competence. So many obvious difficulties surround this circular, self-serving argument that it is probably more useful to consider the usual alternative of surrogate consent mechanism, and utilize a guardian, a committee of protectors, or a court.

Imposing some intervening institutionalized mechanism between the individual's right to be unhealthy and society's right to demand health may make it possible to reconcile these demands. However, one serious objection is that any institutionalized procedure, precisely because it is institutionalized, already loads the dice against the individual. For certain relatively easy cases court intervention may be an acceptable way out. One such case would be the Jehovah's Witness's rejection of a necessary blood transfusion and the hospital's petitions for relief. This type of case is easier than most because the subject is not choosing unhealth, but rather suffers it as a consequence of exercising other rights or privileges. The court, in ordering necessary blood transfusions for an objecting Jehovah's Witness, argued:

> The Gordian knot of this suicide question may be cut by the simple fact that Mrs. Jones did not want to die. Her voluntary presence in the hospital as a patient seeking medical help testified to this. Death, to Mrs. Jones, was not a religiously-commanded goal, but an unwanted side effect of a religious scruple. There is no question here of interfering with one whose religious convictions counsel his death, like the Buddhist monks who set themselves afire. Nor are we faced with the question of whether the state should intervene to reweight the relative values of life and death, after the individual has weighed them for himself and found life wanting. Mrs. Jones wanted to live.[15]

The hard cases, where judicial intervention is clearly less attractive, involve persons who directly and deliberately maintain their wish to be unhealthy. Some of the most difficult cases are middle-ground ones, like the Detroit psychosurgery case, in which the subject argues not that he wants to be unhealthy, but rather that he does not suffer from a disease. Often, whether a person may choose to be unhealthy will turn upon the decision made by the state, or by medicine acting in the name of the state, that what is chosen is to be characterized as a disease. An additional difficulty in the Detroit psychosurgery case stemmed from the possibility that the proposed therapy was objectionable, even if uncontrollable aggressive violence was deemed to be a disease, and even if no one had the right to choose to be unhealthy as regards such a disease.

Concepts of Disease: The Entity Concept and the Behavioral Model

There is a large and rapidly growing literature about the concept of disease.[16] Even traditionalists now recognize alternatives to the "entity" conception, pursuant to which "disease" is regarded as something existing independently of a given observer or a given cultural context. However, the entity conception of disease is still relied upon to determine the extent to which an individual is allowed to be unhealthy. It has probably always been apparent that disease categories are constructions and not discoveries, and that classificatory devices do not report only observable empirical phenomena. Moreover, acknowledging the difference between disease and illness[17] implies that there is a still greater gulf between intersubjectively confirmable reports about reality and the right to be and remain ill. If I were arguing the right to be or remain ill (rather than unhealthy) it would be useful to show how important sociological, psychological, and cultural factors intervene between disease and illness, for even if the symptoms, disorders, and dysfunctions of a disease are not contextual, the "right" to be ill is. However, I will not pursue this matter, for it is more important here to consider whether symptoms, disorders, and dysfunctions are themselves necessarily determined by the cultural context within which they are identified.

Sometimes the entity theory results in viewing the disease not merely as abstract, but as an object—a phenomenon in the real world. But on either interpretation, belief in an entity theory minimizes, if it does not obliterate, the domain within which the right to be unhealthy operates. Disease is viewed as an anatomic or genetic structure or physiochemical process which is dysfunctional in a way which causes pain, discomfort, or disability. Furthermore, dysfunction is not regulated by, or subject to, custom, morality, or law. Sometimes the entity conception is formulated in terms of tissue systems, or interior environment. "*Disease* means at the very least some form of tissue damage or disturbance of function, as in malaria, tuberculosis, arteriosclerosis, chronic brain disorder, etc. That is, in every case of disease there is some disturbance, reversible or irreversible, in the structure or function of tissues. Such disturbances may have wide behavioral and attitudinal ramifications, but the *sine qua non* of disease is the assumption of direct disturbance of tissue structure and function."[18] Horacio Fabrega has pointed out that the common denominator in these organic conceptions of disease is their universalism and absolutism.

> It should be clear that a consequence of applying or using this essentially biologistic framework regarding disease is that specific disease can then be said to be *universal* or transcultural occurrences. . . . There is no reason to doubt that man everywhere is biologically the same individual in most of the important respects that enable physicians to make judgments about disease. Certainly diet, climate, and level of activity have biological effects that are reflected in body chemistries, muscle mass, and even tissue appearance and function; however, scientifically based medical knowledge and experience is such that it enables physicians to confidently interpret biological indicators when they reflect abnormality despite the fact that such "abnormal" indicators may be typical of particular population groups. The use of verbal reports as indicators of disease is not problematic in most instances of disease evaluation.[19]

In a subsequent section of his article, Fabrega develops the contrasting behavioral model of disease.

> It should be stated that in a broader intellectual context, the idea of disease or illness does not logically entail an understanding of bodily function, nor does it require that the users of the concept regard the body's function as a salient consideration. . . . Social scientists are emphasizing that since what patients seek medical advice and care for is expressed *behaviorally,* then it follows that behavioral science is equally relevant to a rational understanding of medical problems of "disease." . . . The manner in which persons perceive, organize, and express disability, *regardless of its origin,* is embedded in behavior, and the form of this behavior, which in many ways is the raw data of medical evaluation, is determined by social, psychological, and cultural factors as well as by biologic, ecologic, or genetic factors. . . . According to these social scientists, then, a physician, in order to make rational and effective use of his knowledge about biological processes, must be aware of the behav-

ioral dimensions and implications of his aims and actions. Stated succinctly, he needs to appreciate the extent to which disease processes link and interconnect with behavioral factors in order to effectively treat patients.[20]

Clearly the biological (tissue-organism-person) model of disease tends to be antiindividualistic, if not dogmatically universalistic, while the behavioral, social construction model can better accommodate the right to be unhealthy. It is equally apparent, however, that the right to be unhealthy is not a logical consequence of the behavioral model; indeed, even with such a model there are at least two powerful forces working to suppress the right to be unhealthy. One results from the pervasive search to find organic validation for any condition that entitles the patient to those "benefits" which flow from the right to be sick. The other results from the general social benefit to almost everyone but the patient which comes from the somatization of his condition.

The current exaggerated use of drugs in America and elsewhere in the world is a consequence of believing that somatic explanations are "better" than sociological or psychological ones. The extent to which Minimal Brain Dysfunction (MBD) children, or so-called hyperactive children, are subjected to organic therapies is a contemporary illustration of this phenomenon.[21] Although probably not more than 12 percent of these children have any organic component in their condition, parents, teachers, and doctors overwhelmingly favor somatization. If the psychological origins and treatments were frankly confronted, they would be much more threatening than somitazation because of the implication that parents, teachers, and doctors had done, and were doing, something that could be corrected if the external environment rather than the internal milieu were altered. It is thus apparent that the tissue-organism-biological-entity model of disease derives much of its attractiveness from the reciprocally reinforcing relationship it establishes between society and those who make disease attributions. Using it, doctors are insulated from the charge of idiosyncratic relativism and society is objectively justified in attaching social consequences to disease attributions, including the individual's duty to make himself, or to be made, normal.

Despite, or perhaps because of, all of the obvious social advantages which flow from reliance upon the disease model, I continue to believe that the right to be unhealthy deserves protection. Even if we do recognize that germs and fractures are natural events, and that the transformation of such natural events into diseases is a function of human or biological "nature," we cannot ignore the fact that the criteria for illness and perhaps also for health are a function of social considerations.

> All departments of nature below the level of mankind are exempt both from disease and from treatment—until man intervenes with his own human classifications of disease and treatment. The blight that strikes at corn or at potatoes is a *human invention,* for if man wished to cultivate parasites (rather than potatoes or corn) there would be no "blight," but simply the necessary foddering of the parasite-crop. Animals do not have diseases either, prior to the presence of man in a meaningful relation with them. . . . Outside the significances that man voluntarily attaches to certain conditions, *there are no illnesses or diseases in nature*. . . . Are there not infectious and contagious bacilli? Are there not definite and objective lesions in the cellular structures of the human body? Are there not fractures of bones, the fatal ruptures of tissues, and malignant multiplications of tumorous growths? Are not these, surely, events of nature? Yet these, as natural events, do not—prior to the human social meanings we attach to them—constitute illnesses, sicknesses, or diseases. . . . Out of his anthropocentric self-interest, man has chosen to consider as "illnesses" or "diseases" those natural circumstances which precipitate the death (or the failure to function according to certain values) of a limited number of biological species: man himself, his pets and other cherished livestock, and the plant varieties he cultivates for gain or pleasure.[22]

In addition to acknowledging that a disease is an attribution and not a description, it should also be noted that any attribution is a function of what is a perceived "disorder" and how that disorder is interpreted. "The same physical condition may be seen as a sign of impending death, as a minor inconvenience, as accidental, as punishment for sins, as a sign of weakness or neuroticism, as a basis for escaping intolerable life tasks, as grounds for demonstrating stoicism, courage or self-sacrifice, etc. Accordingly, the illness behavior which accompanies a disorder follows on the basis of the interpretation given to it, and may even influence the course of the illness via that behaviour."[23] In addition to these compelling reasons for recognizing the contextual relativism of any disease attribution, there is the further fact that "social" conditions—overcrowding, poverty, scarcity of food or water, broken families, stigmatized minority status, divorce, widowhood—themselves "cause" disease. There is also accumulating evidence that important physiological differences are associated with "normal" social factors. For example, hard-driving, competitive and ambitious men have a higher level of noradrenaline in their night urine and a higher rate of heart disease than do men who are more "low-keyed."[24] A major assault on the connection between stress and physiological changes in man is only beginning, although there is interesting animal work to indicate that such links are likely to be found. Rats experience intestinal bleeding, shrinkage of lymph tissue, and heightened adrenal activity when under enough stress. The implication of such a linkage for any theory about the right to be unhealthy should be apparent. Even if man's internal environment (his germs, fractures, etc.) could be the basis for a disease attribution (that is, unmediated by how that environment is perceived, interpreted, and reported), it would still be necessary to acknowledge a causal relation between that environment and the external one.

A Proposal for a Compromised Right to be Unhealthy

If, then, disease is "caused" by the external social world and by how the individual "patient's" symptology is perceived, interpreted, and reported, is it still necessary to argue that a right to be unhealthy deserves legal protection? While my answer is obvious, as is so often the case with controversial moral and legal questions, the hard problem concerns not the existence of some right, but rather the elaboration of criteria by which to establish guidelines. The health anarchist would argue that the right to be unhealthy, like that of free speech, when once established, is absolute: the individual must never be forced to undergo an unwanted therapeutic intervention even if such intervention will make *him* healthier or prevent harm to others. On the other hand, the health traditionalist, who equates "good" with good health, would argue that this right, when once established, does not warrant the individual's refusing any intervention which will make him better or prevent harm to others. John Stuart Mill's famous "one very simple principle" from *On Liberty,* would be the basis for the health liberal's position.

> The object of this Essay is to assert one very simple principle . . . that the sole end for which mankind are warranted, individually or collectively, in interfering with the liberty of action of any of their number, is self-protection. That the only purpose for which power can be rightfully exercised over any member of a civilized community, against his will, is to prevent harm to others. His own good, either physical or moral, is not a sufficient warrant.[25]

Thus, the health liberal would argue that preventing harm to others is the only possible basis for an imposed intervention.

Many sociologically aware, philosophically sensitive, but medically oriented citizens have become increasingly anxious about the price society may have to pay if complete self-realization and moral autonomy is to be each individual's right. I share this concern and what this means in the context of the contemporary Hart-Devlin debate[26] about using law to enforce public morality; indeed, I am increasingly uncomfortable with Hart's defence of Mill while entirely unconvinced by Devlin. Devlin purports to answer the "final" question about who shall watch the watchman by placing his trust in "the man in Clapham omnibus . . . the man in the jury box."[27] My experience as defense counsel in the Detroit psychosurgery case convinced me that for complex, technical, bioethical matters, even a competent three-judge panel, let alone some men from the omnibus, was incapable of comprehending, understanding, or appreciating all the subtleties and significance of relevant scientific material. Moreover, these trained and generally competent judges were highly susceptible to manipulation by public relations techniques. Thus, to deposit our ultimate trust in watchmen taken off a bus, be they judges or jurors (and they do frequently ride the same bus), may well mean placing our confidence in Madison Avenue. Perhaps we will be forced to concede that this is the best we can do, and for some cases it may be the best that should be done, but for a matter like the psychosurgery case it may be no better than rolling dice, and loaded dice at that.

In light of these considerations, and although I am inclined toward the position of the Mill health liberal, I am willing to entertain the possibility that not every and all "medical" alternatives to incarceration, fine, and parole violate the prohibition against cruel and unusual punishment. Indeed, there is nothing in what Mill said to imply that a medical therapeutic intervention is any more suspect than some other ways of exercising power over an individual. That it might be is a modern idea largely due to deeply entrenched notions about the nature of constitutionally permissible punishment. The question I am raising, then, is whether the right to be unhealthy should be compromised when: (1) the chosen unhealthy condition is corrigible; (2) the evidence for that condition is regarded as biological by the relevant scientific community; (3) the curative therapy is not experimental or innovative; (4) the therapy carries no unreasonable degree of organic or psychological risk; (5) the chosen unhealthy condition has previously imposed, and would continue to impose, significant social costs upon the community.

Although imposed therapeutic intervention would violate all five of the conditions required to support my "compromised" right to be unhealthy, such a conclusion in no way implies that an individual found guilty of a crime involving aggressive violence could not "consent" to a therapeutic intervention. Rather, my concern is with imposed therapy in lieu of, in addition to, or regardless of, some other punishment; and on this issue one must notice what the proposed compromised right does and does not imply. It does imply that: (1) despite inevitable social relativism in disease attribution, some such attributions may still support the imposition of therapeutic intervention; (2) even if an intervention is imposed, it is not therefore cruel and unusual. The fifth condition for the compromise further implies that: (3a) before the therapy may be imposed, the individual has been found guilty of a crime which has a significant social cost for the community; (3b) if he had not had the condition, he would not have committed the crime; (3c) if the condition is corrected, the individual would not be more likely than the "normal" population to again commit the crime for which he had been convicted.

The compromised right does not imply that: (1) criminal deviance is a biological disorder; (2) any criminal deviance which is a biological disorder is therefore a condition which warrants an imposed intervention; (3) criminal deviance which is a biological disability therefore imposes significant social costs upon the community; (4) intervention, if therapeutic, cannot constitute cruel and unusual punishment; (5) being found guilty of a crime is sufficient to impose an intervention, even if such a procedure would cure the disorder which "caused" the crime. In other words, the compromised right to be unhealthy is closer to the position of the Mill liberal than to those of the health anarchist or the health traditionalist, in that imposed therapy is neither automatically prohibited nor automatically permitted if therapeutic. There are obviously massive problems in specifying the operational details for the five conditions which must obtain before the right may be compromised. It is equally clear that the compromised right places greater trust in medical watchmen from Park and Fifth Avenues than in those from Madison Avenue. Favoring Park and Fifth over Madison implies much about my own prejudice, even though it would be nice to know how much Madison Avenue, in the service of drug companies, influences Park and Fifth. However, my primary reason for trying to find an operationally viable compromise about health stems from a belief that because the anarchist's position is as unattractive as the traditionalist's, it may be worthwhile to develop a workable liberal position.

I should point out that although the difficulties surrounding the identification or classification of "biological" diseases are great, these problems are considerably greater when the disease concept is expanded to include psychiatric disorders. Although I believe Szasz correctly perceived that psychiatry could and has been used as an instrument of state-determined socialization or resocialization, his famous slogan, "the myth of mental illness," is little more than a metaphor which acquires descriptive plausibility because some psychiatrists unwittingly and others very deliberately have used the medical model as a political instrument. However, we must not therefore conclude that all psychiatric disorder is only a product of deliberate, sociopolitical action.[28] I do not believe, for example, that it is still possible to deny that there is an organic, biological component in schizophrenia, or that there is such a component in at least some types of that disorder, or at some time during the course of that disorder.[29] It is also highly probable that a genetic component is found in at least some forms of schizophrenia, although the proof is still only statistical. Therefore, for these disorders at least, the traditional medical model fits as well as it does for allegedly more paradigmatic nonpsychiatric medical disorders. This is not to say, however, that this medical model is any better in these instances or that it does not suffer all of the sociological relativism previously noted. What is implied, though, is that there are psychiatric disorders which are *no more* mythical than is a malfunctioning prostate. Although a urologist may be a role fascist and give advice about sex, and although a psychiatrist may be a role fascist and give advice about sex, in neither event does it follow that the malfunctioning brain is more or less of a myth than is the malfunctioning prostate. Why the urologist or psychiatrist acts as though his medical training or expertise qualifies him as a sex or marriage counselor is a function of economic, social, and historical factors. But the important point is that there is no intrinsically better justification for compromising the right to be unhealthy because the biological disorder is organic rather than psychiatric.

Let me conclude by constructing a case in which the compromised right to be unhealthy might apply. For ten years, mother has been watching and hearing her son-in-law beat up her daughter when he comes home drunk on Friday and Saturday nights. Every Sunday, for a constellation of social, religious, and other reasons, the daughter forgives her pleading and repentant husband who in turn regularly promises to reform. If the son-in-law has been repeatedly convicted for beating his wife, and the five conditions for compromising the right to be unhealthy I have proposed obtain, this might be an attractive case for an imposed intervention. Of course, interesting questions still remain. Would the intervention be attractive if it involved surgery rather than drugs or operant conditioning? Would the intervention be attractive if it depended on the subject's regularly taking medication? Is the injury which the wife regularly suffered the kind of significant social cost required by the fifth condition? Since the marriage was presumably not consummated under duress, did the wife take the husband for better or for worse? If the son-in-law's biochemistry was like that of most alcoholics and unlike that of nonalcoholics, should he be compelled to become healthy in this respect, even though the basis for compromising his right to be unhealthy was his convictions for wife beating, and not for drunkenness, and even though there is no necessary or even statistical connection between alcoholism and wife beating? If the incidence of wife beating was comparable for drunkards and nondrunkards, could the therapy be imposed in light of (3c) above?

Or, what about a son-in-law who, after ten years of interference by a tormenting mother-in-law, finally dispatches her? Should such one-time family murderers be allowed to remain "unhealthy"? Did he do anything which is biologically or psychiatrically unhealthy? Is murder in any degree evidence of disease? If not, when is murder evidence of disease? Is deliberate, repetitive, interracial murder or rape evidence of disease? Are conventional crimes done for political motives evidence of disease?

I raise these questions to suggest that even the five conditions for compromising an otherwise absolute right to be unhealthy are unlikely to establish easy principles by which to support a compromised right. One clearly missing principle would establish the difference between a "condition" which is possibly unhealthy and a disease which, despite all of its contextual relativism, may still be specific enough to permit one to perceive it as either an illness which we may choose or which, perhaps, ought to be beyond the right to be unhealthy. Yet so long as objectionable deviance is a function of condition and not only of disease, we remain in the uncomfortable position of favoring health anarchy—not because it is so good, but because there may not be anything better.

AFTERWORD

Even during the hearing of the Detroit psychosurgery case it was clear that the questions it raised were too serious and too complex to be answered definitively by the court no matter how it ruled nor how broadly it interpreted its judicial role. To some civil libertarians, the problem "disposed of" in *Kaimowitz v. Dept. of Mental Health* seemed an open and shut case of protecting a powerless individual from harassment by the establishment. To others, perhaps more thoughtful, it was evident that hasty judgments, liberal or conservative, must necessarily be insufficient. The Detroit case attracted international attention, and the extent and intensity of the interest it aroused suggest that many observers saw in it concern for far more than the single John Doe involved. The issue of informed consent by the involuntarily confined, for example, could be seen as only part of a broad general question about the proper relationship between all of the various possible medical interventions and individual liberties.

When the Detroit court did rule, the decision seemed to me wrong, and I undertook the writing of this book in order further to develop and clarify the reasons for my dissent. Others besides myself of course also continued to be concerned with these issues, among them the appointed members of the National Commission for the Protection of Human Subjects of Biomedical and Behavioral Research to which I refer in chapter two. My book was written and in the final stages of being prepared for the printer when a draft of the commission's recommendations on psychosurgery became available.

The commission has to date (October 1976) drafted six specific recommendations, which I quote from the September 29, 1976 unpublished "Report and Recommendations on the Use of Psychosurgery":

(1) The Secretary, DHEW, is encouraged to conduct and support research to evaluate the safety of specific psychosurgical procedures and their efficacy in relieving specific psychiatric symptoms and disorders, provided that the requirements of recommendation (2) are satisfied.

(2) Until the safety and efficacy of any psychosurgical procedure have been demonstrated, such procedure should be performed only at an institution with an institutional review board (IRB) approved by DHEW and only after such IRB has determined that: (a) the surgeon has the necessary competence to perform the procedure; (b) adequate pre- and post-operative evaluations will be performed; (c) patient selection is appropriate; and (d) consent has been given under circumstances which assure that the rights of patients are protected.

(3) Psychosurgery may be performed on an individual under the legal age of consent for medical care provided that: (a) the conditions of recommendation (2) are fulfilled; (b) parental or guardian consent has been given; (c) a court, in which the child has legal representation, has reviewed and approved the performance of the procedure; and (d) if the surgery is performed as part of a research [project], the conditions stipulated in the commission's report on research involving children are fulfilled.

(4) Psychosurgery may be performed on a prisoner or involuntarily confined mental patient provided that: (a) the conditions of recommendation (2) are fulfilled; (b) in the case of an incompetent patient, the legal guardian has consented; (c) a court, in which the patient has been represented by counsel, has reviewed and approved the performance of the procedure on that individual; (d) the candidate is evaluated for surgery, and surgery is performed, in a medical facility separate and apart from the institution in which the mental patient is regularly confined; and (e) if the surgery is performed as part of a research project, all the conditions stipulated in the commission's report on research involving prisoners, or on research involving the institutionalized mentally infirm, or both (as applicable) are fulfilled.

(5) The Secretary should establish a mechanism to compile and assess information regarding the nature, extent and outcomes of psychosurgical procedures performed in this country, the indications for the procedures, and the populations on which they are performed. This mechanism should include stringent provisions to safeguard the privacy of [individual] patients.

(6) The Secretary, DHEW, should withhold all departmental funds

> from any institution which permits psychosurgery to be performed under conditions that are not in compliance with regulations [implementing] these recommendations.

In the course of commenting on recommendation (4), the commission reviews the Detroit decision and finds that the *Kaimowitz* argument, while superficially a defense of individual rights, in effect might be harmful to those rights. The commission observes that "diminished capacity to consent should not exclude prisoners or involuntarily confined patients from the opportunity to benefit from new therapies, if those therapies may be their best (or even, only) possibility for recovering from disabling emotional disorders" (p. 54). The commission further disagrees with the Detroit court as regards the balance of risks and potential benefits of psychosurgery: "Thus, the conclusions of the court in *Kaimowitz* regarding the hazardous nature of psychosurgery, the depersonalizing side-effects, and the lack of benefits, have been sufficiently refuted by new data that the prohibition of psychosurgery as a class of activities no longer seems to be required, even with respect to patients whose capacity to consent may be somewhat diminished" (p. 56).

I have changed nothing in my text since the commission's recommendations were made public. I think a reader may easily discern that the analyses and recommendations which I have made are supported by the independent analyses and recommendations of the commission. I do not, however, intend to sound self-satisfied. No one can afford to assume that any particular guidelines, no matter how carefully reasoned nor how responsive to the needs of the moment, are likely to serve us very long in an area as rapidly developing and changing as that involving the brain.

The *Psychiatric News* (18 February 1977) reports that "The . . . Commission . . . finally approved its report on the use of psychosurgery." The final report, while retaining much of the basic material found in the October draft quoted above, has added two additional requirements and has generally strengthened the conditions pursuant to which psychosurgery may be used, especially when the patient is a minor, a prisoner, or otherwise involuntarily detained.

Appendix A

A Formulation of the First Amendment Argument

By Michael H. Shapiro

"Legislating the Control of Behavior Control: Autonomy and the Coercive Use of Organic Therapies." By Michael H. Shapiro, Associate Professor of Law, University of Southern California. The article appears in Vol. 47 of the *Southern California Law Review,* pp. 237–356 (February 1974). Reprinted by permission of the author and the *Southern California Law Review.*

This short selection from Shapiro's long article furnishes only the outline of his theory about the First Amendment protection of mentation. I have omitted most of the insightful footnotes that accompanied this recent formulation of the mentation argument; those notes which remain have been renumbered.

Let us now consider the thesis that the first amendment protects, as a fundamental right, a person's power to generate thought, ideas and mental activity—his freedom of mentation. The argument can be formulated in this way:

(1) The first amendment protects communication of virtually all kinds, whether in written, verbal, pictorial or any symbolic form, and whether cognitive or emotive in nature.
(2) Communication entails the transmission and reception of whatever is communicated.
(3) Transmission and reception necessarily involve mentation on the part of both the person transmitting and the person receiving.
(4) It is in fact impossible to distinguish in advance mentation which will be involved in or necessary to transmission and reception from mentation which will not.

(5) If communication is to be protected, *all* mentation (regardless of its potential involvement in transmission or reception) must therefore be protected.

The argument thus far establishes that the first amendment protects mentation. The conclusion that the first amendment protects persons against the coercive use of organic therapies follows as a corollary:

(6) Organic therapy intrusively alters or interferes with mentation.[1]

(7) The first amendment therefore protects persons against enforced alteration or intereference with their mentation by coerced organic therapy. (This last proposition would also be a valid inference if it read: "The first amendment therefore protects persons against certain kinds of *denial* of access to organic therapy, or psychoactive agents generally, which are used to alter mentation."

The argument now demonstrates that compelled organic therapies (or, at the very least, the more intrusive organic therapies) generate a threshold claim of infringement of the first amendment. The government can therefore justify such coercion, if at all, only by offering rationales which survive the "compelling state interest" standard of review.

The substance of the first amendment argument articulated here was applied in the recent case of *Kaimowitz v. Department of Mental Health,*

---

1. "Intrusiveness" is a standard invoked *both* to establish whether certain practices create a threshold first amendment claim *and* to determine whether it is constitutionally permissible to use a given organic therapy, rather than a less intrusive one, upon someone lacking the capacity for informed consent. The distinction drawn between certain organic therapies which are effective in a *relatively* nonintrusive way and those which are effective in a highly intrusive way is thus perfectly consistent with premise (6). The distinction is occasionally referred to here as the "effective/intrusive" distinction, but that locution should not be understood to imply that the degree of intrusiveness of any organic therapy is too insignificant to invoke the first amendment's protection. All organic therapies are considerably intrusive and thus probably fall within the scope of the first amendment. For an extended review of organic therapies, *see Comprehensive Textbook supra* note 5, at ch. 35. As used in this Article, the term "intrusive" by definition connotes an interference with personal autonomy: the greater the degree of intrusiveness, the greater the assault on autonomy. For a review of the ways in which choice and opportunity are altered and constricted or enlarged by organic therapy, see text section IV(B)(2) *infra*.

The terms "alteration" and "interference" in premise (6) are intended to be value-neutral. Any given alteration or interference may effect an "improvement" or "deterioration" in mentation and behavior, or both or neither.

in which the trial court held that a patient involuntarily committed in a mental hospital cannot be subjected to psychosurgery:[2]

> A person's mental processes, the communication of ideas, and the generation of ideas, come within the ambit of the First Amendment. To the extent that the First Amendment protects the dissemination of ideas and expression of thoughts, it equally must protect the individual's right to generate ideas.[3]

Some of the more novel propositions set forth in the seven-step argument above, and implicit in the *Kaimowitz* opinion, require further explanation.

1. The Conceptual Connection Between Mentation and Communication.

It should be stressed that the connection between mentation and communication (posited in premise (3) above) is not simply an empirical connection which might put mentation in the same category as *tools* of communication (*e.g.*, printing presses, tympanic membrances, or auditoriums). It is by

---

2. Civil No. 73-19434-AW (Wayne County, Mich., Cir. Ct., July 10, 1973). The court's conclusion seems to be that *in principle* it is impossible to secure informed consent to psychosurgery from a person involuntarily committed in a mental hospital. For a discussion of this somewhat dubious proposition, *see* text section V (A)(3).

3. Kaimowitz v. Department of Mental Health, Civil No. 73-19434-AW (Wayne County Mich., Cir. Ct., July 10, 1973), at 32. The author is obliged to note that the first amendment argument adopted by the court was presented in [Shapiro, "The Use of Behavior Control Technologies: A Response," 7 *Issues in Crim*. 55 at 68–78 (1972)]. That article was cited in the post-trial amicus curiae brief of the American Orthopsychiatric Association. (Brief at 81–84). *See also* Mackey v. Procunier, No. 71-30622 (9th Cir., Apr. 16, 1973). Petitioner there alleged that he had been subjected to the Anectine experiments. In reversing an order dismissing the complaint brought under 42 U.S.C. § 1983 (1970) and related provisions for violation of civil rights, the court said:

> Proof of such matters [*e.g.*, that plaintiff was subjected to a "breath-stopping and paralyzing 'fright drug' " and was treated as a "guinea-pig"] could, in our judgment, raise serious constitutional questions respecting cruel and unusual punishment or impermissible tinkering with the mental processes.

Id. at 2 (footnotes omitted). This author was consulted on the preparation of petitioner's brief before the Ninth Circuit. At no time was this author counsel of record for any party in the *Kaimowitz* or *Mackey* actions.

definition embraced in the term "communication," a term properly defined as involving the expression of ideas, thoughts, and feelings. To affect the nature or content of mentation is thus, as a matter of logical necessity, to affect communication involving or depending upon such mentation. Mentation is not simply a means of or aid for communication; it is a logically prior antecedent of *any* communication. The court in *Kaimowitz* noted this necessary connection between mentation and communication, observing that

> if the First Amendment protects the freedom to express ideas, it necessarily follows that it must protect the freedom to generate ideas. Without the latter protection, the former is meaningless.

The distinction made by the Supreme Court between regulations which "incidentally" rather than "directly" affect communication is therefore inapposite here. We are not concerned with the "tools" or mechanics of communication, nor regulation of its time, place and manner. We are concerned with the very mental processes which are logically prior to communication.

The appropriate inquiry, then, concerns the extent to which a therapeutic regimen affects or intrudes upon mentation. Psychosurgery, for example, may severely affect mentation by permanent destruction of selected areas of the brain. A conditioning or learning program seeking to induce mental and behavioral changes, however, may affect mentation by the use of relatively mild reward or punishment stimuli, and thus would seem to involve a lesser intrusion or assault upon mentation. Since therapies vary in the degree to which we are inclined to view them as intrusive or nonintrusive, we must address some obvious questions: do therapies such as token economies, psychotherapy, moral suasion, or organic behavior modification programs like the Anectine conditioning program fall outside the scope of the first amendment because (unlike, e.g., psychosurgery or ESB) their effects of mentation are in some sense less intrusive? How do we identify among the infinitude of stimuli or conditions which have *some* effect on mentation those which should be deemed so assaultive of our mental autonomy, individuality, or personhood, that the state should be heavily burdened with justifying their use in altering mentation? A legal theory which characterized ordinary instructional methods in public schools, or the psychic effects of confinement *simpliciter,* as raising a threshold first amendment issue would hardly be satisfactory, even though the long run mentational effects may be substantial. Simply walking past a person's field of vision effects a change in his sensorium; but under ordinary circumstances we would not regard this as an instance of coercive mind control. In short, not every effort to change behavior by changing attitudes, emotions, or mentation generally constitutes coercive mind control.

2. Limiting Principles for the Threshold Characterization: Criteria of Intrusiveness.

The limiting principles needed in determining whether a given mode of alteration of mentation raises a threshold first amendment claim seem, at least as a matter of ordinary intuition, to involve notions of the "intrusiveness" of its effects on mentation.

The concept of intrusiveness of a therapy or program in turn seems to involve the following criteria (which, while in the main conceptually distinct, are in fact interdependent): (i) the extent to which the effects of the therapy upon mentation are reversible; (ii) the extent to which the resulting psychic state is "foreign," "abnormal," or "unnatural" for the person in question, rather than simply a restoration of his prior psychic state (this is closely related to the "magnitude" or "intensity" of the change);[4] (iii) the rapidity with which the effects occur; (iv) the scope of the change in the total "ecology" of the mind's functions; (v) the extent to which one can resist *acting* in ways impelled by the psychic effects of the therapy; and (vi) the duration of the change. For present purposes, it is immaterial whether the change effects a construction or amplification of a person's mental functioning, or whether the effects are "good" or "bad". . . .

The rather protean concept of irreversibility may thus, depending upon the circumstances, refer to extended duration of effect; to the fact that the patient alone cannot eliminate the psychotropic agent; to the fact that the effects of a given psychotropic agent may be immune from "will power," and may thus hold for a substantial time unless neutralized by some means unavailable to the patient; or to the fact that the therapy may erase any desire to avoid the effects of that therapy. Psychosurgery may produce effects irreversible in several of these senses. Although some of its effects may dissipate or be compensated for through the use of drugs, other effects seem to be permanent.
Since the procedure destroys brain tissue which cannot regenerate, neither patient nor therapist has an option to "withdraw" the psychotropic agent. The "bleaching of the personality" or "blunting of emotions" effected by psychosurgery may in any event destroy the desire to alter one's newly-acquired psyche.

A second index of the intrusiveness of a mind-altering technique is the "unnatural" or "foreign" quality of its effects for the person in question, at least under normal circumstances. Consider, for example,

4. A further distinction might be drawn between "foreign" and "abnormal" mood states. Under the influence of a mind-altering drug, for example, a person may be propelled into a state of mind strikingly different from any he has experienced before (say, a compulsive urge). Or, he may experience a familiar feeling—anxiety, for example—but to a degree which for him is unprecedented. . . .

the effects of ESB in producing word aphasia, or an orgasmic feeling without the customary erotic stimuli. The exhortations of a psychotherapist, however, do not generally produce highly abnormal states of mind, and since the subject ordinarily has an opportunity to accept or reject the suggestions or hortatory efforts of his mentors, it is rather an overstatement to talk of intrusive or coerced changes in mentation.[5] Compare also the highly euphoric result of a stimulant drug in relieving—by a "masking" effect—a depressive state, with the effect of antidepessants such as the tricyclic compounds or MAO-inhibitors. Such antidepressants may in many cases simply "cancel out" the depressive mood, restoring the subject to an earlier state which he would regard as normal for him. It seems appropriate to consider the latter therapy as being an *effective* cure for an illness, but a less intrusive one than would be generated by stimulants.

The rapidity with which the changes in mentation occur may be another index of the intrusion upon mentation and autonomy. The more gradual the change, the more likely we are to regard it as voluntary and consistent with the maintenance of the integrity of individuality. Although confinement alone may produce profound changes in mentation, it generally does so gradually, and we normally would not consider such confinement a direct intrusion on mentation.[6]

The degree of intrusion may also be a function of the range or extent of the change in mentation. The change may be quite "limited," *e.g.*, a transient mood change induced by a simple tranquilizer. Contrast such an effect with the creation of a profound and extended depressive episode and its attendant psychic ramifications brought on as a side-effect of a phenothiazine drug. Such a complex array of mentational effects suggests the

5. There is a fourth and final difference [between psychotherapeutic techniques and] the biological therapies. . . . Drugs or the surgeon's scalpel represent intrusive assaults against which we feel prevention is the only defense. It is different with psychotherapy; we imagine ourselves as patients to be free agents throughout the process, free to reject it and free to leave with no more scar than in any other human transaction.

Michels, "Ethical Issues of Psychological and Psychotherapeutic Means of Behavior Control: Is the Moral Contract Being Observed?," 3 *Hast. Center Rep.* 11 (Apr. 5, 1973). . . .

6. Although confinement considered as a tool of altering mentation would not generally make for a strong first amendment argument, confinement might violate the first amendment if it were the result, say, of holding and expressing particular political views *simpliciter*. Most diagnoses of mental illness do involve analysis of speech and mentation ("flight of ideas" is said to be a frequent characteristic of mania . . .; and diagnostic criteria may be so vague that official "discretion" is virtually unbounded. In principle, then, commitment or any other governmental restriction based upon a diagnosis of mental illness may implicate the first amendment.

episode's intrusiveness. (The extensive/limited and intrusive/nonintrusive distinctions are not coextensive. Extensive changes in mentation and behavior may be the result of a prolonged, nonintrusive psychotherapeutic regimen; and very limited effects may be produced by ESB, or various psychotropic drugs.)

Still another gauge of intrusiveness is the ability to resist the impulse to act or move in certain ways while under the influence of an organic therapy's psychic effects. A rather striking example is the inducing of involuntary motor effects by ESB—although one may decline to call such movements "acts." A euphoric or panic state induced by stimulants may generate strong urges to act in uncharacteristic ways—*e.g.*, to recklessly spend large sums of money.

Finally, the duration of a psychic effect is relevant to assessing its intrusiveness. Even a limited change in mentation might be considered intrusive if it were to last for an indefinite period. ESB which produces nothing but a mild sensation of odor might well be regarded as a serious intrusion upon mentation if there were no way for the subject to remove the electrode or deactivate it. A profound drug-induced mood change which readily yields to chemotherapy, or remits within a very short time, may be a less serious assault than a less striking change which turns out to be permanent.

These criteria of intrusiveness may be roughly captured in part by some notion of voluntariness or self-help in altering thought and behavior patterns. If such alterations seem to be more the joint product of the therapy and the person's voluntary efforts in changing himself rather than the product mainly of mentational effects over which the person has no control, then a conclusion that the regimen (forcibly imposed though it may be) is beyond the first amendment's protection seems justified. Something was done *for* the person with his help, and not *to* him, or to his mind or personality. . . .

3. The Protection of Solitary Thought.

It has been argued that mentation must be protected because it is necessary for communication. It might be urged, however, that not all mentation is directed toward or intended for purposes of communication or association. But it appears impossible to distinguish in advance between thought which will ultimately be expressed in communication, and thought which will not. Communication and expression are such constant, ongoing activities of virtually everyone that all mentation must be protected because of a strong likelihood that it will be important or necessary for such communication and expression. Any attempt to segment out instances of "isolated" mentation which are unlikely to be of value in communication would clearly jeopardize by overkill the values protected by the first amendment. As Professor Kalven noted in a related context,

> a reason implicit in the breadth of the protection afforded speech is due to the judicial recognition of its own incapacity to make nice discriminations. It reflects a strategy that requires that speech be overprotected in order to assure that it is not underprotected.[7]

Even if such mentation could be identified and "segregated" for "treatment," however, it would appear to be constitutionally protected under a doctrine of mental privacy.

4. The Protection of Disordered Thought.

The first amendment argument structure presented thus far may appear suspect because it entails protection of lunatic thought and behavior. Since "insane" or "disordered" thought possesses no value, intrinsic or instrumental (so the argument might go), it is not worth sheltering under the first amendment. The next step of that argument might require that a constitutional rule be established according first amendment protection only to "normal" or "sane" thought, and not insane mentation. . . .

One obvious response to this argument is that it remains extremely difficult to explicate a distinction between sane and disordered thought that will clearly apply to any but a few paradigm cases. One of the reasons for the difficulty is that there may be a strong element of moral evaluation in any given conclusion that someone is, or is not, mentally ill in some respect. This difficulty of articulating an adequate "general theory of insanity" strongly suggests that all mentation should be considered presumptively protected by the first amendment.

Consider, however, this exemplar: the thought and behavior of someone hardly functional and unable to care for himself. Such mentation has little, if any, utility, and hardly seems to represent the kind of interest the first amendment was targeted to protect—*i.e.,* both cognitive and emotive communication. Indeed the term "communication" seems distinctly inapt when applied to the behavior of one so thoroughly ill. But clearly there is a continuum from the "vegetable" paradigm through all gradations of disorder to "normalcy." This difficulty of diagnosis suggests the awkwardness of invoking the *Roth* model of "protected expression" and "non-protected expression." As a matter of *threshold* first amendment protection, a theory of "protected mentation" and "non-protected mentation" would

7. Kalven, "The New York Times Case: A Note on 'The Central Meaning of the First Amendment,' " 1964 *Sup. Ct. Rev.* 191, 213.

probably fare no better than the *Roth* model.[8] As will be seen later, the same sort of difficulty will plague us in attempting to demarcate a concept of capacity for informed consent within the domain of the first amendment. But within that domain all thought—even disordered thought—is protected by first amendment standards, and a conclusion that someone lacks the capacity for informed consent does not give the state carte blanche to treat him in any way it sees fit.

The rejection of the *Roth* model does not, of course, mean that the state can never compel organic therapy to control mental illness or deviant behavior. It does mean that the state's discretion in choice of therapy for those lacking the capacity for informed consent is constricted by constitutional standards. The argument here is simply that the *presumption* favors personal autonomy—which includes the right to be mad, if you will.

---

8. It should be emphasized that if "disordered" mentation were considered to be a form of "nonprotected" mentation, one result would be that persons involuntarily confined in mental institutions would, in order to secure threshold first amendment protection against organic therapy, bear the burden of demonstrating that their condition was in fact not one of "disorder." If they were unable to attain that threshold, then they would be left with only the "rational basis" test for attacking any therapy as excessively intrusive, or attacking it on any basis whatever. The first amendment requires greater protection for freedom of mentation. However, in McCabe v. Illinois, 49 Ill. 2d 338, 275 N.W.2d 407 (1971), the court, under the "rational basis" test, closely scrutinized the state's classification of marijuana as a narcotic, and concluded that such a classification was constitutionally impermissible under the equal protection clause of the fourteenth amendment.

Appendix B

Opinion of the Court in the Detroit Case

Kaimowitz v. Department of Mental Health

Civil Action No. 73-19434-AW (Wayne County, Michigan, Cir. Ct. July 10, 1973). Not officially reported but available in 2 *Prison Law Reporter* 433 (Aug. 1973), and excerpted in 42 *United States Law Week* 2063 (July 31, 1973). I have omitted some introductory comments and renumbered footnotes.

John Doe signed an "informed consent" form to become an experimental subject prior to his transfer from the Ionia State Hospital.[1] He had obtained signatures from his parents giving consent for the experimental and innovative surgical procedures to be performed on his brain, and two separate three-man review committees were established by Dr. Rodin to review the scientific worthiness of the study and the validity of the consent obtained from Doe. . . .

---

1. "Since conventional treatment efforts over a period of several years have not enabled me to control my outbursts of rage and anti-social behavior, I submit an application to be a subject in a research project which may offer me a form of effective therapy. This therapy is based upon the idea that episodes of anti-social rage and sexuality might be triggered by a disturbance in certain portions of my brain. I understand that in order to be certain that a significant brain disturbance exists, which might relate to my anti-social behavior, an initial operation will have to be performed. This procedure consists of placing fine wires into my brain, which will record the electrical activity from those structures which play a part in anger and sexuality. These electrical waves can then be studied to determine the presence of an abnormality.

"In addition electrical stimulation with weak currents passed through these (continued)

The facts concerning the original experiment and the involvement of John Doe were to be considered by the Court as illustrative in determining whether legally adequate consent could be obtained from adults involuntarily confined in the state mental health system for experimental or innovative procedures on the brain to ameliorate behavior, and, if it could be, whether the State should allow such experimentation on human subjects to proceed. . . .

Throughout this Opinion, the Court will use the term psychosurgery to describe the proposed innovative or experimental surgical procedure defined in the questions for consideration by the Court.

At least two definitions of psychosurgery have been furnished the Court. Dr. Bertram S. Brown, Director of the National Institute of Mental Health, defined the term as follows in his prepared statement before the United States Senate Subcommittee on Health of the Committee on Labor and Public Welfare on February 23, 1973:

> "Psychosurgery can best be defined as a surgical removal or destruction of brain tissue or the cutting of brain tissue to disconnect one part of the brain from another, with the intent of altering the

---

wires will be done in order to find out if one or several points in the brain can trigger my episodes of violence or unlawful sexuality. In other words this stimulation may cause me to want to commit an aggressive or sexual act, but every effort will be made to have a sufficient number of people present to control me. If the brain disturbance is limited to a small area, I understand that the investigators will destroy this part of my brain with an electrical current. If the abnormality comes from a larger part of my brain, I agree that it should be surgically removed, if the doctors determine that it can be done so, without risk of side effects. Should the electrical activity from the parts of my brain into which the wires have been placed reveal that there is no significant abnormality, the wires will simply be withdrawn.

"I realize that any operation on the brain carries a number of risks which may be slight, but could be potentially serious. These risks include infection, bleeding, temporary or permanent weakness or paralysis of one or more of my legs or arms, difficulties with speech and thinking, as well as the ability to feel, touch, pain and temperature. Under extraordinary circumstances, it is also possible that I might not survive the operation.

"Fully aware of the risks detailed in the paragraphs above, I authorize the physicians of Lafayette Clinic and Providence Hospital to perform the procedures as outlined above."

October 27, 1972	/S/ Louis M. Smith
Date	Signature
Calvin Vanee	/S/ Emily T. Smith/Harry L. Smith
Witness	Signature of responsible relative or guardian

behavior, even though there may be no direct evidence of structural disease or damage to the brain."

Dr. Peter Breggin, a witness at the trial, defined psychosurgery as the destruction of normal brain tissue for the control of emotions or behavior; or the destruction of abnormal brain tissue for the control of emotions or behavior, where the abnormal tissue has not been shown to be the cause of the emotions or behavior in question.

The psychosurgery involved in this litigation is a subclass, narrower than that defined by Dr. Brown. The proposed psychosurgery we are concerned with encompasses only experimental psychosurgery where there are demonstrable physical abnormalties in the brain. Therefore, temporal lobectomy, an established therapy for relief of clearly diagnosed epilepsy is not involved, nor are accepted neurological surgical procedures, for example, operations for Parkinsonism, or operations for the removal of tumors or the relief of stroke.

We start with the indisputable medical fact that no significant activity in the brain occurs in isolation without correlated activity in other parts of the brain. As the level of complexity of human behavior increases, so does the degree of interaction and integration. Dr. Ayub Ommaya, a witness in the case, illustrated this through the phenomenon of vision. Pure visual sensation is one of the functions highly localized in the occipital lobe in the back of the brain. However, vision in its broader sense, such as the ability to recognize a face, does not depend upon this area of the brain alone. It requires the integration of that small part of the brain with the rest of the brain. Memory mechanisms interact with the visual sensation to permit the recognition of the face. Dr. Ommaya pointed out that the more we know about brain function, the more we realize with certainty that many functions are highly integrated, even for relatively simple activity.

It is clear from the record in this case that the understanding of the limbic system of the brain and its function is very limited. Practically every witness and exhibit established how little is known of the relationship of the limbic system to human behavior, in the absence of some clearly defined clinical disease such as epilepsy. Drs. Mark, Sweet and Ervin have noted repeatedly the primitive state of our understanding of the amygdala, for example, remarking that it is an area made up of ninc to fourteen different nuclear structures, with many functions, some of which are competitive with others. They state that there are not even reliable guesses as to the functional location of some of the nuclei.[2]

The testimony showed that any physical intervention in the brain must

2. Mark, Sweet and Ervin, "The Affect of Amygdalotomy on Violent Behavior in Patients with Temporal Lobe Epilepsy," in Hitchcock, Ed. *Psycho-Surgery: Second International Conference* (Thomas Pub. 1972), 135 at 153.

always be approached with extreme caution. Brain surgery is always irreversible in the sense that any intrusion into the brain destroys the brain cells and such cells do not regenerate. Dr. Ommaya testified that in the absence of well defined pathological signs, such as blood clots pressing on the brain due to trauma, or tumor in the brain, brain surgery is viewed as a treatment of last resort.

The record in this case demonstrates that animal experimentation and non-intrusive human experimentation have not been exhausted in determining and studying brain function. Any experimentation on the human brain, especially when it involves an intrusive, irreversible procedure in a [non] life-threatening situation, should be undertaken with extreme caution, and then only when answers cannot be obtained from animal experimentation and from non-intrusive human experimentation.

Psychosurgery should never be undertaken upon involuntarily committed populations, when there is a high-risk low-benefit ratio as demonstrated in this case. This is because of the impossibility of obtaining truly informed consent from such populations. The reasons such informed consent cannot be obtained are set forth in detail subsequently in this Opinion.

There is widespread concern about violence. Personal violence, whether in a domestic setting or reflected in street violence, tends to increase. Violence in group confrontations appears to have culminated in the late 60's but still invites study and suggested solutions. Violence, personal and group, has engaged the criminal law courts and the correctional systems, and has inspired the appointment of national commissions. The late President Lyndon B. Johnson convened a commission on violence under the chairmanship of Dr. Milton Eisenhower. It was a commission that had fifty consultants representing various fields of law, sociology, criminology, history, government, social psychiatry, and social psychology. Conspicuous by their absence were any professionals concerned with the human brain. It is not surprising then, that of recent date, there has been theorizing as to violence and the brain, and just over two years ago, Frank Ervin, a psychiatrist, and Vernon H. Mark, a neurosurgeon, wrote *Violence and the Brain*[3] detailing the application of brain surgery to problems of violent behavior.

Problems of violence are not strangers to this Court. Over many years we have studied personal and group violence in a court context. Nor are we unconcerned about the tragedies growing out of personal or group confrontations. Deep-seated public concerns [beget] an impatient desire for miracle solutions. And necessarily, we deal here not only with legal and medical issues, but with ethical and social issues as well.

Is brain function related to abnormal aggressive behavior? This, fundamentally, is what the case is about. But, one cannot segment or simplify that

3. Mark and Ervin, Violence and the Brain (Harper and Row, 1970).

which is inherently complex. As Vernon H. Mark has written, "Moral values are social concerns, not medical ones, in any presently recognized sense."[4]

Violent behavior not associated with brain disease should not be dealt with surgically. At best, neurosurgery rightfully should concern itself with medical problems and not the behavior problems of a social etiology.

The Court does not in any way desire to impede medical progress. We are much concerned with violence and the possible effect of brain disease on violence. Much research on the brain is necessary and must be carried on, but when it takes the form of psychosurgery, it cannot be undertaken on involuntarily detained populations. Other avenues of research must be utilized and developed.

Although extensive psychosurgery has been performed in the United States and throughout the world in recent years to attempt change of objectionable behavior, there is no medically recognized syndrome for aggression and objectionable behavior associated with nonorganic brain abnormality.

The psychosurgery that has been done has in varying degrees blunted emotions and reduced spontaneous behavior. Dr. V. Balasubramaniam, a leading psychosurgeon, has characterized psychosurgery as "sedative neurosurgery," a procedure by which patients are made quiet and manageable.[5] The amygdalotomy, for example, has been used to calm hyperactive children, to make retarded children more manageable in institutions, to blunt the emotions of people with depression, and to attempt to make schizophrenics more manageable.[6]

---

4. Mark, "Brain Surgery in Aggressive Epileptics," The Hastings Center Report, Vol. 3, No. 1 (February, 1973).

5. See Defendant's Exhibit 38, Sedative Neurosurgery by V. Balasubramaniam, T. S. Kanaka, P. V. Ramanuman, and B. Ramaurthi, 53 Journal of the Indian Medical Association, No. 8, page 377 (1969). In the conclusion, page 381, the writer said:

> "The main purpose of this communication is to show that this new form of surgery called sedative neurosurgery is available for the treatment of certain groups of disorders. These disorders are primarily characterized by restlessness, low threshold for anger and violent or destructive tendencies.
>
> "This operation aims at destruction of certain areas in the brain. These targets include the amygdaloid nuclei, the posteroventral nuclear group of the hypothalamus and the periaqueductal grey substance. . . ."
>
> "By operating on the areas one can make these patients quiet and manageable."

6. The classical lobotomy of which thousands were performed in the 1940's and 1950's is very rarely used these days. The development of drug therapy pretty well did away with the classical lobotomy. Follow-up studies show that the lobotomy procedure was overused and caused a great deal of damage to the persons who were subjected to it. A general bleaching of the personality occurred and the operations were associated with loss of drive and concentration. Dr. Brown in his testimony before the United States Senate, supra, page 9, stated: "No responsible scientist today would condone a classical lobotomy operation."

As pointed out above, psychosurgery is clearly experimental, poses substantial danger to research subjects, and carries substantial unknown risks. There is no persuasive showing on this record that the type of psychosurgery we are concerned with would necessarily confer any substantial benefit on research subjects or significantly increase the body of scientific knowledge by providing answers to problems of deviant behavior.

The dangers of such surgery are undisputed. Though it may be urged, as did some of the witnesses in this case, that the incidents of morbidity and mortality are low from the procedures, all agree dangers are involved, and the benefits to the patient are uncertain.

Absent a clearly defined medical syndrome, nothing pinpoints the exact location in the brain of the cause of undesirable behavior so as to enable a surgeon to make a lesion, remove that portion of the brain, and thus effect undesirable behavior.

Psychosurgery flattens emotional responses, leads to lack of abstract reasoning ability, leads to a loss of capacity for new learning and causes general sedation and apathy. It can lead to impairment of memory, and in some instances unexpected responses to psychosurgery are observed. It has been found, for example, that heightened rage reaction can follow surgical intervention of the amygdala, just as placidity can.

It was unanimously agreed by all witnesses that psychosurgery does not, given the present state of the art, provide any assurance that a dangerously violent person can be restored to the community.[7]

Simply stated, on this record there is no scientific basis for establishing that the removal or destruction of an area of the limbic brain would have any direct therapeutic effect in controlling aggressivity or improving tormenting personal behavior absent the showing of a well defined clinical syndrome such as epilepsy.

To advance scientific knowledge, it is true that doctors may desire to experiment on human beings, but the need for scientific inquiry must be reconciled with the inviolability which our society provides for a person's mind and body. Under a free government, one of a person's greatest rights is the right to inviolability of his person, and it is axiomatic that this right necessarily forbids the physician or surgeon from violating, without permission, the bodily integrity of his patient.[8]

---

7. Testimony in the case from Dr. Rodin, Dr. Lowinger, Dr. Breggin, and Dr. Walter, all pointed up that it is very difficult to find the risks, deficits and benefits from psychosurgery because of the failure of the literature to provide adequate research information about research subjects before and after surgery.

8. See the language of the late Justice Cardozo in *Schloendorff v. Society of New York Hospitals,* 211 N. Y. 125, 105 N. E. 92, 93 (1914) where he said, "Every human being of adult years or sound mind has a right to determine what shall be done with his own body. . . . "

Generally, individuals are allowed free choice about whether to undergo experimental medical procedures. But the State has the power to modify this free choice concerning experimental medical procedures when it cannot be freely given, or when the result would be contrary to public policy. For example, it is obvious that a person may not consent to acts that will constitute murder, manslaughter, or mayhem upon himself.[9] In short, there are times when the State for good reason should withhold a person's ability to consent to certain medical procedures.

It is elementary tort law that consent is the mechanism by which the patient grants the physician the power to act, and which protects the patient against unauthorized invasions of his person. This requirement protects one of society's most fundamental values, the inviolability of the individual. An operation performed upon a patient without his informed consent is the tort of battery, and a doctor and a hospital have no right to impose compulsory medical treatment against the patient's will. These elementary statements of tort law need no citation.

Jay Katz, in his outstanding book "Experimentation with Human Beings" (Russell Sage Foundation, N. Y. (1972)) points out on page 523 that the concept of informed consent has been accepted as a cardinal principle for judging the propriety of research with human beings.

He points out that in the experimental setting, informed consent serves multiple purposes. He states (page 523 and 524):

> " . . . Most clearly, requiring informed consent serves society's desire to respect each individual's autonomy, and his right to make choices concerning his own life.
>
> "Second, providing a subject with information about an experiment will encourage him to be an active partner and the process may also increase the rationality of the experimentation process.
>
> "Third, securing informed consent protects the experimentation process by encouraging the investigator to question the value of the proposed project and the adequacy of the measures he has taken to protect subjects, by reducing civil and criminal liability for nonnegligent injury to the subjects, and by diminishing adverse public reaction to an experiment.
>
> "Finally, informed consent may serve the function of increasing society's awareness about human research . . . "

It is obvious that there must be close scrutiny of the adequacy of the

---

9. See "Experimentation on Human Beings," 22 Stanford Law Review 99 (1967); Kidd, "Limits of the Right of a Person to Consent to Experimentation Upon Himself," 117 Science 211 (1953).

consent when an experiment, as in this case, is dangerous, intrusive, irreversible, and of uncertain benefit to the patient and society.[10]

Counsel for Drs. Rodin and Gottlieb argues that anyone who has ever been treated by a doctor for any relatively serious illness is likely to acknowledge that a competent doctor can get almost any patient to consent to almost anything. Counsel claims this is true because patients do not want to make decisions about complex medical matters and because there is the general problem of avoiding decision making in stress situations, characteristic of all human beings.

He further argues that a patient is always under duress when hospitalized and that in a hospital or institutional setting there is no such thing as a volunteer. Dr. Ingelfinger in Volume 287, page 466, of the New England Journal of Medicine (August 31, 1972) states:

> ". . . The process of obtaining 'informed consent' with all its regulations and conditions, is no more than an elaborate ritual, a device that when the subject is uneducated and uncomprehending, confers no more than the [semblance] of propriety on human experimentation. The subject's only real protection, the public as well as the medical profession must recognize, depends on the conscience and compassion of the investigator and his peers."

Everything defendants' counsel argues militates against the obtaining of informed consent from involuntarily detained mental patients. If, as he argues, truly informed consent cannot be given for regular surgical procedures by noninstitutionalized persons, then certainly an adequate informed consent cannot be given by the involuntarily detained mental patient.

We do not agree that a truly informed consent cannot be given for a regular surgical procedure by a patient, institutionalized or not. The law has long recognized that such valid consent can be given. But we do hold that informed consent cannot be given by an involuntarily detained mental patient for experimental psychosurgery for the reasons set forth below.

The Michigan Supreme Court has considered in a tort case the prob-

---

10. The principle is reflected in numerous statements of medical ethics. See the American Medical Association, "Principles of Medical Ethics,["] 132 JAMA 1090 (1946); American Medical Association, "Ethical Guidelines for Clinical Investigation["] (1966); National Institute of World Medical Association, "Code of Ethics" (Declaration of Helsinski) reprinted in 2 British Medical Journal, 177 (1964). It is manifested in the code adopted by the United States Military Tribunal at Nuremberg which, at the time, was considered the most carefully developed precepts specifically drawn to meet the problems of human experimentation. See Ladimer, "Ethical and Legal Aspects of Medical Research in Human Beings," 3 J. Pub. I. 467, 487 (1954).

lems of experimentation with humans. In *Fortner v. Koch,* 272 Mich. 273, 261 N. W. 762 (1935), the issue turned on whether the doctor had taken proper diagnostic steps before prescribing an experimental treatment for cancer. Discussing medical experimentation, the Court said at page 282:

> "We recognize the fact that if the general practice of medicine and surgery is to progress, there must be a certain amount of experimentation carried on; but such experiments must be done with the knowledge and consent of the patient or those responsible for him, *and must not vary too radically from the accepted method of procedure*.["] (Emphasis added).

This means that the physician cannot experiment without restraint or restriction. He must consider first of all the welfare of his patient. This concept is universally accepted by the medical profession, the legal profession, and responsible persons who have thought and written on the matter.

Furthermore, he must weigh the risk to the patient against the benefit to be obtained by trying something new. The risk-benefit ratio is an important ratio in considering any experimental surgery upon a human being. The risk must always be relatively low, in the non-life threatening situation to justify human experimentation.

Informed consent is a requirement of variable demands. Being certain that a patient has consented adequately to an operation, for example, is much more important when doctors are going to undertake an experimental, dangerous, and intrusive procedure than, for example, when they are going to remove an appendix. When a procedure is experimental, dangerous, and intrusive, special safeguards are necessary. The risk-benefit ratio must be carefully considered, and the question of consent thoroughly explored.

To be legally adequate, a subject's informed consent must be competent, knowing and voluntary.

In considering consent for experimentation, the ten principles known as the Nuremberg Code give guidance. They are found in the Judgment of the Court in *United States v. Karl Brandt.*[11]

There the Court said:

> " . . . Certain basic principles must be observed in order to satisfy moral, ethical and legal concepts:

---

11. Trial of War Criminals before the Nuremburg Military Tribunals. Volume 1 and 2, "The Medical Case," Washington, D. C.; U. S. Government Printing Office (1948) reprinted in "Experimentation with Human Beings," by Katz (Russell Sage Foundation (1972)) page 305.

[“]1. The voluntary consent of the human subject is absolutely essential.

This means that the person involved should have legal capacity to give consent; should be so situated as to be able to exercise free power of choice, without the intervention of any element of force, fraud, deceit, duress, overreaching, or other ulterior form of constraint or coercion; and should have sufficient knowledge and comprehension of the elements of the subject matter involved as to enable him to make an understanding and enlightened decision. This latter element requires that before the acceptance of an affirmative decision by the experimental subject, there should be made known to him the nature, duration and purpose of the experiment; the methods and means by which it is to be conducted; all inconveniences and hazards reasonably to be expected; and the [effects] upon his health or person which may possibly come from his participation in the experiment.

The duty and responsibility for ascertaining the quality of the consent rests upon each individual who initiates, directs, or engages in the experiment. It is a personal duty and responsibility which may not be delegated to another with impunity.

“2. The experiment should be such as to yield fruitful results for the good of society, unprocurable by other methods or means of study, and not random and unnecessary in nature.

“3. The experiment should be so designed and based on the results of animal experimentation and a knowledge of the natural history of the disease or other problem under study that the anticipated results will justify the performance of the experiment.

“4. The experiment should be so conducted as to avoid all unnecessary physical and mental suffering and injury.

“5. No experiment should be conducted where there is an a priori reason to believe that death or disabling injury will occur; except, perhaps, in those experiments where the experimental physicians also serve as subjects.

“6. The degree of risk to be taken should never exceed that determined by the humanitarian importance of the problem to be solved by the experiment.

“7. Proper preparations should be made and adequate facilities provided to protect the experimental subject against even remote possibilities of injury, disability, or death.

“8. The experiment should be conducted only be scientifically qualified persons. The highest degree of skill and care should be required through all stages of the experiment of those who conduct or engage in the experiment.

"9. During the course of the experiment the human subject should be at liberty to bring the experiment to an end if he has reached the physical or mental state where continuation of the experiment seems to him to be impossible.

"10. During the course of the experiment the scientist in charge must be prepared to terminate the experiment at any stage, if he has probable cause to believe, in the exercise of the good faith, superior skill, and careful judgment required of him that a continuation of the experiment is likely to result in injury, disability, or death to the experimental subject."

In the Nuremberg Judgment, the elements of what must guide us in decision are found. The involuntarily detained mental patient must have legal capacity to give consent. He must be so situated as to be able to exercise free power of choice without any element of force, fraud, deceit, duress, overreaching, or other ulterior form of restraint or coercion. He must have sufficient knowledge and comprehension of the subject matter to enable him to make an understanding decision. The decision must be a totally voluntary one on his part.

We must first look to the competency of the involuntarily detained mental patient to consent. Competency requires the ability of the subject to understand rationally the nature of the procedure, its risks, and other relevant information. The standard governing required disclosure by a doctor is what a reasonable patient needs to know in order to make an intelligent decision. See Waltz and Scheunenman, "Informed Consent Therapy," 64 Northwestern Law Review 628 (1969).[12]

Although an involuntarily detained mental patient may have a sufficient I. Q. to intellectually comprehend his circumstances (in Dr. Rodin's experiment, a person was required to have at least an I. Q. of 80), the very nature of his incarceration diminishes the capacity to consent to psychosurgery. He is particularly vulnerable as a result of his mental condition, the deprivation stemming from involuntary confinement, and the effects of the phenomenon of "institutionalization."

The very moving testimony of John Doe in the instant case establishes this beyond any doubt. The fact of institutional confinement has special force in undermining the capacity of the mental patient to make a compe-

12. In Ballentine's Law Dictionary (Second Edition) (1948), competency is equated with capacity and capacity is defined as "a person's ability to understand the nature and effect of the act in which he is engaged and the business in which he is transacting."

tent decision on this issue, even though he be intellectually competent to do so. In the routine of institutional life, most decisions are made for patients. For example, John Doe testified how extraordinary it was for him to be approached by Dr. Yudashkin about the possible submission to psychosurgery, and how unusual it was to be consulted by a physician about his preference.

Institutionalization tends to strip the individual of the support which permits him to maintain his sense of self-worth and the value of his own physical and mental integrity. An involuntarily confined mental patient clearly has diminished capacity for making a decision about irreversible experimental psychosurgery.

Equally great problems are found when the involuntarily detained mental patient is incompetent, and consent is sought from a guardian or parent. Although guardian or parental consent may be legally adequate when arising out of traditional circumstances, it is legally ineffective in the psychosurgery situation. The guardian or parent cannot do that which the patient, absent a guardian, would be legally unable to do.

The second element of an informed consent is knowledge of the risk involved and the procedures to be undertaken. It was obvious from the record made in this case that the facts surrounding experimental brain surgery are profoundly uncertain, and the lack of knowledge on the subject makes a knowledgable consent to psychosurgery literally impossible.

We turn now to the third element of an informed consent, that of voluntariness. It is obvious that the most important thing to a large number of involuntarily detained mental patients incarcerated for an unknown length of time, is freedom.

The Nuremberg standards require that the experimental subjects be so situated as to exercise free power of choice without the intervention of any element of force, fraud, deceit, duress, overreaching, or other *ulterior form of constraint or coercion*. It is impossible for an involuntarily detained mental patient to be free of ulterior forms of restraint or coercion when his very release from the institution may depend upon his cooperating with the institutional authorities and giving consent to experimental surgery.

The privileges of an involuntarily detained patient and the rights he exercises in the institution are within the control of the institutional authorities. As was pointed out in the testimony of John Doe, such minor things as the right to have a lamp in his room, or the right to have ground privileges to go for a picnic with his family assumed major proportions. For 17 years he lived completely under the control of the hospital. Nearly every important aspect of his life was decided without any opportunity on his part to participate in the decision-making process.

The involuntarily detained mental patient is in an inherently coercive atmosphere even though no direct pressures may be placed upon him. He finds himself stripped of customary amenities and defenses. Free movement is restricted. He becomes a part of communal living subject to the control of the institutional authorities.

As pointed out in the testimony in this case, John Doe consented to this psychosurgery partly because of his effort to show the doctors in the hospital that he was a cooperative patient. Even Dr. Yudashkin, in his testimony, pointed out that involuntarily confined patients tend to tell their doctors what the patient thinks these people want to hear.

The inherently coercive atmosphere to which the involuntarily detained mental patient is subjected has bearing upon the voluntariness of his consent. This was pointed up graphically by Dr. Watson in his testimony (page 67, April 4.) There he was asked if there was any significant difference between the kinds of coercion that exist in an open hospital setting and the kinds of coercion that exist on involuntarily detained patients in a state mental institution.

Dr. Watson answered in this way:

> "There is an enormous difference. My perception of the patients at Ionia is that they are willing almost to try anything to somehow or other improve their lot, which is—you know—not bad. It is just plain normal—you know—that kind of desire. Again, that pressure—again—I don't like to use the word 'coercion' because it implies a kind of deliberateness and that is not what we are talking about—the pressure to accede is perhaps the more accurate way, I think—the pressure is perhaps so severe that it probably ought to cause us to not be willing to permit experimentation that has questionable gain and high risk from the standpoint of the patient's posture, which is, you see, the formula that I mentioned we hashed out in our Human Use Committee."

Involuntarily confined mental patients live in an inherently coercive institutional environment. Indirect and subtle psychological coercion has profound effect upon the patient population. Involuntarily confined patients cannot reason as equals with the doctors and administrators over whether they should undergo psychosurgery. They are not able to voluntarily give informed consent because of the inherent inequality in their position.[13]

---

13. It should be emphasized that once John Doe was released in this case and returned to the community he withdrew all consent to the performance of the proposed experiment. His withdrawal of consent under these circumstances should be compared with his response on January 12, 1973, to questions placed to him by

(continued)

It has been argued by defendants that because 13 criminal sexual psychopaths in the Ionia State Hospital wrote a letter indicating they did not want to be subjects of psychosurgery, that consent can be obtained and that the arguments about coercive pressure are not valid.

The Court does not feel that this necessarily follows. There is no showing of the circumstances under which the refusal of these thirteen patients was obtained, and there is no showing whatever that any effort was made to obtain the consent of these patients for such experimentation.

The fact that thirteen patients unilaterally wrote a letter saying they did not want to be subjects of psychosurgery is irrelevant to the question of whether they can consent to that which they are legally precluded from doing.

The law has always been meticulous in scrutinizing inequality in bargaining power and the possibility of undue influence in commercial fields and in the law of wills. It also has been most careful in excluding from criminal cases confessions where there was no clear showing of their completely voluntary nature after full understanding of the consequences.[14] No lesser standard can apply to involuntarily detained mental patients.

Prof. Slovenko, one of the members of the Human Rights Committee. These answers are part of exhibit 22 and were given after extensive publicity about this case, and while John Doe was in Lafayette Clinic waiting the implantation of depth electrodes. The significant questions and answers are as follows:

1. Would you seek psychosurgery if you were not confined in an institution?

A. Yes, if after testing this showed it would be of help.

2. Do you believe that psychosurgery is a way to obtain your release from the institution?

A. No, but it would be a step in obtaining my release. It is like any other therapy or program to help persons to function again.

3. Would you seek psychosurgery if there were other ways to obtain your release?

A. Yes. If psychosurgery were the only means of helping my physical problem after a period of testing.

14. See, for example, *Miranda v. Arizona,* 384 U. S. 436 (1966) and *Escobedo v. Illinois,* 378 U. S. 478 (1964).

Prof. Paul Freund of the Harvard Law School has expressed the following opinion:

> "I suggest . . . that [prison] experiments should not involve any promise of parole or of commutation of sentence; this would be what is called in the law of confessions undue influence or duress through promise of reward, which can be as effective in overbearing the will as threats of harm. Nor should there be a pressure to conform within the prison generated by the pattern of rejecting parole applications of those who do not participate. . . . " P. A. Freund, "Ethical Problems in Human Experimentation," New England Journal of Medicine, Volume 273 (1965) pages 687–92.

The keystone to any intrusion upon the body of a person must be full, adequate and informed consent. The integrity of the individual must be protected from invasion into his body and personality not voluntarily agreed to. Consent is not an idle or symbolic act; it is a fundamental requirement for the protection of the individual's integrity.

We therefore conclude that involuntarily detained mental patients cannot give informed and adequate consent to experimental psychosurgical procedures on the brain.

The three basic elements of informed consent—competency, knowledge, and voluntariness—cannot be ascertained with a degree of reliability warranting resort to use of such an invasive procedure.[15]

To this point, the Court's central concern has primarily been the ability of an involuntarily detained mental patient to give a factually informed, legally adequate consent to psychosurgery. However, there are also compelling constitutional considerations that preclude the involuntarily detained mental patient from giving effective consent to this type of surgery.

We deal here with State action in view of the fact the question relates to involuntarily detained mental patients who are confined because of the action of the State.

Initially, we consider the application of the First Amendment to the problem before the Court, recognizing that when the State's interest is in conflict with the Federal Constitution, the State's interest, even though declared by statute or court rule, must give way. See *NAACP v. Button,* 371 U. S. 415 (1963) and *United Transportation Workers' Union v. State Bar of Michigan,* 401 U. S. 576 (1971).

A person's mental processes, the communication of ideas, and the generation of ideas, come within the ambit of the First Amendment. To the extent that the First Amendment protects the dissemination of ideas and the expression of thoughts, it equally must protect the individual's right to generate ideas.

As Justice Cardozo pointed out:

> "We are free only if we know, and so in proportion of our knowledge. There is no freedom without choice, and there is no choice without knowledge,—or none that is illusory. Implicit, there-

15. It should be noted that Dr. Vernon H. Mark, a leading psychosurgeon, states that psychosurgery should not be performed on prisoners who are epileptic because of the problem of obtaining adequate consent. He states in "Brain Surgery in Aggressive Epileptics," the Hastings Center Report, Vol. 3, No. 1 (February, 1973: "Prison inmates suffering from epilepsy should receive only medical treatment. [S]urgical therapy should not be carried out because of the difficulty in obtaining truly informed consent."

fore, in the very notion of liberty is the liberty of the mind to absorb and to beget . . . The mind is in chains when it is without the opportunity to choose. One may argue, if one please, that opportunity to choice is more an evil than a good. One is guilty of a contradiction if one says that the opportunity can be denied, and liberty subsist. At the root of all liberty is the liberty to know. . . .

"Experimentation there may be in many things of deep concern, but not in setting boundaries to thought, for thought freely communicated is the indispensable condition of intelligent experimentation, the one test of its validity. Cardozo, *The Paradoxes of Legal Science,* Columbia University Lectures, reprinted in *Selected Writings of Benjamin Nathan Cardozo*" (Fallon Publications (1947)), pages 317 and 318.

Justice Holmes expressed the basic theory of the First Amendment in *Abrams v. United States,* 250 U. S. 616, 630 (1919) when he said:

" . . . The ultimate good desired is better reached by free trade in ideas—that the best test of truth is the power of the thought to get itself accepted in the competition of the market, and that truth is the only ground upon which their wishes safety can be carried out. That at any rate is the theory of our Constitution. . . . We should be eternally vigilant against attempts to check expressions of opinions that we loathe and believe to be fraught with death, unless they so imminently threaten immediate interference with the lawful and pressing purposes of the law that an immediate check is required to save the country . . . "

Justice Brandeis in *Whitney v. Cal.* 274 U. S. 357, 375 (1927), put it this way:

"Those who won our independence believed that the final end of the State was to make men free to value their faculties; and that in its government the deliberative force should prevail over the arbitrary . . . They believed that freedom to think as you will and to speak as you think are means indispensible to the discovery and spread of political truth; that without free speech and assembly discussion would be futile; that with them, discussion affords ordinarily adequate protection against the dissemination of noxious doctrine; that the greatest menace to freedom is an inert people; that public discussion is a political duty; and that this should be a fundamental principle of the American government . . . "

Thomas Emerson, a distinguished writer on the First Amendment, stated this in "Toward a General Theory of the First Amendment," 72 Yale Law Journal 877, 895 (1963):

> "The function of the legal process is not only to provide a means whereby a society shapes and controls the behavior of its individual members in the interests of the whole. It also supplies one of the principal methods by which a society controls itself, limiting its own powers in the interests of the individual. The role of the law here is to mark the guide and line between the sphere of social power, organized in the form of the state, and the area of private right. The legal problems involved in maintaining a system of free expression fall largely into this realm. In essence, legal support for such a society involves the protection of individual rights against interference or unwarranted control by the government. More specifically, the legal structure must provide:
>
> "1. Protection of the individual's right to freedom of expression against interference by the government in its efforts to achieve other social objectives or to advance its own interests . . .
>
> "3. Restriction of the government in so far as the government itself participates in the system of expression.
>
> "All these requirements involve control over the state. The use of law to achieve this kind of control has been one of the central concerns of freedom-seeking societies over the ages. Legal recognition of individual rights, enforced through the legal processes, has become the core of free society."

In *Stanley v. Georgia*, 397 U. S. 557 (1969), the Supreme Court once again addressed the free dissemination of ideas. It said at page 565–66:

> "Our whole constitutional heritage rebels at the thought of giving government the power to control men's minds . . . Whatever the power of the state to control dissemination of ideas inimical to public morality, it cannot constitutionally premise legislation on the desirability of controlling a person's private thoughts."

Freedom of speech and expression, and the right of all men to disseminate ideas, popular or unpopular, are fundamental to ordered liberty. Government has no power or right to control men's minds, thoughts, and expressions. This is the command of the First Amendment. And we adhere to it in holding an involuntarily detained mental patient may not consent to experimental psychosurgery.

For, if the First Amendment protects the freedom to express ideas, it necessarily follows that it must protect the freedom to generate ideas. Without the latter protection, the former is meaningless.

Experimental psychosurgery, which is irreversible and intrusive, often leads to the blunting of emotions, the deadening of memory, the reduction of affect, and limits the ability to generate new ideas. Its potential for injury to the creativity of the individual is great, and can impinge upon the right of the individual to be free from interference with his mental processes.

The State's interest in performing psychosurgery and the legal ability of the involuntarily detained mental patient to give consent must bow to the First Amendment, which protects the generation and free flow of ideas from unwarranted interference with one's mental processes.

To allow an involuntarily detained mental patient to consent to the type of psychosurgery proposed in this case, and to permit the State to perform it, would be to condone State action in violation of basic First Amendment rights of such patients, because impairing the power to generate ideas inhibits the full dissemination of ideas.

There is no showing in this case that the State has met its burden of demonstrating such a compelling State interest in the use of experimental psychosurgery on involuntarily detained mental patients to overcome its proscription by the First Amendment of the United States Constitution.

In recent years, the Supreme Court of the United States has developed a constitutional concept of right of privacy, relying upon the First, Fifth and Fourteenth Amendments. It was found in the marital bed in *Griswold v. Conn.* 381 U. S. 479 (1962); in the right to view obscenity in the privacy of one's home in *Stanley v. Georgia,* 395 U. S. 557 (1969); and in the right of a woman to control her own body by determining whether she wishes to terminate a pregnancy in *Rowe v. Wade,* 41 L W 4213 (1973).

The concept was also recognized in the case of a prison inmate subjected to shock treatment and an experimental drug without his consent in *Mackey v. Procunier, ________ F 2d ________, 71-3062 (9th Circuit, April 16, 1973).*

In that case, the 9th Circuit noted that the District Court had treated the action as a malpractice claim and had dismissed it. The 9th Circuit reversed, saying, inter alia:

> "It is asserted in memoranda that the staff at Vacaville is engaged in medical and psychiatric experimentation with 'aversion treatment' of criminal offenders, including the use of succinycholine on fully conscious patients. It is emphasized the plaintiff was subject to experimentation without consent.
>
> "Proof of such matters could, in our judgment, raise serious constitutional questions respecting cruel and unusual punishment or

> *impermissible tinkering with the mental processes.* (Citing Stanley among other cases) In our judgment it was error to dismiss the case without ascertaining at least the extent to which such charges can be substantiated . . . " (Emphasis added).

Much of the rationale for the developing constitutional concept of right to privacy is found in Justice [Brandeis's] famous dissent in *Olmstead v. United States,* 277 U. S. 438 (1928) at 478, where he said:

> "The makers of our Constitution undertook to secure conditions favorable to the pursuit of happiness. They recognized the significance of man's spiritual nature, of his feelings and of his intellect. They knew that only a part of the pain, pleasure, and satisfaction of life are to be found in material things. They sought to protect Americans in their beliefs, their thoughts, their emotions and their sensations. They conferred, as against the Government, the right to be let alone—the most comprehensive of rights and the right most valued by civilized men."

There is no privacy more deserving of constitutional protection than that of one's mind. As pointed out by the Court in *Huguez v. United States,* 406 F 2d 366 (1968), at page 382, footnote 84:

> " . . . Nor are the intimate internal areas of the physical habitation of mind and soul any less deserving of precious preservation from unwarranted and forcible intrusions than are the intimate internal areas of the physical habitation of wife and family. Is not the sanctity of the body even more important, and therefore, more to be honored in its protection than the sanctity of the home? . . . "

Intrusion into one's intellect, when one is involuntarily detained and subject to the control of institutional authorities, is an intrusion into one's constitutionally protected right of privacy. If one is not protected in his thoughts, behavior, personality and identity, then the right of privacy becomes meaningless.[16]

Before a State can violate one's constitutionally protected right of privacy and obtain a valid consent for experimental psychosurgery on involuntarily detained mental patients, a compelling State interest must be shown. None has been shown here.

To hold that the right of privacy prevents laws against dissemination of contraceptive material as in *Griswold v. Conn.* (supra), or the right to view obscenity in the privacy of one's home as in *Stanley v. Georgia* (supra),

16. See Note: 45 So. Cal. L R 616, 663 (1972).

but that it does not extend to the physical intrusion in an experimental manner upon the brain of an involuntarily detained mental patient is to denigrate the right. In the hierarchy of values, it is more important to protect one's mental processes than to protect even the privacy of the marital bed. To authorize an involuntarily detained mental patient to consent to experimental psychosurgery would be to fail to recognize and follow the mandates of the Supreme Court of the United States, which has constitutionally protected the privacy of body and mind.

Counsel for John Doe has aruged persuasively that the use of psychosurgery proposed in the instant case would constitute cruel and unusual punishment and should be barred under the Eighth Amendment. A determination of this issue is not necessary to decision, because of the many other legal and constitutional reasons for holding that the involuntarily detained mental patient may not give an informed and valid consent to experimental psychosurgery. We therefore do not pass on the issue of whether the psychosurgery proposed in this case constitutes cruel and unusual punishment within the meaning of the Eighth Amendment.

For the reasons given, we conclude that the answer to question number one posed for decision is no.

In reaching this conclusion, we emphasize two things.

First, the conclusion is based upon the state of the knowledge as of the time of the writing of this Opinion. When the state of medical knowledge develops to the extent that the type of psychosurgical intervention proposed here becomes an accepted neurosurgical procedure and is no longer experimental, it is possible, with appropriate review mechanisms,[17] that involuntarily detained mental patients could consent to such an operation.

Second, we specifically hold that an involuntarily detained mental patient today can give adequate consent to accepted neurosurgical procedures.

In view of the fact we have answered the first question in the negative, it is not necessary to proceed to a consideration of the second question, although we cannot refrain from noting that had the answer to the first question been yes, serious constitutional problems would have arisen with reference to the second question.

---

17. For example, see Guidelines of the Department of Health, Education and Welfare, A C Exhibit 17.

Appendix C

Selections from the Posttrial Briefs on the Question of Legally Adequate Consent by One Involuntarily Committed to a Mental Facility

The materials presented below are matters of public record. I have omitted some material, deleted some footnotes, and renumbered the remaining ones.

1. From the Posttrial Brief of Petitioners-Plaintiffs.

On this brief were Gabe Kaimowitz, Michigan Legal Services Assistance Program, Wayne State University Law School, and Corey Y. S. Park, Legal Aid Office, Detroit, Michigan.

1. The very nature of being involuntarily confined vitiates the ability to give a truly voluntary consent.

No one would argue that voluntariness is not an essential element of the process in question. Indeed, it is assumed by the very definition of obtaining consent. However, the evidence makes clear that true voluntariness, and the absence of coercion, are never possible in the situation of a confined patient who is approached to be the subject of an invasive and dangerous experimental procedure. There are just too many inducements and coercive factors that impinge upon both the conscious and unconscious to permit a truly willful consent.

The most obvious inducement is that of obtaining freedom. It is not unreasonable to assume that many of those presently confined want to get out. Dr. Ayub K. Ommaya, of the National Institute of Neurological Diseases and Stroke, in testifying that he would never use the involuntarily confined as experimental subjects, stated:

A. Well, personally—and I think ethics is a very personal matter, there are certain standards for morality and ethics which are well-defined in philosophy, but I think one's testimony can best be given as personal. And that is that I find it difficult to believe that a person who is incarcerated, with an indefinite sentence, will—can really be a volunteer in such a test, because there is a very strong motivation which is always present that he is going to reap some benefit from this in terms of his personal freedom, and unless a person is completely removed from reality, is very paranoid, has such total disruption of his personality that he has no concept of freedom, then, you know that fact doesn't arise, and if such a state exists, that is not a candidate for any type of surgery.

Dr. Peter Breggin, of Washington, D.C., reached the same conclusion against the use of confined subjects, and also noted the high degree of uncertainty caused by the indeterminate nature of the confinement (Breggin, TR., 18–19 (4/5)):

Q. Very briefly, first of all, is there a difference between involuntarily confined mental patients, in your opinion, and prison inmates, which is the only thing Mark specifically describes?

A. I don't think there is any difference between prison inmates and mental patients other than the mental patients are still more vulnerable. A prison inmate who has a determinate sentence of say 10 years, he knows how long he will be in there before he gets out, depending on how determinate the sentence is. Whereas, if he is committed involuntarily, he is in a position like John Doe so clearly describes himself in. He never knows when he will get out. Therefore, the issue of freedom becomes so important that I think consent is considerably more difficult when you are under civil committment than when you are under conviction for a criminal proceeding.

A second important factor is the highly coercive nature of mental institutions. One commentator has noted that

> the nature of the institutional setting and its various features, e.g., the garb of the staff, giving the appearance of authority which demands obedience, may intimidate the inmate.

Note, R. Spece, "Conditioning and Other Technologies Used to 'Treat' 'Rehabilitate?' 'Demolish?' Prisoners and Mental Patients," 45 *S. Cal. L.*

Rev. 616, at 670 (1972) (hereinafter cited as Note, 45 *S. Cal. L. Rev.* 616). This is not surprising since, as several witnesses testified, mental hospitals are extremely conservative institutions whose primary task is that of management or control. For instance, Dr. Andrew Watson stated (Watson, TR., A29 (4/4)):

> Q. Let me ask you a more general question. Do you have any fear that if experimental brain surgery of the sort we are talking about in this case to control aggressive conduct is permitted to take place on the population involuntarily detained in mental hospitals, that that brain surgery will be grossly overused?
>
> A. I would be afraid so, because again one of the big characteristics of institutions is conservatism, and if you don't know what somebody is going to do and you have a technique which you knows promises to invoke control, then why shouldn't you use it . . . ?

These institutions have performed their management function all too well. They have established a strict regimen to closely regulate the minute details of life and have deprived the patient of his autonomy. Dr. Paul Lowinger testified (Lowinger, TR., A33 (4/3)):

> Well, very often all the circumstances in a patient's life in such an institution depend upon the decisions of the doctor and the superintendent, including where he lives, what he does during the day, the garb he wears, the food he eats and the other details of his life. He is totally dependent.

Professor Erving Goffman, in his excellent description of the dynamics of life in "total institutions," *Asylums,* Anchor Books, Garden City, New York (1961), reaches a like conclusion, at p. 38:

> In a total institution, however, minute segments of a person's life of activity may be subjected to regulations and judgments by staff; the inmate's life is penetrated by constant sanctioning interaction from above, especially during the initial periods of stay before the inmate accepts the regulations unthinkingly. Each specification robs the individual of an opportunity to balance his needs and objectives in a personally efficient way and opens up his line of action to sanctions.

Goffman further notes that this high degree of control invests itself in the granting and denial of minor privileges and to the ultimate question of freedom, pp. 50–51:

> The building of a world around these minor privileges is perhaps the most important feature of inmate culture, and yet it is something that cannot easily be appreciated by an outsider, even one who has previously lived through the experience himself.
>
> * * *
>
> In any case, conditions in which a few easily controlled privileges are so important are the same conditions in which their withdrawal has a terrible significance.
>
> * * *
>
> [T]he question of release from the total institution is elaborated into the privilege system. Some acts become known as ones that mean an increase, or no decrease, in length of stay, while others become known as means for shortening the sentence.

Directly related to this highly controlled environment is the fear that patients have of the staff. Total institutions are characterized by rigid deference patterns, stratification, and excessive stereotyping. . . .

A third important factor is that of the dependency that is created in the patient-therapist relationship. It has been observed that

> The position of the therapist and inmate in this setting is arguably akin to that of parent and child—the inmate may feel that he must consent. Or, though not feeling compelled to consent, the inmate may do so to curry favor with the therapist who may later give him a break.

Note, *supra,* 45 *S. Cal. L. Rev.,* at p. 672. Dr. Lowinger's experience supports this observation (Lowinger, TR., A32-33(4/3)):

> Q. Let me ask you this with specific reference to a mental institution now—there has been [s]ome indication in testimony when we're talking about informed consent, generally, that when a doctor proposes to a patient that that patient should undergo some kind of procedure, with attendant risks or not, that a patient desires to please that doctor for a variety of motives, and motives that can indeed cloud or diminish the notion of a fully rational, informed consent and that this is a typical characteristic of doctor-patient relationships across the board. Would [that] be your observation?
>
> A. Yes. And this is especially true if the patient is ill with an illness that—you know—makes him—or puts him in pain. He has a fear—you know—some kind of visible or striking manifestation of sickness.

In fact, Dr. Yudashkin's experience is no different. He admitted that there is a tendency for confined mental patients to tell their therapists what the therapists want to hear (Yudashkin, TR., C32 (3/28)).

There are many other inducements that can act to detract from the ability to give truly voluntary consent. The problem of monetary compensation was discussed at length. While these sums may appear to be paltry to those on the outside, to the confined they represent a comparatively substantial buying power. (Lowinger, TR., A27-28 (4/3); see, also *Baldwin v. Smith,* 316 F. Supp. 670, at 675 (D.Vt. 1970); and Mitford, "Experiments Behind Bars," *Atlantic Monthly,* January, 1973, p. 64). While this particular problem of monetary compensation is not presented in this case, this phenomenon does illustrate that the granting or denial of what may appear to the outsider to be small privileges can take on great significance and import to the deprived inmate of a total institution. (see Goffman, *Asylums,* at pp. 50–51). Other inducements include security and physical safety, and the approval of officials, which can lead to numerous side-benefits (Lowinger, TR., A28, A30, (4/3)).

2. The very nature of being involuntarily confined vitiates the ability to give a truly educated and informed consent.

Dr. Ingelfinger discusses the most difficult problem of imparting sufficient information to an experimental subject and concludes that it is practically an insoluble problem. "Informed (But Uneducated) Consent," 287 *New England Journal of Medicine* 465 (Aug. 31, 1972). . . . In the case before the Court, there is the added complicating factor of the subject being confined, which raises serious problems concerning the patient's ability to perceive and understand all that is disclosed to him.

The best reasoned discussion of the inability of an involuntarily confined patient to perceive accurately the data disclosed was presented by Dr. Lowinger (Lowinger, TR, A31-32, and B3-5 (4/3)):

> Q. Now, why can't one simply say—well, a rational balance can be struck there or can one say that there is simply a rational balancing of risks on the one hand and risks on the other or is there something about the institutional setting and the immediate pressures that overweigh rational choice?
>
> A. Yes. Well, I don't think the context or mental frame of the prisoner within the institution is such that he can rationally predict what is going to happen to him. He is in a state of mind where he doesn't know what is going to happen from day to day. He is very frightened, has good reason to be, and finds his jail or guards or attendants often unpredictable or irrational. There is in his behavior towards him—he may or may not re-

gard his presence there as justifiable. Often he regards it as unjustifiable. So he is not in a frame of social behavior or situation in which he can make rational judgments because he regards his status and circumstances as subject to whim and fancy and circumstances outside of his control.

* * *

Q. Now, this paragraph [from John Doe's consent form] begins by saying that any operation on the brain carries a number of risks which may be slight or which could be potentially dangerous, and then there are listed a number of the risks that we have talked about here, such as infection, bleeding, paralysis of one of the legs or arms, difficulty with speech and then it ends by saying that under extraordinary circumstances it is also possible that he might not survive the operation; and that was part of the Informed Consent Form signed by John Doe.

Now, on its face that recitation and the fact that John Doe signed it would appear to be a wholly rational recitation of the magnitude of risk that is being run. Is there reason to believe that someone involuntarily institutionalized for eighteen years would not perceive risk to himself in a way that a person on the outside would perceive it?

A. Yes. I think one's presence in an institution under deprived and often unpleasant circumstances and the deprivation of the freedom which is almost always unpleasant might lead one to a negative view of one's self-worth so that one would not really have the perspective of enjoyment of life and activity so that he wouldn't really have the perspective of choosing between good and bad. He might just be choosing the lesser of two evils by signing that.

Q. You were speaking about self-worth—

A. (Interposing) Yes, the [depreciated] view of self-worth.

Q. And when you say the [depreciated] view of self-worth that this person might have, are there specific things in a total situation of being institutionalized that feed that depreciated view that one is not worth very much by ordinary standards?

A. Yes. The most obvious and common one is the fact that the community, the people who work there, have often—and also the people who are patients or prisoners there—regard it as a crazy house or a bad place to be.

I think that is a fundamental or universal view of institutions or asylums or hospitals which still affects all of us whether we work in them or not. I think the lack of freedom and activity, voluntarily chosen activity, by people who live there is another. They think their lives are not as worth-while or as full or as creative as if they were on the outside.

I think the other common experience they have is that they wear old clothes, eat second class food, are often dealt with, summarily dealt with by rules or arbitrary and unpleasant regulations such as getting up at a certain time and working doing menial or uncreative things, often beneath or below their capacity.

They have no free choice in much of their daily activity; and that stands in direct contrast to people on the other side of the walls, members of their own family who are more fortunate than they.

They have this matter brought to their attention every day by visitors and television and the circumstances of their lives.

Q. Am I right in thinking that you are saying that this depreciated sense of self, that sense of relative worthlessness could lead someone in this setting to not prize his own bodily integrity as much as someone on the outside?

A. Yes, I think that could be and often is the case.

The diminution of self-worth referred to by Dr. Lowinger is called the "process of mortification" by Professor Goffman. Goffman, however, views the process as much more pervasive and invidious, in effect finding that the entire socialization of the new patient into the total institution is a conscious process of mortification or the creation of a negative view of one's self-worth, *Asylums,* beginning at p. 12.

Finally, there is the added problem that the full risks and consequences of an experimental procedure, by definition, are not completely known or understood. . . .

The standard procedure utilized in medical research and experimentation delegates to the principal investigator a large degree of power and control over all aspects of the experiment. This is amply demonstrated by the testimony and other evidence in this case. For instance, there is no provision in the Michigan Department of Mental Health to monitor or review medical research, including experimentation on human subjects, carried out within the Department's various facilities. In fact, the Lafayette Clinic proposal that was the original subject of this litigation was submitted to Dr. Gordon E. Yudashkin, Director of the Department, only because it required the Department to seek funds from the state legislature. Otherwise, the proposal may never have been presented to the Director. (Yudashkin, TR., p. C13 (3/28).) However, even when he did receive the proposal, he did not review it for its medical or scientific validity, but merely approved it even though the procedure was experimental and involved surgery on the brain (Yudashkin, TR., 90 (3/13). With respect to experimentation in the Department's other facilities, Dr. Yudashkin testified at length that there is no review or monitoring of these projects, that he did not even know what particular kinds of research [were] being performed, that he may never find out, and that he was not even sure that each institution had its own system of internal controls (Yudashkin, TR., C12 to C18 (3/28)).

Dr. Rodin described his almost total and unchecked authority over his research (Rodin, TR., A16–17 (3/27)):

> Q. Dr. Gottlieb testified that senior staff at Lafayette Clinic had considerable leeway in the formulation of their research projects: Did you hear his testimony to that effect?
> Q. When you formulate a new research project, Dr. Rodin, do you have to have it cleared by anybody within the clinic?
> A. I inform Dr. Gottlieb.
> Q. But you are one of the senior researchers of whom he spoke?
> A. That's correct.
> Q. And you inform Dr. Gottlieb of what you intend to do?
> A. Well, we discuss it between the two of us.
> Q. Is there any—is there any committee of your peers that has to pass on your research projects?
> A. No: We're it.
> Q. You're it. And there's no requirement that it be discussed?
> A. No, sir.
> Q. Is that true when you're using animal research subjects?
> A. That is true all over the country, among senior investigators.
> Q. It's true of human research subjects, as well?
> A. Oh, yes.
> Q. There's no routine procedure for clearing—
> A. No, sir.
> Q. —such cases? That leaves you on your own, then, to determine the shape of a research program, in consultation with Dr. Gottlieb?
> A. Yes, that is correct. If I'm a bad boy, I'm being fired.
> Q. That's really the—the control on you: Is—is firing?
> A. Yes. If my scientific work does not measure up to scientific standards, then I'm cut.

Combining this near absolute autonomy over research with the responsibility for obtaining consent from the subject vests substantial power in the investigator. Of course, the requirement of obtaining consent is supposed to be designed to protect the rights and interests of the subject. The problems of role conflict and objectivity are immediately apparent in such a situation. As discussed above, there is a coercive and manipulative force inherent in the therapist-patient relationship, see Note, 45 *S. Cal. L. Rev.* 616, at 672. The possibility of the skewing of the data, whether intentionally or not, by the very person who has a vested interest in seeing that the project continue is always present. The California Supreme Court recognized this in a related situation,

> A problem may also be presented by the possibility of role conflict arising from the entrusting of the notice and explanation of rights function to the same agency which undertakes to perform the therapeutic function.

Thorn v. Superior Court, 1 Cal. 3d 666, at 675, 83 Cal. Rptr. 600, 464 P. 2d 56. An example of the possible abuse that can arise out of this situation was presented in the Mark and Ervin book, *Violence and the Brain,* Harper and Row, New York, N.Y. (1970), at pp. 96–97:

> However, it was obviously impractical to keep doing this [stimulate the patient's brain to alleviate facial pain] for the rest of Thomas's life, and so we suggested to him that we make a destructive lesion in the medial portion of both his amygdalas—that is, in the area where stimulation elicited facial pain and rage. He agreed to this suggestion while he was relaxed from lateral stimulation of the amygdala. However, 12 hours later, when this effect had worn off, Thomas turned wild and unmanageable. The idea of anyone making a destructive lesion in his brain enraged him. *He absolutely refused any further therapy, and it took many weeks of patient explanation before he accepted the idea of bilateral lesions' being made in his medial amygdala.* Four years have passed since the operation, during which Thomas has not had a single episode of rage. He continues, however, to have an occasional epileptic seizure with periods of confusion and disordered thinking.

Besides being appalled at the attempt to obtain consent from a patient in an artificially stimulated, unnatural state, one must wonder what was involved in the "many weeks of patient explanation." See also, Note, 45 *S. Cal. L. Rev.* 616, at 671, discussing the presentation of data to obtain consent from California prisoners to participate in a drug program that induced a death-like state.

4. There can be no mechanism, whether it be an independent consultant or committee, capable of protecting an involuntarily confined patient against actual or perceived psychological inducements, dur-

> ess, and coercion so as to permit the needed consent for an innovative or experimental surgical procedure upon the brain.

It has been suggested by some of the witnesses in this case that although serious problems exist in attempting to obtain consent from involuntarily confined patients for experimental surgery, safeguards can be established to protect the rights of the patient. The above discussion should make clear, however, that this is impossible. The subtle, and not so subtle, pressures inherent in our mental institutions, the doctor-patient relationship, the desire for freedom, and other kinds of physical and psychological inducements all combine to raise substantial questions as to whether a confined patient can truly give an uncoerced, uninduced, voluntary agreement based on an accurate perception of the data presented to him. There are the further questions of whether the information imparted to him is, or can be, complete, since an experimental procedure is contemplated, and whether data are accurately portrayed. These questions raise such serious doubts as to the validity of any consent that no mechanism can alleviate these problems.

One of the alternative suggestions made was the appointment of uninvolved consultants to aid the patient. However, this is an inadequate suggestion not only because of the questionable independence of such a party, but more importantly because this person really cannot aid the patient in obtaining the perspective of himself and life necessary to the decision making. . . .

A second alternative that has been suggested is that an independent committee, with or without lay representation, be appointed. Obviously, the problems of independence of this committee are presented, and in greater degree, and this committee would be in no better position to perform the important and necessary function of giving the patient the perspective of himself and life, discussed above, that is necessary.

There is another, practical, objection to the use of such a committee. This is that,

> Now in practice, the advisory councel [the "independent" committee with lay representation] usually—seldom disagrees with what the study section [the medical committee] says.

(Ommaya, TR., 48 (3/28)).

The committees involved in the proposal originally before this Court highlight some of the practical problems. The Human and Animal Experimentation Committee was not empowered to make an independent review of the proposal (Gottlieb, TR., 1–19 (3/27)). The Medical Review Committee members were all appointed by the principal investigator, Dr. Rodin (Luby, TR., 13 (4/2)). Its chairman stated,

> We must depend upon Dr. Rodin's integrity, his professional ability, his knowledge of the literature, to provide us with information upon which we can act.
>
> * * *
>
> The committee depends upon the information provided by its investigators. It can function in no other way.

(Luby, TR., 26–27, and 35).

The human rights committee was also appointed by Dr. Rodin, or under his direction, and this committee also relied quite heavily on the investigator as its source of information. (E.g., Sawher, TR., 9 (4/3)). This committee never really functioned as a committee. One of its members never submitted a written confirmation of his approval (Slovenko, TR., C60 (4/2)), but expressed doubts since the patient felt indebted to the doctors and had "the desire to do something useful, as a means of expiating for the crime that he committed" (Slovenko letter to Rodin, January 15, 1973). . . . Another committee member, who never attended any meetings but sent a "second", felt "unqualified to judge the medical, psychological, legal, religious and philosophical aspects of this project," but found no problems anyway (Moran letter to Rodin, November 17, 1972, attached as part of exhibits to complaint). Perhaps the greatest telling point of the inability of such a committee to effectively function was its failure to discover all of the dynamics that were working on John Doe during this process (see discussion below at A,5). This committee really should not be faulted since, as the John Doe case illustrates, no committee, however constituted, directed and run, could have discovered and understood all the conscious and unconscious forces at work.

5. The good faith efforts to obtain consent from John Doe illustrate graphically the impossibility of obtaining meaningful consent from an involuntarily confined person and the inability of any mechanism to assure such consent.

The entire process of obtaining consent from John Doe points out the impossibility of assuring a truly informed and voluntary consent. In light of the above discussion, it is not surprising to see such a drastic reversal of positions from anxious determination to go through with the operation to a questioning and inquisitive refusal. John Doe's experience fits nicely the above analysis, and he really is no different from most other involuntarily confined patients as they are molded by their closed institutions.

John Doe's initial intent to proceed with the operation was clearly linked to his desire to obtain his freedom. This inducement operated on both the conscious and subconscious levels. . . .

The pressures of institutionalization and the total control exercised, discussed above, were vividly described by John Doe in his testimony (Doe, TR., beginning at 3 (4/4)):

> Q. Could you tell us what your current attitude toward that procedure is? Whether today you are willing to have that happen to you?
>
> A. Well, as I understand it right today, I am not willing to go through with this. Do you want me to elaborate?
>
> Q. Sure. Please do.
>
> A. Well, I have went through a number of changes and I would like to be able to pursue a convalescent status and be able to go out on this type of thing because I am finding out that since I have been out from under the pressure of Ionia and I see that I have gotten a future and I have settled down quite a bit and the feelings that I was constantly going through have decreased a considerable amount. And I think that when I am out from under the institutional life and policies that I think that I will become even more stable. And I have become even less with problems of nervousness and so forth. [P. 3–4].
>
> * * *
>
> Q. Could you describe in a general way for us your feelings about Ionia and about your confinement there?
>
> A. Well, overall, it is not a very good attitude. I must truthfully say that. The hospital was set up for detention, and as far as I am concerned, the attitude and the policies towards patients when I first went there were very nil. I have the feeling that when I was put there that it was just nothing but for detention and to get rid of me and, well, a place to stay. And this is the way it has been over the years. And, of course, I have never been mistreated really physically, but the emotional treatment has been like—as far as I am concerned—it has been like a dog in a pen. And that is about it. [Pp. 4–5]. . . .

It has already been noted that the patient-therapist relationship is a highly dependent one akin to that of parent and child and that the patient may feel [coerced] into consenting or

> though not feeling compelled to consent, the inmate may do so to curry favor with the therapist who may later give him a break.

Note, 45 *S. Cal. L. Rev.* 616, 672. John Doe fits remarkably well into this analysis. John Doe described at length how pleased he was that, after years of deprivation and being treated "like a dog in a pen," Dr. Yudashkin treated him with care and respect, and gave him many privileges previously denied (Doe, TR., 13–15 (4/4)). Having someone care about him was important to John Doe, as it would be to any human being, and it was important that this relationship continue (Doe, TR, 22 (4/4)):

> Q. Were you concerned that Dr. Yudashkin continued to have this good attitude of you?
> A. Was I concerned?
> Q. Was it important to you that Dr. Yudashkin have this—
> A. Oh, absolutely, it was very important to me.

John Doe's attitude towards Dr. Rodin was similar (Doe, TR, 23 (4/4)):

> I went down [to Lafayette Clinic] that Monday is what it was. Dr. Rodin came in the hospital and we had—oh, we talked for a good hour, anyway. And, again, I was very pleased with Dr. Rodin's attitude and the way he also talked to me on a one-to-one basis.

The fostering of this dependency relationship ties in closely with the presentation of the information on the procedure to the patient and the patient's ability to fully perceive that data. John Doe first discussed the proposed operation with Dr. Yudashkin (Doe, TR., 13–15 (4/4)):

> A. [Dr. Yudashkin] called me in. He talked to me. And this is after I went down to the Lafayette for two EEG's. And he said that, "I would like to send you down to Lafayette for surgery." And I got real excited and I was just about ready to tell him to forget it. And he interjected and he said, "Let me explain to you what the situation is." And Dr. Yudashkin told me that he wanted—
> Q. Yes?
> A. He explained that I would not be hurt physically or it would impair my emotionally ability. And that they would like to send me down to Lafayette to see what they could do for me. And we discussed other things about Lafayette. And I told Dr. Yudashkin—I said—
> Q. What other kinds of things did you discuss?
> A. Well, just generally about going down there and getting help, to see what they can do for me and on a treatment basis—you know.
>
> And we sat there and we discussed. And I told him—I said, well, I thought that he was very fair in discussing this whole thing with me and calling me in and all and asking me about it. I

said that I would like to have time to think about it and to have other people discuss this with me—you know—before I make my decision. And he said, "Well, Louis," he says, "that is fair enough."

And I was quite surprised by it.

Q. Quite surprised by what?

A. By him asking me this—you know—going down to Lafayette to have the surgery.

Q. Why did it surprise you?

A. Well, you are just not asked these types of questions every day. This is something that is brand new in my life.

Q. Yes.

A. And I felt that Dr. Yudashkin was—you know really trying to do something for me—you know. And he told me that it was—that I wouldn't be seriously hurt—you know—physically.

Q. Why did it please you [?]

A. Well, because I don't think that there had been too many people in my institutional life that approached me the way Dr. Yudashkin has.

The presentation of the risks by Dr. Rodin was described by John Doe (Doe, TR., 25–26 (4/4)):

Q. So, [Dr. Rodin] read this whole paper [the consent form] to you?

A. Yes. We went over that item by item. And the question that you asked me about the dangers, the bleeding, the infection—you know—he described me the blood—if a vein was cut or something—that they had to go in and tie this off—you know—it could cause damage and you are liable to lose the movement of your arm or something. But that is something that just might happen at that particular time or—you know—

Q. How high a risk did you think that was?

A. Well, I was really concerned. When anybody starts to mess with the brain, it is a risk. And, I mean, a very serious one. And I think that I was aware of this risk. But, again, Dr. Rodin as well as Dr. Yudashkin led me to believe that I would be coming through this operation with very little difficulty. And they—Dr. Rodin described himself as a very competent individual, and since that he had treated me as an individual and I trusted Dr. Rodin and I took him for what he had to say, I was very pleased in the way that he talked to me. Again, I was pleased with the way this man handled himself and the way he talked to me and the way he treated me generally.

Q. Have you subsequently learned that there might have been more risk to the diagnostic implant than you had thought about before?
A. Yes, I have.
Q. How did you learn it?
A. Well, as this thing [this litigation] went on, I have done some reading.

Upon learning that there were many more substantial risks involved than he thought, John Doe was not bitter towards Drs. Rodin and Yudashkin. He felt that they were both acting ethically at all times, and pointed out, quite perceptively, that the information imparted may depend on whom you are talking to. . . .

The confusion and inability of the patient to perceive what is going on is further illustrated by John Doe's understanding of the procedures as contrasted to what he agreed to in the consent form. That form indicated that the surgery would take place if certain medical conditions were met. However, it was John Doe's understanding, and his Mother's and Father's, that no surgery would take place until a further extensive discussion was held with John Doe and further consent had been obtained. (In fact, it appears that both Mother and Father were completely opposed to any surgery beyond implantation (Doe's parents, TR., 45, and 51, 4/4).) When this discrepancy, between whether the surgery was a one or two step procedure, was pointed out at trial, John Doe appeared confused and stated that he really had not thought about it (Doe, TR., 32–33 (4/4)):

Q. Now, what was your exact understanding of what would happen after the diagnostic implantation?
A. Well, Dr. Rodin told me that we would go through the implant. Well, then, when the implants were finished, that he and whoever was involved with this would sit down with me and my mother and father—you know—and discuss this whole thing—you know. And I was under the impression that we would make another decision as far as going on with the surgery itself. They would give their recommendations for or against this type of thing.
Q. Well, now, as we have talked about it, have shown you this language, am I correct in saying that it doesn't explicitly state this?
A. Yes, it doesn't.
Q. When you say—
A. I realize it now.
Q. When you say you realize it now, what do you mean?
A. I really don't think I gave it that much thought at the time. The

> way it is stated, it is exactly—you know—all the—our main concern was that the implant would be given and that afterwards that we would have a long discussion or we would have a serious discussion about the implants, what they showed and what they didn't show and so fourth. And about the operation itself, success, whatever it may be—you know—whatever they thought should be done and so forth—you know. They would give their recommendations and so forth.

The extensive quotes from the testimony of John Doe and Dr. Watson [little of which has been included here] are used . . . in an attempt to portray, though grossly inadequately, the complex dynamics of the human mind and the utter frustration and desperation created by our mental institutions as they affect those dynamics. However, this Court should not consider what appears to be an extreme situation as aberrational, but rather, as the numerous experts make clear above, as wholly typical of life molded by even some of our better total institutions.

Recognizing this, the Court can only conclude that involuntarily confined patients cannot give a truly voluntary consent that is based on a full and accurate perception of the data. The investigator's ease and convenience in securing an adequate patient population, and that is what it all boils down to, cannot by any stretch of the imagination outweigh the rights of the confined patient.

2. *From the Posttrial Brief of Petitioner-Intervener.*

On this brief were Robert A. Burt and Francis A. Allen of the University of Michigan Law School.

> The taint of state compulsion cannot be adequately dispelled from any involuntary mental patient's decision to accept experimental neurosurgery for aggressivity.

John Doe testified in this Court, concerning the reasons that he agreed to the contemplated surgery while involuntarily confined in state custody, and the reasons he withdrew his consent after—and only after—this Court had ruled unconstitutional the Criminal Sexual Psychopath statute under which Doe was confined. Dr. Andrew Watson, a psychiatrist who had seen Doe both before and after this Court's opinion, confirmed in his testimony the dramatic change in psychological capacity that accompanied this change in legal status. In response to Mr. Burt's question whether the

Court's action regarding the CSP statute "was a quite significant part of this psychological mechanism" that led John Doe to withdraw his consent, Dr. Watson stated, "Absolutely. He sees himself now as an entirely different person. And he comes into the process in an entirely different way." (April 4, pp. 65–66). John Doe's testimony establishes that the pressures on an institutionalized person are both pervasive and impossible to allay while that person remains involuntarily confined.

These pressures do not, of course, affect all persons in the same way. Some persons, for example, fight institutional pressures to the last ditch. Others, like John Doe, bow to institutional pressures in order to prove themselves "cooperative" and therefore worthy for freedom, or even more trivially, for minor privileges (such as a reading lamp for one's bedroom or ground passes to have picnic lunches with visiting parents). But since the state is constitutionally obliged to assure that no one is compelled by the state to accept experimental neurosurgery for aggressivity, it is insufficient to argue that since *some* can resist state pressures, it is permissible to overlook the existence of others—such as John Doe—who cannot so resist.

There are two possible responses to the reality that some persons, at least, involuntarily confined by the state will not have psychological capacity to exercise free choice regarding the contemplated surgery. One response, apparently pursued by defendants in this case, is to design mechanisms that screen out those in the institutionalized population who do and those who do not have the necessary capacity. But that response, we submit, is patently inadequate. John Doe, for one, was subjected to as extensive a screening procedure—to test the reality of his consent—as is ever likely to be carried out. That screening procedure failed; it did not identify the inappropriate motives that led Doe to consent to the operation. Dr. Yudashkin, who first presented the contemplated surgery to Doe and who interviewed him several times on this question, stated as follows: "I doubt that a person would submit themselves to unnecessary surgery in order to gain their release." (March 28, p. C5). Regarding his contacts with John Doe, specifically, the following questioning took place with Dr. Yudashkin:

Q. Did you indicate to him that if he volunteered, and it was found that he was not suitable for the surgery . . . that simply that volunteering act would increase his chances of being released?

A. No.

Q. You did not?

A. No.

Q. Did you think that he believed that? That is to say, that volunteering alone would increase his chances?

A. I have no way of knowing what he was thinking. You would have to ask John Doe.
Q. You would have no way of knowing at all?
A. How would I know what he was thinking about his motivation.
Q. Well, let me take a moment.
A. It never occurred to me to ask that question.

* * *

Q. If he were to have told you, doctor, that an important motive of his was to volunteer just to increase his chance to get out, whether or not the surgery would be done, would that have affected your opinion?
A. I would have advised him against it. (March 29, pp. A65–A66)

The fact is, however, that this was a central motivation for John Doe in consenting to the surgery. The fact emerged with considerable clarity in the course of his testimony in this trial:

Q. You mentioned a minute ago when I said what were they looking for in terms of giving you privileges like going on the outside—you mentioned that you had participated in all the therapeutic programs?
A. Yes.
Q. Did you think that that was one of the things that—one of the conditions that the people in charge of the hospital were imposing on you as a way of earning these privileges?
A. Well—
Q. Let me rephrase it to be clear. Did you think that this would help you earn privileges?
A. Well, no doubt about it. Everyone that they suggested group therapy or this type of therapy and so forth, it was expected for that individual to go. But on the other hand, as far as I am concerned, I went to my therapy because I was trying to—you know—get help and I needed it. And I took active part and everything in everything that I went to. And I got a great deal out of my therapy. But still this didn't seem to have much weight on what was as far as them going to let me out for extra privileges and stuff like this—you know. It was discouraging. I was disgust[ed]. I often thought why should I even go through with these things because I just hit my head against the wall and it was very frustrating at times. Extremely so.

* * *

Q. Did you believe that if Dr. Yudashkin ordered you released that he had the power to do that?

A. Oh, yes, I realized what Dr. Yudashkin was an if he wanted me released, he could [do] so. If he wanted me held there, he could keep me there. . . .

For purposes of understanding John Doe's motivation, it is not dispositive whether Dr. Yudashkin indicated any desire that Doe agree to the surgery. Indeed, Dr. Yudashkin has testified that he meant to exercise no influence one way or the other with Doe, and when directly asked the question, Doe stated, "I wouldn't say he was really advising me. I would say that he was really asking me. You know—there was no pressure." (April 4, p. 14). But this statement by Doe illustrates why the institutional setting is so powerful in undermining truly voluntary consent. The pressure need not come from the individuals' conscious intent. In perfect good faith, Dr. Yudashkin could believe that he was leaving John Doe free to accept or reject the surgery. In perfect [good] faith, John Doe could believe that he was in fact free on this matter. But the circumstance, the total environment, in which both men acted kept from John Doe both his freedom, and his capacity to see how coerced and inappropriate his motives were in agreeing to the surgery. Even more importantly, that coercive environment gave John Doe a powerful motive to hide from himself, and from all others, the real, inappropriate motives that led to his consent.

Dr. Watson's testimony clearly establishes this, as follows:

> In my first contact with him [John Doe], he was still believing that his destiny was linked with getting that surgery. And he got angry with me when I threatened that by challenging that. As I said earlier, [I said to him], if everything is going so fine, why do you want to get this surgery? And you see, that is a threat psychologically. And he wanted to get it because that is how he was going to get the end he wished to achieve. . . .

The institutional pressures that led John Doe to hide from himself and others the true character of his consent to the surgery had an even more treacherous impact in this case, according to Dr. Watson's testimony. Those pressures also likely led John Doe to present a false or exaggerated picture of the intensity of his "emotional surges." Because John Doe had not engaged in any violently aggressive acts for eighteen years—during the entire period of his confinement at Ionia—these self-reported "surges" were the central basis for the doctors' judgment that he was a proper candidate for the contemplated surgery. Dr. Watson testified as follows:

He also told me, . . . during the point where he was still justifying surgery to me and to himself and to everyone else—he told me—whenever he feels some emotion, he feels it more intensively than other people. . . . [H]e was endeavoring then to prove to me on that first interview that he was a violent person who has these episodic rages.

By the way, I thought it was a catechism which they had him recite over and over.

Q. What would have motivated him—I am sure it was against his interest to portray himself as you describe, as a violent, aggressive, uncontrollable individual—what would have motivated him to try to do that?

A. It sounds like that, but [if] his motivation is to get himself this surgery so as to get him out of Ionia, then it is not against his interest. . . .

Q. So, are you saying that in the way he presented himself, he falsely,—although unconsciously—falsely tried to distort the diagnostic impression that the diagnoser would get in order to qualify for this surgery?

A. By the point of time I saw him, he wanted that surgery because he thought that was going to serve his end and that was what he was talking about. He had described that very thoroughly.

Q. Is it possible that this conduct on his part that you are describing could fool some diagnosticians?

A. Oh, yes. People fool people all the time in the sense, you know, that they are misled, especially, if they have done something like kill somebody. That mere idea instantly potentiates everybody's misperception, and, indeed, I think I could trace through the record of Ionia for year after year after year precisely that type of non-perception of John. . . . (April 4, pp. 70–72, A1)

John Doe's testimony, and Dr. Watson's explanation of Doe's state of mind in his testimony, thus establishes two propositions:

first, that John Doe's consent to the experimental surgery was for "social gain . . . not medical gain." As Dr. Watson testified, "he was tying his major motivation to the wish to please—to cooperate—and, therefore he would get treatment. Now, that is not the same linkage at all as going for a medical—a dangerous medical procedure in order to change something in order to be able to behave differently." (April 4, p. 59); and

second, that the environmental pressures of the institution which pushed John Doe to this inappropriate consent also led him to conceal, from himself and from others, the real basis for his consent and, perhaps even more importantly, the real reason for his descriptions of the "emotional surges'' that made him appear appropriate for the operation. This second proposition establishes the virtual impossibility of designing effective screening mechanisms to differentiate among involuntarily confined persons who should and should not participate in experimental neurosurgery for aggressivity.

This second proposition is further proven by considering the elaborateness of the procedural screening mechanisms that John Doe passed through, to the point that the implantation of depth electrodes would have occurred if this litigation had not been filed. In this screening mechanism, the Director of the State Department of Mental Health interviewed Doe several times. Doe was interviewed by three members of a Consent Committee, composed of a clergyman, a layman and a lawyer. The latter, Ralph Slovenko, Professor of Law and Psychiatry at Wayne State University testified regarding John Doe's motives as follows:

> We all have various motives, and . . . the major one in this case is that this person was concerned about his self-control over his aggression. (April 2, p. C44);
>
> In other words, he had put aside whether or not this was a consideration for discharge. It was a matter—he looked upon it entirely as therapeutic, as a means of dealing with his aggressive outbursts. (April 2, p. C49)

The propriety of the medical diagnosis in John Doe's case was reviewed by a three-man professional committee chaired by Dr. Luby of the Lafayette Clinic, and they concluded that John Doe was a suitable candidate. Dr. Rodin, the principle investigator, testified as follows:

> Q. In your judgment, did he consent as you have described it in order to assure that he would be released from institutional confinement.
>
> A. No, he wanted to be relieved of his uncontrollable urges. (March 27, p. A26)

Dr. Gottleib, the director of the Lafayette Clinic, talked with John Doe, and testified to his motivation as follows:

> A. Well, I think he expressed that pretty clearly, that he has surges from time to time that he would like to be relieved of that are disturbing to him. And this offered an opportunity for him to be relieved of these surges and urges so that he could regain his position in society. (March 27, pp. 1–39)

In this trial, however, we have had a quite unique and fortuitous opportunity to conduct a "controlled experiment" (better controlled, we would note, than the experimental surgery contemplated in this case). We have had extensive testimony of John Doe's attitudes toward surgery while he was involuntarily confined in the state mental hospital system. Then, because on March 23, 1973, this Court ruled that John Doe was illegally detained, John Doe testified in this Court on April 4 as a free man (though still residing in a state mental hospital while community placement was being arranged). In that testimony, the following exchange took place:

> Q. . . . Now, in January, before this suit was filed, we understand from the doctors that they were prepared—they were ready—they had done everything up to the point of actually implanting these electrodes deep in your brain. Is that your understanding?
> A. Yes.
> Q. Could you tell us what your current attitude toward that procedure is? Whether today you are willing to have that happen to you?
> A. Well, as I understand it right today, I am not willing to go through with this. Do you want me to elaborate?
> Q. Sure. Please do.
> A. Well, I have went through a number of changes and I would like to be able to pursue a convalescent status and be able to go out on this type of thing because I am finding that since I have been out from under the pressure of Ionia and I see that I have gotten a future and I have settled down quite a bit and the feelings that I was constantly going through have decreased a considerable amount. And I think that when I am out from under the institutional life and policies that I think that I will become even more stable. And I have become even less with problems of nervousness and so forth. (April 4, pp. 3–4)

John Doe's experience, and his testimony, proves that the state cannot discharge its constitutionally required obligation to demonstrate that no taint of compulsion would accompany the decision of an involuntarily detained person to agree to experimental neurosurgery for aggressive conduct. . . . Because that taint of compulsion cannot be removed, because it is inescapable in the coercive setting of a state confinement institution, it is "cruel and unusual punishment" and an invasion of the constitutionally protected "right to privacy" for the state to sponsor such surgery on its captive population.

This holding need not mean that no conventional medical treatment can be provided to a captive population. For those committed to mental institutions, conventional treatment at least related to cure of mental illness can be offered without regard to consent. . . . Conventional treatment for other purposes to those committed to mental institutions, and conventional treatment of all sorts for those confined in prisons, are—by their very conventionality—much less likely to be viewed by commitment patients or prisoners as keys to their freedom or even to increased privileges.

More difficult questions are presented for medical experimentation on these captive populations. Consent to experimentation, for example, for malaria or cancer cures might be viewed by inmates as leading toward earlier parole or better institutional treatment. But the most troubling, the least assuredly consensual of all possible experiments, is an experimental procedure directly related to the reason that originally brought the potential subjects to be committed. That is, medical experiments related to "cures for aggressivity" are likely to be viewed by institution inmates and staff alike as particularly pressing concerns. John Doe might or might not prove his worth for release, his "cooperativeness" by agreeing to an experiment that might cure malaria. Whether he would consent to an experiment that might cure his "aggressivity" is, however, much more patently relevant to his view, and staff views, of Doe's worth for release, his "cooperativeness." Accordingly, this Court's ruling that the contemplated surgical procedure cannot be performed on involuntarily confined persons in state mental institutions would not necessarily imply that no medical experiments of any sort can be performed on state mental hospital or prison populations.

Further, this ruling would not necessarily mean that neurosurgery for aggressivity could never be performed in the future on state mental hospital or prison populations. The specially stringent standards, to assure no taint of compulsion, are imposed by constitutional norms. But if this neurosurgery becomes widely accepted conventional therapy for aggressive conduct, the constitutional norm would not apply with full force to it. If, that is, the neurosurgery in question becomes conventional therapy practiced by a broad range of reputable physicians, it will no longer be arbitrary in application: a clearly identifiable, and diagnosable, patient population will be defined. It will no longer have unknown risks and uncertain benefits: risks and benefits will be clearly and persuasively identified in the course of its wider use in the medical profession. And community dismay and unease at this procedure will be substantially allayed; the acceptance of this neurosurgical technique as conventional treatment by the medical community generally will amply testify on this score. Accordingly, the basis for ruling that compelled neurosurgery for aggressivity is constitutionally impermissible may, in the future, be so attenuated that it will be permissible to perform this surgery in institutional settings notwithstanding the inescapably coercive pressures of those settings. . . .

3. From the Posttrial Brief of Amicus Curiae.

On this brief were Charles R. Halpern, Alix H. Sanders, Benjamin W. Heineman, Jr., and Cheryl Curciana, The Mental Health Law Project, Washington, D.C.

II. As a Matter of Tort Law, Legally Adequate Consent to Dangerous, Irreversible, and Experimental Psychosurgery Cannot be Given by Involuntarily Confined Mental Patients.

A. Experimental Surgical Procedures Are Legal Only If There is Informed Consent by the Subject.

[Amicus here develop this topic with citation to much of the relevant literature.]

B. To be Legally Adequate a Subject's Consent Must be Competent, Knowing and Voluntary.

[Amicus here deal with these criteria in relation to any subject—whether or not confined.]

C. Involuntarily Confined Mental Patients Cannot Give Legally Adequate Consent to Experimental Psychosurgery.

If the doctors at the Lafayette Clinic were to perform experimental psychosurgery on an involuntarily committed mental patient, they would commit the tort of battery. This is so, amicus submits, because involuntarily confined mental patients cannot give a legally adequate consent to psychosurgery. We contend that, in the special circumst[a]nces of this case, when an involuntarily confined population is being asked to consent to an experimental, dangerous, and irreversible procedure, the legal adequacy of all three elements of consent—competence, knowledge and voluntariness—is "suspect" and, as a matter of law, these [suspicions] when taken in combination, should render the consent of *any* mental patient invalid within the framework of tort law. Hence, the state cannot conduct psychosurgery experimentation on that population.

In developing this argument, we shall draw on the fact[s] surrounding the case of John Doe to illustrate the consent problem. It is clear from the record in this case that Doe's competence for making the decision concerning psychosurgery was impaired by the environment in which he has lived for so long and by the complexity of the issues; that Doe did not have sufficient information to consent knowingly; and that his consent was not voluntary because the hospital setting was inherently coercive and the desire for release inevitably shaped his decision. An indication of how suspect is the consent of an involuntarily confined mental patient is found in the fact that, as soon as Doe obtained release, on other constitutional grounds, and was "out from under the pressure of Ionia" he withdrew his previously tendered "consent". . . .

The problems with Doe's consent are not uniquely his. They are symptomatic of the problems which vitiate a consent to experimental psychosurgery by any involuntarily confined patient.

(1) *Legal Competence.* Under Dr. Rodin's proposal, all research subjects to be used in the psychosurgery experiments must be competent. The "Criteria for Inclusion in the Aggression Project" requires that each subject have an I.Q. of at least 80 and that he "be mentally competent to the extent that he fully comprehends the procedure of depthelectrography and possibly stero-tactic surgery." A.C. Ex. 1. During the course of the trial, the possibility was raised that incompetent patients, in particular the severly retarded, might also become experimental subjects with the consent of a guardian. . . .

Amicus does not rest its argument about the invalidity of consent on a general theory of the legal incompetence of mental patients to make rational decisions. On the contrary, the competence of mental patients to exercise their civil rights, even when institutionalized, should be recognized. Brakel and Rock, *The Mentally Disabled and the Law* 155–172 (1971). And amicus assumes that some patients will be identified, who have the general capacity to understand rationally the nature of a medical procedure, its risks and other relevant information. *Winters* v. *Miller,* 446 F.2d 65 (1971), *cert. denied* 404 U.S. 985 (1972); Note, *Conditioning and Other Technologies Used to "Treat?" "Rehabilitate?" "Demolish?" Prisoners and Mental Patients,* 45 So.Cal. L.R. 616, 674 (1972).

However, amicus asks the court to recognize that, with respect to this decision, legally competent mental patients have diminished capacity and are peculiarly vulnerable, as a result of their mental condition, the deprivations stemming from involuntary confinement, and the effects of the phenomenon of "institutionalization."[1] These factors undermine their capacity both to resist external institutional pressures which will undermine their *voluntariness,* and to cope with the confusions engendered by the extremely abstract and complex questions regarding psychosurgery that will affect their ability to make a *knowing* decision. J. Katz, Experimentation With Human Beings 1013 (1972).

The fact of institutional confinement has special force in undermining the capacity of the mental patient to make a competent decision on this

[1] John Doe described the conditions of confinement as being "like a dog in a pen." Doe, pp. 5, 40. Vail, *Dehumanization and the Institutional Career* (1966, C. Thomas); Goffman, *Asylums* (1961); Lowinger, Watson, *passim.*

issue. In the routine of institutional life all decisions are made for the patient. John Doe testified how extraordinary it was, when he was approached about possible submission to psychosurgery, to be consulted by a physician about his preferences. Institutionalization strips the individual of the supports which permit him to maintain his sense of self in the oustide world. Goffman has described this phenomenon:

> Like the neophyte in many of these total institutions, the new inpatient finds himself cleanly stripped of many of his accustomed affirmations, satisfactions, and defenses, and is subjected to a rather full set of mortifying experiences: restriction of free movement, communal living, diffuse authority of a whole echelon of people, and so on. Here one begins to learn about the limited extent to which a conception of oneself can be sustained when the usual setting of supports for it are suddenly removed. *Asylums,* p. 148.

In addition, institutionalization causes the patient to have a diminished sense of his own worth and the value of his physical and mental integrity. John Doe's decision to participate in the psychosurgery experiment and the process by which he reached that decision, illustrate the process by which the mental patient's capacity is undermined by being institutionalized for many years.

Amicus, therefore, is asking the Court to recognize that involuntarily confined mental patients who are legally competent to make a host of important decisions, have diminished capacity for making a decision about irreversible, experimental psychosurgery, which raises questions so complex that most lay persons have difficulty untangling them. The suggestion that each prospective research subject will "fully comprehend the procedure of depthelectrography and possibly stereo-tactic surgery" only highlights the problem of securing competent consent to such procedures. Doubts about a mental patient's capacity to make a legally competent decision about experimental psychosurgery may not, in and of themselves, constitute a ground for holding that consent, in these circumstances, cannot be legally adequate. But they are, as will be argued [below] an important factor to be noted when deciding that all three elements of consent cannot be sufficiently satisfied so as to render a consent to experimental psychosurgery by involuntarily confined mental patients legally adequate.

(2) *Knowledge.* It is extremely difficult for an involuntarily confined patient to give a *knowing* consent to experimental psychosurgery. See Shapiro, *The Uses of Behavior Control Technologies: A Response,* 7 Issues in Criminol. 55, 57, (1972). All the participants in this trial—doctors, lawyers and judges—appreciate how profoundly uncertain is the state of the facts surrounding experimental brain surgery, facts which are basic

to a knowing consent. There is substantial confusion, for example, about the following vital matters:

—Whether physical abnormality in the brain causes aggressive behavior?
—Whether alternative treatments have been exhausted?
—What the likelihood is that substantial personality change will occur?
—What are the risks of unknown harms?
—What is the likelihood that objectionably aggressive behavior can be eradicated for the long term?
—What is the likelihood that the subject's behavior will be sufficiently "ameliorated" so that he may be released to the community?

Of course, any experimental procedure has elements of uncertain harm and benefit. But, at some point the uncertainties concerning an experimental procedure are so great that consent is no longer a *rational* decision, where one can even approximately evaluate the probabilities of harms and benefits, or weigh these against each other. Rather such a decision is a purely arbitrary one, based on faith, or irrational drives. Under the facts of this case, it is hardly a *knowing* decision to consent to psychosurgery when there are so many unknowns and virtually no reliable statements regarding the probable occurrence of even the uncertain aspects of the operation. The decision to undergo psychosurgery, to be blunt, must be characterized as a blind gamble, a rolling of unmarked dice with no understanding of what combinations cause a "loss" or a "win" and with extremely high but uncertain stakes.

It should also be noted that the knowledge obtained by the involuntarily confined mental patient is likely to be particularly limited. He must rely on the information provided to him by the researcher who seeks his participation in the experiment. Without impugning the motives of research scientists, under these circumstances, the presentation of the information is unlikely to be wholly objective. In John Doe's case, after this case was filed and Doe had access to information from a variety of sources (including reports of the testimony of expert witnesses, a lengthy article in *Ebony* on psychosurgery, and *Violence and the Brain,* he developed a fuller understanding about the uncertainties of the procedure. After the court ruled that he was unconstitutionally confined, he withdrew his consent.

In these circumstances and at this point in the development of psychosurgery, can we say, as a matter of law, that consent to psychosurgery is "knowing," within any sensible meaning of that term, especially the consent of involuntarily confined mental patients whose capacity to make such a decision has been diminished by factors stemming from his institutionalization? The "knowledge" component of consent largely turns on what is—or *can be*—disclosed about an experimental procedure, and not primarily on the person's capacities under the circumstances (although the two factors are obviously intertwined). Although arguably, knowing consent to experimental psychosurgery can, therefore, never be given,[2] we do not rest our case solely on the ground that such consent is not knowing.

Suffice to say, rather, that there are substantial doubts whether consent is "knowing" when a procedure is as experimental as psychosurgery—and these doubts should be given great weight when the procedure is also dangerous, intrusive and irreversible and threatens the subject's autonomy and personality.

(3) *Voluntariness*. There are also substantial doubts, stemming primarily from the potential subject's involuntary confinement in a state mental hospital, that any consent can be free from subtle but potent forms of psychological coercion.

First, patients who are involuntarily confined for an indefinite term are often desperate to obtain their freedom. The prospect of release will, inevitably, shape their thinking about psychosurgery and make it extremely difficult for them to appreciate the likelihood and the dimensions of benefits and harms involved in so experimental, dangerous, and irreversible a procedure. Even if hospital authorities do not explicitly promise the patient that he will be released if he consents to and undergoes psychosurgery, the promise may be implicit—or the patient may simply create such a hope in his own mind because of his involuntary, indefinite confinement. In John Doe's case, consent to psychosurgery was part of an effort to show the doctors at the hospital that he was, beyond argument, a cooperative patient who should be released. In an analogous situation, courts have held that consent is not voluntary when a willingness to undergo sterilization is a prerequisite of release from prison, and professional societies have similarly questioned the voluntariness of consent to sterilization by involuntarily confined mental patients, because such patients are so often eager to be discharged. And, unlike sterilization, the claimed changes resulting from psychosurgery can hardly be said to occur with any certainty; [ironically], the hoped release is not only an intolerable pressure but also an irrational one.

Second, doctors who are administering experimental "therapies" to research subjects have a conflict of interest which means that they may not

---

[2] Some scholars have raised questions about knowing consent to experimental medical techniques, since *no* subject can fully understand the nature and implications of such technical procedures. 2 British Medical Journal 1119 (1962); Beecher, *Consent in Clinical Experimentation: Myth and Reality,* 195 A.M.A.J. 34 (1966); Beecher, *Experimentation in Man,* 169 A.M.A.H. 461, 473 (1959); Guttentag, *The Problem of Experimentation on Human Beings,* 117 Science 207, 209–210 (1953); Note, *Experimentation on Human Beings,* 20 Stan.L.R. 99, 104 (1967).

be able to act solely in the patient's interest. Although they will want the patient to improve, they will, inevitably, also wish to advance science through pursuit of their own research interests. Accordingly, they may, consciously or unconsciously, exert psychological pressure on the potential subject to induce him to undergo an experimental medical procedure or cut corners in administering procedures designed to secure a fully voluntary consent. Such pressure may be especially prevalent when, as is the case here, the doctors are trying to fit patients into a research design, rather than simply making an individual judgment that for a particular patient an experimental procedure is the last resort. Moreover, the possibilities of improper pressure are heightened when, as here, the research institution has received funds especially appropriated by the legislature for the particular research project and when trained staff and costly equipment await experimental subjects. See generally, Waltz and Scheuneman, *Informed Consent to Therapy,* 64 Nw. U.L.R. 628, 645–646 (1969); Note, *Experimentation on Human Beings,* 20 Stan.L.R. 99, 106, 114; *Editorial,* 270 New England J. Medicine 1014–1015 (1964).

Third, and related to the point immediately above, all patients, and especially those confined in mental hospitals, may be unduly susceptible to pressures to please their doctor. This too impairs the ability to make a voluntary decision about the costs and benefits of participation in a particular experimental project. Note, *Experimentation on Human Beings,* 20 Stan.L.R. 99, 106; Freund, *Ethical Problems in Human Experimentation,* 273 New England J. Medicine 687, 691 (1965); J. Katz, *Experimentation with Human Beings* 635–650. The supervising physicians in a mental hospital control even the most intimate details of the patient's life, and the patient is extraordinarily dependent on them. As Dr. Yudashkin testified, involuntarily confined patients tend to tell the people in charge what the patient thinks those people want to hear. Patients may also fear that there will be reprisals within the institution if they do not consent to the profferred procedure. S. Brakel and R. Rock, *The Mentally Disabled and the Law* 161–164 (1971).

In sum, involuntarily confined mental patients live in an inherently coercive institutional environment. The types of possible psychological coercion mentioned above have profound adverse effects on a vulnerable patient population. This means that involuntarily confined patients cannot "bargain" as equals with the doctors and administrators over whether they should undergo psychosurgery. They cannot reason or argue with authorities about costs and benefits. It is precisely this inequality in bargaining power and the possibility of undue influence which has led courts to invalidate apparent voluntary action in the commercial field and with regard to wills on the ground that the concept of the individual as a free agent is irreconcilable with the realities of commercial life or the particular testimentary context. See, e.g., *Williams* v. *Walker-Thomas Furniture Co.,* 350 F.2d 445 (D.C.Cir. 1965). See Driver, *Confessions and the Social Psychology of Coercion,* 82 Harv.L.R. 42 (1968).

Judicial protection of the potential research subject who is not able to act in a fully voluntary manner from dangerous and irreversible experimental psychosurgery is surely more important than holding that a contract term is unconscionable and void because of inequality in bargaining power. It is this doubt about the voluntariness of a mental patient's consent that has led expert witnesses in this trial to state that experimental psychosurgery should not be undertaken on involuntarily confined mental patients.

(4) *No Legally Adequate Consent.* Amicus submits that, in this case of first impression, a new rule should be established within the framework of the common law of battery. We respectfully urge the Court to hold that, as a matter of law, there cannot be a legally adequate consent by an involuntarily confined mental patient to dangerous, irreversible and experimental brain surgery which threatens the patient's personality and autonomy. Hence, the state cannot legally fund such experimental procedures.

The substantial doubts, which have been discussed above, about whether consent by an involuntarily confined mental patient can be competent, knowing and voluntary should, when combined, yield a judgment that consent, for patients so confined, cannot be legally adequate. Obviously, one cannot, with mathematical precision, establish the limits of competence, knowledge and voluntariness. The perimeters of those concepts are defined, utlimately, by legal judgments—judgments which may be hard to make, but which must be made by judges under our scheme of law. The cumulation of substantial doubts about the validity of the various components of consent leads to the holding that there cannot be legally adequate consent.

D. Policy Considerations Buttress the Conclusion that Involuntarily Confined Mental Patients Cannot Give Legally Adequate Consent to Experimental Psychosurgery.

In addition to the preceding legal analysis which leads to the conclusion that involuntarily confined mental patients cannot give legally adequate consent to experimental psychosurgery, there are several policy factors which buttress the conclusion that the judicial ban on such state-funded experimentation is appropriate.

First, such judicial action would *not* deny to involuntary mental patients access to a procedure which would give them a substantial chance of prompt release to the community. This would be a more difficult case if involuntarily confined patients were given a stark choice between continued confinement, on the one hand, and the likelihood of freedom with a possibility of injury, on the other. Such a choice could exist if some disease entity had been defined, and if there were a clear likelihood that psychosurgery would treat such disease, ameliorating behavior and allowing mental patients to obtain release from the institution. But this is *not* such a situation. As the record shows . . . the benefits of psychosurgery to the research subject are highly uncertain, *at best.* There is no assurance that any behavior changes will remain effective in the long run, thereby justifying the subject's release. Moreover, there are substantial risks of harms—both known and unknown. And these harms . . . threaten the individual's autonomy and personality, in addition to posing a danger to physical well-being and possibly causing pain. Accordingly, where there is so little likelihood of personal benefit to the subject, this is one of those rare cases when the court should, at this stage in psychosurgery development, prohibit the state from soliciting participation of involuntarily confined mental patients in psychosurgery experimentation. The purpose of curtailing the range of surgical procedures the state may offer the patient is, thus, to enhance the person's autonomy and welfare by protecting him from experimental, dangerous, and irreversible brain surgery.

Second, the other purposes of the informed consent requirement . . . will be served by a holding that informed consent cannot be given in these circumstances. The rationality of the experimentation process will not be advanced (and it may be harmed) when psychosurgery is performed on involuntarily confined patients, who may not be able to participate as freely in the flow of information which might surround experimentation on other, "non-captive" subjects. "The controls on the scientific validity and the useful purpose of the experiments are much less likely to be present when they are conducted in total institutions, for example, than they are in a broader community."

Further, the experimentation process could be seriously harmed through significant adverse public reaction when the state uses experimental, dangerous and irreversible brain surgery on a captive population. As a number of defense witnesses observed, there is already widespread social concern about the practice of psychosurgery. There is some fear that use of psychosurgery is not just medical experimentation. Rather, it is the medicalization of a social problem. This means that medical therapies are impermissibly being used to control aggressive behavior when there is *no* demonstration that such behavior results from illness and that the behavior is thus an appropriate subject for medical, as opposed to political or social, responses. In the Detroit setting this anxiety is fed by the statements to Dr. Rodin suggesting that psychosurgery may be an appropriate societal response to the Detroit riots. In addition, there are overtones of eugenic engineering in Dr. Rodin's suggestion of castration experiments involving the violence prone "dumb young male," paired with psychosurgery. . . .

E. Guardians of Incompetent Patients Cannot Give Legally Adequate Consent to Psychosurgery.

Amicus further submits that the guardians of those judged legally incompetent to make decisions about psychosurgery cannot give legally adequate consent to the medical procedure.

First, and most fundamentally, it will, for the reasons developed above . . . be extremely difficult for the guardian to make a *knowing* choice. It is extremely difficult to make a rational judgment about whether or not to undergo psychosurgery, given the limits of present knowledge. And it is, thus, far from clear what is the "best interest" of the patient—especially when the "benefits" claimed are so uncertain. We should not let guardians gamble with the lives of their wards, when the risks are so high and the results so uncertain—and potentially dangerous. Such speculative leaps of faith should only be taken by a potential research subject himself, not by a guardian who cannot, no matter how hard he tries, act, as would a "reasonable person" in his own "best interest."

Second, when guardians of mental patients are parents or close relatives, there may be a conflict of interest which would vitiate the validity of any guardian consent on behalf of the patient. In juvenile law and the law of incompetents, it is recognized that there is not necessarily an identity of interest between child and parent. The parent (or close relative) may be motivated to consent to psychosurgery for a variety of reasons other than the best interests of the patient himself, e.g., mental frustration, economic stress, hostility toward the patient. In such a setting, the law cannot presume that the parent's voluntary act is also the patient's voluntary act. See, *e.g., Frazier* v. *Levi,* 440 S.W.2d (Tex.Civ.App. 1969) (mother cannot consent to sterilization of child); *In re Seifurth,* 309 N.Y. 80, 127 N.E.2d 820 (1955) (minor can object to operation for cleft palate even though parents wish it); *Strunk* v. *Strunk,* 445 S.W.2d 145 (Ct.Appl.Ky. 1969) (parent needs court consent to donate incompetent son's kidney for transplant to competent brother).

Finally, if the goals of increasing the rationality of the experimentation process and protecting that process from harm would not be served by allowing an involuntarily confined but legally competent patient to give an informed consent, *a fortiori,* they will not be served by allowing a guardian to consent for an incompetent, involuntarily confined patient. Obviously, there can be little rational interchange with an incompetent patient. And, more importantly, to allow the state to try an experimental, dangerous and intrusive medical procedure on an incapacitated patient, when it is not allowed to do so on a competent patient, would create an impression of over-bearing and exploitation of the helpless that can only injure the experimental process.

4. From the Posttrial Brief of Respondents-Defendants.

On the brief were Hon. Frank J. Kelley, Attorney General, and Milton I. Firestone, Thomas R. Wheeker, and Terrence P. Grady, Assistant Attorneys General.

The fundamental question in this case is the ability of involuntarily detained patients to consent to innovative surgical procedures on the brain. It is impossible to discuss that question without examining the functions of consent. Why do we insist in the vast majority of cases that a patient consent to the use of a medical procedure on his person?

One function of consent is to recognize that the inviolability of a person's body is a fundamental tenet of Western legal thought. No man has the right to touch or invade the body of another without the other's permission. . . .

Closely related to the concept of inviolability is the concept of humanity. The would-be patient is a human being and insofar as possible should have the right to make his own decisions regarding his affairs. He should not be treated as a mere object upon which the physician practices his art. As one writer has said:

> "The written consent is important, however, because it accords to the patient the status of a person, not an experimental animal, and provides a degree of assurance that he is being considered as an end, not merely a means."

Gellhorn, *Experimental Treatment of Cancer Patients,* 98 Daedalus, 361, 375 (1969).

A recognition of the patient's humanity requires not only that he consent to a medical procedure, but that that procedure be explained to him prior to that consent. The patient is entitled to know what is going to happen to him and to participate in any decisions regarding his health and wellbeing.

In an innovative or experimental situation consent serves other functions as well. It increases the rationality of the procedure by informing the patient of the nature of the procedure and encouraging him to be as active a participant as is possible.

More importantly, the requirement of consent serves as a check on the innovator or experimentor. The interplay between doctor and patient requires the doctor to examine the value of his own procedure. . . .

The Plaintiffs' argument that an involuntarily detained person cannot consent to a surgical procedure of the type before this Court is based on three assumptions: 1) That the atmosphere surrounding the giving of such a consent is inherently coercive; 2) That the mental illness itself makes the person unable to properly and rationally evaluate the factors involved in a consent decision; and 3) That a patient who is not in a mental institution is free of such complicating factors. All of those assumptions are false.

When a person is ill and hospitalized, his ability to freely consent to a medical procedure is affected by several important factors. First, in the case of any seriously ill patient, the atmosphere surrounding the consenting to an innovative medical procedure is "coercive". Very often the patient is faced with the ultimate coercive factor—death. A person faced with certain death due to cancer will consent to virtually any innovative procedure which offers hope. In fact, the patient often approaches the doctor and "volunteers." He often seeks out fraudulent practioners offering miracle "cures," some of which are quite painful and expensive, even though he would never have thought of consulting such a person before the discovery of his illness. The pressures on such a patient, and his doctor, are enormous. . . . Fox, *A Sociological Perspective on Organ Transplantation and Hemodialysis,* 169 *Annals of the New York Academy of Sciences* 406, 413–415 (1970).

Nevertheless, no one would suggest that a person in such a desperate mental state should be prohibited from consenting to a legitimate, innovative medical procedure, even though such consent would be coerced and probably not based on rational consideration. Nor, is there any lawsuit seeking to prohibit the accepting of such a consent.

Even in a less desperate situation, a person who is ill and hospitalized is not in the same position as he was when healthy and his capacity to truly consent is diminished. . . . Payne, *Teaching Medical Psychotherapy in Special Clinical Settings,* in *Psychiatry and Medical Practice In a General Hospital* (Zinberg, ed) pp. 135, 143–144 (1964).

A second factor which diminishes the voluntariness of a patient['s] consent is found in the nature of the doctor-patient relationship. When a person is sick he turns to his doctor for help. In almost any doctor-patient relationship, the doctor dominates and the patient does little more than acquiesce in the recommended treatment. "Doctor knows best" is the prevailing attitude of the patient. . . .

A third factor which lessens the rationality of the consent concept is the fact that patients rarely, if ever, really understand the medical alternatives posed to them. A patient who is asked to submit to a pneumoencephalogram cannot be expected to grasp the methodology of the test, what results it may produce, what those results would mean, why they would have that meaning, etc. That does not excuse a physician from attempting to explain such facts, but it does impose a barrier to, rational decision-making on the part of the patient. Some writers have concluded that the patient is simply not qualified to evaluate the true risks and expected benefits of any innovative medical procedure. Rheingold, *Products Liability—The Ethical Drug Manufacturer's Dilemma,* 18 *Rutgers Law Rev.* 947 (1964); Note, *Experimentation on Human Beings,* 20 *Stanford L. Rev,* 99 (1967).

A fourth factor which affects the integrity of the consent concept is that people do not always react rationally. The requirement of the patient's consent to a medical procedure presumes that he acts rationally. Often, however, a patient acts out of emotion or as a result of internal or external compulsions. For example, a kidney donor may consent to the donation of his kidney because of his emotional attachment to the donee or because of overt or subtle family pressure to donate. At least one study has shown that the donors make up their minds to consent or not to consent long before they are given the facts upon which to make a rational decision. Fellner and Marshall, *Kidney Donors—The Myth of Informed Consent,* 126 *American Journal of Psychiatry,* 1245 (1970). . . .

There is no valid reason why a mental patient should be *per se* excluded from any medical treatment solely because of his status as a mental patient. The law has retreated from the position that a mentally ill person can never contract or consent. Instead, the modern approach is to look at the facts of each case individually and to decide if the person possessed sufficient mental capacity to understand the nature, the terms and the effect of the transaction. *Grannum* v *Berard,* 422 P 2d 812 (Wash. 1967). To accept the position of the Plaintiffs and "amicus curiae" would be to retreat from that principle by deciding in advance that *no* mentally person could *ever* consent to certain ill-defined procedures.

Furthermore, the position of Plaintiffs and "amicus curiae" reflects a lack of comprehension of the population of the state mental hospitals. A person does not magically become a passive, docile creature, unable to resist or to think for himself, when he enters a mental hospital. He will essentially retain the personality traits which he had when he came into the hospital.

Witnesses for the Plaintiff testified that all mental patients suffered a loss of "self-worth" upon entering the doors of a mental hospital and therefore were not in a position to evaluate the risks and benefits, especially the risks, of a procedure of the type in question in this case. Such a proposition has several defects.

First, if a mental patient cannot evaluate the risks and benefits of this type of medical procedure, then he cannot realistically evaluate the risks and benefits of any medical procedure, including his own psychotherapy. Most medical procedures entail risks and promise benefits. In many cases, those risks are quite substantial and the benefits are real but difficult to predict easily. For example, surgery for some suspected cancers is extremely risky, often leads to unanticipated complications and may or may not benefit the patient. Should a mental patient be prohibited from consenting to such an operation, where it is a last resort and death may result without the surgery? If in fact Plaintiffs' witnesses are correct, the mental patient should not be allowed to consent, because he does not appreciate the risks and cannot evaluate the possible benefits. If in fact there is a loss of self-worth, that loss does not manifest itself in one situation only.

The loss of self-worth theory would apply equally to the mental patient's psychotherapy. There again he cannot appreciate the risks and benefits. (And as Dr. Yudashkin testified, psychoanalysis, for example, can involve serious risks). It logically follows that the patient should not be treated or that he should be treated without any attempt to obtain his consent. The former alternative is illegal as a denial of the "right to treatment" and the later alternative is a step backwards in the treatment of mental patients. . . .

A second fallacy of the self-worth theory is that it assumes that a person who is not a mental patient can fully appreciate the risks and benefits of a proposed medical procedure and make a rational decision regarding consent. As noted above, however, patients do not evaluate risks and benefits, but rather tend to accept or reject proposed treatment for irrational reasons. A non-mental patient who is seriously ill tends to regress and to feel helpless. He is much more apt to suffer a loss of self-worth than a person admitted to a mental hospital. Nevertheless, no one seriously suggests that his consent should be prohibited.

A third fallacy of the loss of self-worth theory is that it makes false assumptions about the nature of a mental hospital. It presumes long commitments, lack of therapy, inhumane conditions. None of Plaintiffs' witnesses had any broad or recent exposure to the state mental hospitals. The average stay on commitment in Michigan is 40 days. . . .

The major fallacy of the loss of self-worth theory, however, is that it just does not reflect reality.

Commitment to a mental institution does not cause a loss of self-worth. Rather a person's self-worth is a reflection of his basic mental background and outlook. If anything, the mental hospitals increase a patient's self-worth:

> "I think that a degree of self-worth of any individual comes from his total life experience, and most important in that life experience is his very early life experience.
>
> "I think most psychotherapists, especially the psychoanalysts, hold that view that the early years of life are the most formative in terms

> of the individual's picture of his self-worth. My experience has been if a patient comes in to the institution with a low self-worth, the function of the institution, that is what our therapy is all about, is to try to raise his image of himself so that he can live in harmony with himself, and this is what we call getting the patient better, that is, his self-worth improves to a point where he no longer has to act aberrantly and get into difficulties, and can function.
>
> "He has that internal strength to be able to live in harmony with himself and others. That he no longer has to hallucinate or have a delusion that he is Jesus Christ or God or something like that, which makes up for his low self-worth in his illness.
>
> "As his self-worth increases, the delusions diminish because he doesn't need it any more.
>
> "Judging from the one great example currently is all of the veterans coming back from Vietnam who have been incarcerated, many five or six years under even more deplorable conditions than we have at Ionia, and their self-worth from what I could see on television didn't seem to be damaged by that experience. I think the same is true about patients who are incarcerated in our institutions.
>
> "I would say we improve the self-worth of a patient in his eyes more than we diminish it. . . . " (Dr. Yudashkin R 23 to 25-A 9)

Plaintiffs and "amicus curiae" also contend that a mental patient should not be allowed to consent to an innovative surgical procedure on the brain because the "inherently coercive" character of a mental institution compels that consent. The Defendants submit that such a conclusion is fallacious.

First, the Plaintiff[s'] argument is unsupported by any credible testimony. As noted above, none of their witnesses [has] any recent *or* substantial experiences upon which they based their testimony or their conclusions.

Second, as in the case of the arguments involving self-worth, the inherently coercive argument assumes a homogeneous population of docile, suggestible patients which doesn't exist. The only witness who testified at the trial who has any substantial experience with the population of the state mental hospitals, Dr. Yudashkin, responded to the inherently coercive theory:

> " . . . There are people who are passive and dependent. There are people who are negativistic and aggressive and hostile. . . .
>
> "Some people are sort of obsessive and compulsive. Other people

> tend to deal with things in broad, general ways of when approached with informed consent they approach informed consent like they approach anything, so that some patients will ask the doctor every cotton-picking detail, let's say a paranoid patient who is particularly concerned with details. He loses the broad general picture because he is so concerned with details many times, but he would want to know every little aspect of what was involved in this procedure if he was going to give informed consent.
>
> "Whereas, a patient who was more expansive and dealt with generalities, he would just take it with one blanket statement. A patient who was passive-dependent would consent to almost anything. A patient who was hostile and aggressive like the kind of patient we are talking about, have proven time and time again that they do not conform, that they do not submit to society's standards, that they do not easily agree with things that are put to them, in fact, the particular criminal sexual psychopath group." (R 32, 33-A 9)

Again, as has been pointed out frequently in this brief, each mental patient is an individual and should be treated as such. Attempting to treat them as a class who are all of a like personality is to do a tremendous disservice to those patients.

Furthermore, the type of patient contemplated as a potential candidate for neurosurgery is the aggressive patient. By nature, such patients tend to be hostile, antagonistic and aggressive. Their nature is to dissent, not to passively consent. . . .

The Defendants submit that as a matter of public policy this Court should not prospectively prohibit a mental patient from consenting to any medical procedure.

Such a holding would in effect be a step *backwards* in the quest for dignity for mental patients. As the testimony of Dr. Yudashkin quoted earlier indicates, enlightened professionals have spent years fighting for the proposition that a mental patient should have the right to consultation and consent regarding his treatment. To deny that right for any one treatment modality inevitably deals a setback to that right, particularly where the denial is based on alleged factors such as loss of self-worth or inherent coerciveness, which would apply to any form of psychiatric treatment.

A decision which denies a mental patient the right to consent (and, accordingly, to dissent) to innovative surgery will inevitably provide fodder for those who would trample on the dignity of the patient in the name of "treatment". The Court would be providing a judicial precedent which continues to recognize the unfortunately prevalent attitude that mental patients (and former mental patients) are second-class citizens. . . .

5. From the Posttrial Brief of Respondents-Defendants, Drs. Gottlieb and Rodin.

On this brief was S. I. Shuman. I have freely edited the brief since it was my own material; however, the substance of the arguments has in no way been changed.

I. General Problems Regarding Informed Consent.

A. The Existing State of the Law. The cardinal point in the development of any rational treatment of the subject of consent is to distinguish between experimental therapeutic interventions and experimental interventions. While it would be something of an exaggeration to say that there is an abundance of state law applicable to the control of experimental therapeutical interventions, compared to the state of the law on the control of medical experimentation with human subjects there is indeed an abundance of relevant precedents. While there is no statutory law in any state that deals with a doctor's liability for nontherapeutic experimental research, and almost no case law, there are a number of important decisions which affect both liability and the matter of consent when the experimental intervention is therapeutic. The only possible exception to the generalization about the absence of case law controlling experimentation is *Hyman v. The Jewish Chronic Disease Hospital,* 251 N.Y.S.2d 818, Rev'd 258 N.Y.S.2d 397 (1965). In addition, there is a Canadian case of some relevance and possibly one or two other American decisions which may bear on the question of a doctor's liability to a volunteer for medical research.

The paucity of decisional material for the regulation and control of medical experimentation need not imply that the common law is incapable of regulating this field. As one commentator has observed: "Viewed in its most favorable interpretation . . . the law concerning human experimentation could be expected to develop on a case-by-case basis in traditional common law fashion. The courts would look to expert witnesses drawn from the research field to testify as to common, accepted practices in clinical research." (Curran, "Governmental Regulation of the Use of Human Subjects in Medical Research: The Approach of Two Federal Agencies," *Daedalus* 542 at 545 (Spring 1969).) Or as another law professor has suggested: "A court exercising its common-law jurisdiction in a suit for damages could condemn experiments of high risk if there had been no committee approval of the protocol. To reach this result, the most likely recourse would be to the concept of negligence, which subjects the injury-producing action of an individual or corporate body to the test of 'due care.' It is particularly relevant that 'due care' is a continually evolving concept. . . . Absorbed into the law in this way the committees and the procedures that they develop become a functioning part of the legal system of control." (Jaffe, "Law As a System of Control," *Daedalus* 406 at 412 (Spring 1969).) Professor Jaffe continues his analysis of the development of common law as a mechanism for the control of medical experimentation involving humans by observing: "Judges are sensitive to the ethos of the times. Our society places a high premium on scientific experimentation and the pursuit of knowledge. To a greater extent than was formerly true, judges will be conscious of the conflict of interests and will seek to give due weight to each of them in any case involving experimentation carried on pursuant to current standards of propriety. . . . We should proceed on the hypothesis, therefore, that in framing our ethical principles, the common law will be hospitable to procedures that recognize the social value of human experimentation without sacrificing the interests of patients and subjects." (*Id.* at 416.)

We mention these suggestions for the development of common law mechanisms for the control of medical experimentation with human subjects not because this is precisely our problem, but rather to indicate that in the area of our present concern there is great need for the courts to exercise considerable restraint in light of the dearth of precedential material available, and in view of the complexities of the problems which have been generated by the explosion in medical research. But just as this truth may emerge from these suggestions on how the common law may further develop in this field, a further insight also emerges. The courts do have a role to play, and the history of the development of the common law reveals quite precisely that when the courts are made aware of problems which require judicial intervention they then proceed cautiously so that the appropriate and necessary regulation of the problem area is achieved without undue suppression of important interests.

It was suggested above that the material concerning the development of common law judicial mechanisms for the institutionalized control of human experimentation is not directly relevant. It is not directly relevant because the subject area with which we are concerned in the so-called consent question concerns a therapeutic rather than a purely experimental intervention. No matter what other considerations are relevant to this matter, it cannot be denied that the intervention is intended to be therapeutic for the individual subject and that the investigation is undertaken precisely with this subject and not some other "normal subject," just because this subject is believed to be capable of benefiting from the particular intervention proposed. We shall return to this point below because it is of overriding importance in much of the analysis which follows. But for the present, we develop the distinction between a therapeutic experimental innovation and one which is purely experimental in order to make clear that although there may not be an abundance of precendential material for cases of therapeutic intervention, there are decisions of considerable importance. Consequently, even if it were true, as some have argued, that the traditional common law of medical malpractice is not adequate for the protection of volunteers in medical experiments, there may nonetheless be a great deal of continuing utility in the common law precedents when the situation concerns an experimental but therapeutic intervention.

Writing in 1969 about this matter, Frank Grad, Professor and Director of the Legislative Drafting Fund at Columbia University Law School, observed: "When we deal with therapeutic research, we are operating essentially in the long-established and traditional field of regulation of medical practice, with the well-known liabilities placed on the physician for his malpractice. A medical practitioner under generally accepted rules is expected to follow the standards of medical practice prevailing at that time and place. If he decides to deviate from such a standard practice, and if injury results to the patient, the legal issue is almost invariably cast in terms of medical malpractice. Was the deviation from standard practice justified by the circumstances of the case, and did the patient give his informed consent to the unorthodox treatment pursued? The situation in which major departures from established medical procedures accrue may be extreme or emergency situations that justify heroic measures. The law and the medical profession have gone far to recognize that the nature of the informed consent may differ, depending on the particular situation. Thus, there is obviously no requirement that a physician disclose to a timid, feeble patient or to one who is *in extremis* the full details of the procedure or the full range of the risks that may have to be taken. But it should be remembered that in the therapeutic situation, withholding of information or avoidance of a full disclosure of the risk may be justified because such a holding back is not for the protection of the physician but for the benefit of the patient.

"Although, on the whole, it is increasingly being recognized that new procedures must be tried in order to establish their safety, the field of therapeutic research is likely to continue to remain subject to the regulation of the common law doctrines of medical malpractice.

"The protection of the patient in therapeutic research lies usually in the state's regulatory apparatus for medical practice generally. The licensing of physicians and other health professionals, the licensing and supervision of clinical and x-ray laboratories, the licensure of hospitals and other institutions, assures that only persons with adequate knowledge and background and only institutions with adequate facilities and staff will engage in any research effort incidental to therapy. Such a research effort then becomes part and parcel of regulated medical practice, and it is only in situations where damage or injury to a patient is alleged that medical malpractice rules become applicable. *Thus there appears to be little immediate need for new legislation or new methods of control of the field of therapeutic research.* Improvements and advancements in medical practice generally and better regulatory supervision of medical practice will raise the level of competence of the medical researcher and will provide assurances of sound treatment in the overwhelming number of instances. Where departures from accepted and established treatment procedures occur, and where these result in injury, the physician as well as the institution will continue to be faced with malpractice suits subject to usual common law rules. Where consent to a new procedure has been obtained, the argument will generally revolve around the question whether or not the consent was sufficiently 'informed.' *In view of the broad variety of unforeseeable situations that may have to be faced, and in view of the rather well-established body of case law on informed consent that is undergoing almost daily development, a new legislative definition of informed consent in the therapeutic situation is hardly called for. It would serve no particular purpose to require 'informed consent' by statute, or even to try to spell out in statutory form what informed consent means in particular situations . . .* " [Italics added] (Grad, "Regulation of Clinical Research By the State," 169 *N.Y. Acad. of Sciences, Annals* 533 at 534–35 (1970).)

As concerns our immediate problem, much of the law in the area is derived from a decision of the Michigan Supreme Court which is generally regarded as one of the most important in the field of therapeutic medical experimentation. Indeed, it is quite probably the most important case in that it marks the beginning of the development of the modern law on therapeutic experimentation with human subjects. In *Fortner v. Koch,* Mr. Justice Sharpe for the Court laid down dictum which has been very widely relied upon and quoted. He said: "We recognize the fact that, if the general practice of medicine and surgery is to progress, there must be a certain amount of experimentation carried on; but such experiments must be done with the knowledge and consent of the patient, or those responsible for him, and must not vary too radically from the accepted method of procedure. . . . " (272 Mich. 273, 261 N.W. 762 (1935).) A lawyer especially experienced in medical juisprudence said of this decision: "It removed experimentation in a clinical situation from the 'outlaw' category. Up to this time, experimentation in medical practice was considered an intentional transgression on the person of the patient. . . . The *Fortner* case also brought into the open the two assumptions underlying most of the earlier decisions—the matters of patient consent and accepted standards of practice." (Curran, *supra* at 543–44). Commenting further upon this decision, Curran points out: "The court's application of the first assumption would seem to be quite proper under past and current common law. Though the requirements of consent are still far from clear, it would currently seem to be accepted as obligatory among responsible medical investigators. This cannot be said, however, for the court's treatment of the second assumption. The court imposes an obligation on the investigator-clinician not to deviate 'too radically' from accepted methods even though he is conducting an investigation and even though he has informed the patient and received his consent to the investigational procedure. This restriction would seem clearly unacceptable to research interests, at least in many instances. Almost by definition, clinical investigaion must deviate from the normal or traditional in some *significant* degree. . . . What . . . did the Michigan Court mean by its restrictive language? I submit that it can only mean to contain experimentation within the bounds of reasonableness as judged by other colleagues engaged in similar practice involving clinical research. In research, acceptable standards would be determined by examining the practice and procedure followed by reputable and qualified clinical investigators. Today, even more than in 1935 when *Fortner v. Koch* was decided, a 'researcher's test' of reasonableness should be applied to clinical medical investigation." (*Id. 543–44.)*

B. When Is a Patient a Patient? Throughout the proceeding before this Court, it has been presumed that the standards for consent and the standards for judging the propriety with which Dr. Rodin dealt with John Doe were to be derived from the domain of experimental medicine. Why we have so presumed is one of the most interesting questions in this case and furnishing an answer to this question is one of the most difficult matters before this Court. It would be fair to say that no witness called by any party in this matter gave testimony which was relevant, let alone decisive, on the question of what distinguishes a patient from a volunteer in a medical experiment involving human subjects. It is worthwhile recognizing that there is almost no relevant common law on this question and no statutory law. Nor are there answers available from federal guidelines nor in the coes which led up to them, such as the Nuremburg Code or the Helsinki Declaration.

One of the few things that is clear, is that in this action no effort was made to make the distinction and the trial proceeded on the presumption that John Doe was a volunteer. That this presumption underlies the attitude of the Court as well as counsel in the case became especially obvious in the almost hostile reaction to Professor Slovenko's suggestion that the traditional common law of medical malpractice might be adequate for dealing with certain classes of cases involving innovative or experimental medical procedures. Yet it is perfectly clear that Professor Slovenko was quite right in suggesting that there is a rather well-entrenched body of common law (mentioned above), and that this is available for dealing with those cases where a doctor *treats* a patient by an innovative or experimental medical procedure.

While the answer to the question of when is a patient a patient is hardly obvious, the one thing that is obvious is that an answer which is thought to be clear because dictated by common sense is almost certain to be misleading. As is characteristically the case in matters which are either highly technical or ethically subtle, common sense is just not enough. Look at this case by way of illustration: John Doe did "volunteer" and Dr. Rodin is a physician. Is this therefore a physician-volunteer relation? On the other hand, what was considered for John Doe was clearly not a medical experimentation or investigaion as those expressions are traditionally used. It was not proposed that John Doe be used to test some new substance or procedure, nor was John Doe to be used as a control for such testing. John Doe in this case was nothing like the usual college student or prison inmate who in response to an advertisement on a local bulletin board makes himself available for medical experimentation in return for a certain sum of money or for other considerations. Nor did John Doe in this case come forward in response to any such advertisement. Rather John Doe was asked to consider this innovative procedure precisely because he was not just another member of the normal population. The prisoner or college student volunteers and is acceptable precisely because he is symptom-free and therefore can be tested in a particular situation. In this case, were John Doe symptom-free, he would have been on that very ground an unsuitable candidate.

However, we may ask, was not John Doe nonetheless a volunteer? He was surely not a patient in the sense in which that expression is used in the paradigm case of an individual who has been seen by a given doctor over a period of several years, and who then is asked by that doctor to consider some innovative or experimental procedure because the therapies administered over that period of years have not been successful. Rather, it would seem that John Doe and Dr. Rodin, in the instant case, illustrate a position somewhere between these two paradigm cases.

As Dr. Rodin testified, perhaps somewhat immodestly, but accurately and by testimony which has been neither challenged or even questioned, he is the court of last resort in this area for those difficult or doubtful cases involving unclear or indefinite EEG reports. And in that capacity, as a physician whose specialty is neurology and whose acknowledged expertise is in the field of EEG, he is asked to see a Mr. X who for the past five years has been seen and treated by Dr. Y for suspected epilepsy. Now Dr. Rodin sees Mr. X and does a neurological workup on him, including an EEG, and makes a diagnosis of psychomotor epilepsy and then recommends a temporal lobectomy. Is Mr. X a patient to Dr. Rodin or is he a volunteer? Why? Did Mr. X voluntarily come to Dr. Rodin? And if so, does that make him a volunteer for an innovative or medical experiment? (We presume for purposes of this hypothetical analysis that the temporal lobectomy was recommended at a time when it might still have been considered a nonstandard procedure.) Did just the one fact that Dr. Rodin sought out John Doe for a *therapeutic* intervention make John Doe a volunteer, whereas X, in the above hypothetical case, is a patient if he seeks out Dr. Rodin for the same therapeutic intervention? Indeed, in analyzing the comparison between the hypothetical case and John Doe's, it is worth bearing in mind that now the temporal lobectomy is a standard procedure and a considerably more drastic intervention than an amygdalotomy. A temporal lobectomy now involves the removal or destruction of the amygdala as well as the temporal lobe and thus considerably larger area and structures are affected by such a procedure.

It is clear that neither John Doe nor Mr. X were volunteers in the sense in which the college student or prisoner volunteer for an experiment, even though both X and Doe "voluntarily" consent to be seen, evaluated, and diagnosed by Dr. Rodin. It is also clear that neither X nor Doe "expect" to be subjected to the surgical intervention which Dr. Rodin may recommend, whereas the college student and prisoner, by volunteering, expect that they will be subjected to the new drug or procedure.

We have dwelt upon this matter of the difficulty of distinguishing John Doe the volunteer from John Doe the patient because it is of cardinal importance in understanding the whole range of problems generated by this case and by the hypothetical one which arose out of the so-called agression study. If Dr. Rodin were on the staff at Ionia rather than on the staff of Lafayette, although both are within the Department of Mental Health, and had he been seeing and treating John Doe since, say, 1965, and then in 1972 recommended a depth EEG workup, would that be a different case from the one now before us? If so, why? What is the magic by which this case has become a *cause célèbre?* Is it because John Doe was asked by Dr. Rodin to consider becoming his patient rather than having been asked by some other doctor to become Dr. Rodin's patient? Is the magic that made this case a *cause célèbre* due to the fact that Dr. Rodin asked John Doe to become his patient because the doctor believed there was an innovative therapeutic modality which had not yet been considered for Doe? It is submitted that even though all of the technical problems would be just the same for Mr. X or John Doe (that is, questions about side effects, causal connections, etc.) there would not be this case had Dr. Rodin merely considered treating John Doe as hundreds of patients have been treated by doctors who ultimately recommended neurosurgical procedure. The "magic" which converted this doctor-patient relationship, in which the contemplated intervention was admittedly intended to be therapeutic, into a *cause célèbre*, came about because Dr. Rodin wanted to do more than just treat this patient. He wanted to do what doctors should always do, especially with relatively new procedures; he wanted to learn from it so that something could be added to medical knowledge! The "magic," in other words, was that Dr. Rodin made the "mistake" of hoping to help John Doe within the context of a proposal to study uncontrollable aggression, rather than treating him as merely another sick patient! The message of this case to the medical profession then is just this: treat your patients and when necessary treat them by innovative or experimental procedures, but keep it dark! Do not, in advance, announce what you hope to learn or how you hope to learn it, but instead (if you do learn anything) after learning it, publish the results. Encouraging such an attitude towards medical research moves medicine back fifty years. Professionally incompetent extremists, acting in the name of civil liberties, should not be permitted to push medical research underground and thus suppress those very fundamental human and social rights which courts are supposed to protect.

C. Some General Considerations About the Problem of Consent. Without having decided the question, and it is clearly the case that the quesion has not been argued to the court, let us presume, as the court and counsel have, that we are concerned with a matter in which the doctor-volunteer standards are more readily applicable than are those of doctor-patient. And let us do so despite the fact that there are relatively well-entrenched common law standards regarding the doctor-patient relations and that these standards do provide considerable guidance on questions as to informed consent as well as liability. Proceeding then on the assumption that we are not to be guided by these precedents, and that we are dealing with the novel and as yet undecided questions about consent for medical experimentation, we turn to some general problems in the field of consent. However, in doing so we must stress again that both the problem of John Doe in the actual case which precipitated the present matter, and the John Doe who might be the subject considered in hypothetical question No. 1, are not volunteers for a medical experimentation or investigation (as those expressions are used in the literature), and that the court has not decided, and does not have the question before it, of whether or not the traditional common law is applicable to an instance of the kind we are considering.

Such answers as may be relevant to the general question about what constitues "legally adequate consent" gravitate around three general propositions: (1) nothing is going to be settled by cliches or slogans, but rather by weighing costs and benefits; (2) in the transition from duress to submission through acquiescence to consent, there is no hard and fast line and no way of quantifying the kinds of considerations which could then provide a litmus paper test for deciding when there is consent rather than duress, submission, or acquiescence; and (3) in varying degrees, consent by the patient himself is essentially a symbolic act.

It is worth noticing at the outset that the test proposed in the hypothetical question was deliberately framed as "legally adequate consent" rather than "informed consent" precisely because it was recognized that patient consent is largely symbolic. Even though informed consent doctrines as developed in the common law cases on medical malpractice may have relevance in connection with human subjects of medical experimentation, meeting the requirements of proper information is not sufficient for determining the propriety of the consent. That "informed" is necessary but not sufficient becomes perfectly clear, for example, when we recognize that no amount of "informed" will convert duress or submission into consent. It may be doubtful whether complete knowledge and information converts even acquiescence into consent. Indeed, one could very plausibly argue that having complete knowledge and being thoroughly informed effectively destroy consent. Dr. Louis Lasagna, one of the most frequently quoted writers in the field of human experimentation, says this: "Much has been written, for example, on the need for 'informed consent,' but little research has been conducted on what this term actually means. What do we consider a 'fair shake' as far as the subject is concerned? How much tailoring of our presentation is required by differences in age, personality, or I.Q. among patients? What minimal information do we want conveyed before we ask whether a subject is willing to participate in an experiment? In one experiment, we have found that lengthy, detailed expositions of risks and purposes may defeat the process of communication, with less comprehension of the problems and dangers than if one uses a brief, straightforward statement." (Lasagna, "Special Subjects in Human Experimentation", *Daedalus* 449 at 461 (Spring 1969).) In the study referred to, sixty-six subjects were asked to take either a specific tablet or a placebo when they next had a headache. They received varyingly detailed descriptions of the actions and hazards of the drug. "The results of this study reveal how important the way in which information is presented can be in determining comprehension and providing truly 'informed' consent. Subjects who read the short form of the protocol in which the pertinent information was included without detailed elaboration retained significantly more of the important facts than did subjects shown either the intermediate or long protocol forms. In many cases, the detailed descriptions of the side effects or toxic actions of aspirin apparently served to frighten the subject, who then was unable to classify the information usefully. . . . Indeed, five of the twenty-two subjects in the long-form group did not even realize, after reading the protocol, that the drug could produce death. . . . Thus while the lengthier forms, which tended to stress the toxic effects and provide extra information and detail about them, seemed to discourage volunteering, they also failed to give a clear picture of the risks." (Epstein and Lasagna, "Obtaining Informed Consent: Form or Substance," 123

Archives of Internal Medicine 682 at 684–85 (June 1969).) However, in another study Alfidi points out: "When this statistical study of informed consent was begun, it was expected to prove that patients would indeed refuse angiography after they were informed of its possible complications. Much to my surprise it proved the opposite." Alfidi then describes in some detail the complications and risks involved in the procedure and the way in which this information was conveyed to the subjects, and concludes: "The straightforward and perhaps even harsh statements of the possible complications of angiography were accepted and desired by the majority of patients." (Alfidi, in Katz, *Experimentation with Human Subjects* 584 and 586 (1972).) (The Katz collection of materials contains many of the important papers relevant to our problem, and since it is easier to use this single volume than to locate the individual items, we will frequently make reference to the Katz volume.)

We cited these two seemingly contradictory empirical investigations not to prove some specific point about "informed" consent, but rather only to support the propositions suggested at the outset, that no cliche or crass generalization is likely to suffice in this area and that "informed" is not an adequate test for determining what constitutes legally adequate consent. Further, the quantity of information conveyed is probably irrelevant in determining whether the consent is legally adequate. Perhaps "irrelevant" is too harsh, and it might be fairer to say that the degree or quality or extent of information conveyed is unlikely to be crucial in determining whether or not consent is legally adequate.

If then the degree or quality or quantity of information conveyed is hardly likely to exhaust the requirements for adequacy as to consent, why the overwhelming concern with consent? It is perfectly clear that in many important areas of social relations we do not require consent of the individual who is to be subjected to an intervention or procedure. Particularly is this the case in regard to children, and (at least in the past), in some instances even to women, and certainly it is also the case in regard to adults regardless of sex as, for example, in connection with compulsory blood samples from suspected drunk drivers and as with compulsory vaccination. (See *Schmerber v. California,* 384 US 757 (1956); and, for example, also see *O'Brien v. Cunard Steamship Lines,* 154 Mass. 272, 28 N.E. 266 (1891).) Thus we see both that there are important exceptions to the otherwise general requirement that consent is required before a bodily invasion may be undertaken, and secondly, that the legal adequacy of consent is unlikely to be affected significantly by a determination as to the degree or quality of the information conveyed. There is an even more important third difficulty about "informed consent" which makes one wonder why so much emphasis is placed upon this one doctrine. It is the fact that it is quite easy in most cases to "engineer" consent. As Edmond

Cahn, a distinguished lawyer and legal philosopher, has written: "Consent may be 'engineered' by the kind of psychologist who takes it for granted that his assistants and students will submit to experiments and implies a threat to advancement if they raise questions. Or the total community may 'engineer' a consent, as when the president, the generals, and the newspapers call with loud fanfare for a heroic crew of astronautical volunteers to attempt some ultrahazard exploit." (Cahn, in Katz at 634). If these three factors were not reason enough to question placing so much reliance upon "informed consent," there is the further, perhaps overriding, reservation about the utility of consent which will be considered below. It is undeniable that in order to require anything more than submission, let alone consent, we must presume some real freedom on the part of the patient. Yet we know that this is conceivable (let alone realizable) only with the emotionally mature, well-integrated patient who is functioning normally. Yet what person is functioning "normally" when he is a patient—let alone a patient sick enough to be hospitalized?

Given all of these problems, and the further consideration that patients, like other people in even nonmedical situations, have deep and grave anxieties about being free to make choices because we all do suffer from what Fromm calls "the dizziness of freedom," why do we continue to insist upon consent as almost a litmus paper test for propriety in the field of medical experimentation? One would have thought that any one of these several considerations which mitigate against any real consent would have sufficed to reveal the symbolic character of the act and thus to diminish its importance. Where so much is at stake, as it is in cases where an experimental therapeutic intervention is considered, it seems almost irrational to place so much confidence upon an act which is often entirely symbolic and, at best, is likely to be largely so. It would seem that the answer must be that the symbol itself is important even if the act of consenting is not functionally adequate to the job for which it was intended.

In part, the answer to the symbolic importance of consent is found in the fact that consent serves not one function but two. It is intended not only to protect the patient and his health and bodily integrity, but also, even more, to protect the integrity of his humanity. It is this latter element for which consent is symbolically important and it requires the most careful consideration in dealing with the subject before us. Here the important considertion is not that the patient knowingly consents or even acquiesces in what is to be done, nor is it that the patient even wishes to "choose," let alone has the kind of information, talent, education, and emotional stability requisite for understanding the matter before him. Rather, it is just that the patient is human, and unlike an animal, must have his humanity recognized, and that there is no better way of recognizing that humanity than by requiring his "participation" in, rather than his subjection to, the procedure which is involved. It is probably considerations such as these which led Paul Ramsey from the Department of Religion at Princeton to write: "The convenantal bond between consenting man and consenting man makes them 'joint adventurers' in medical care and progress, joint adventurers also in the moral history of mankind, in the exigencies of a convenant or fiduciary relation of man with man in which they resolve to live faithfully even while not knowing the future outcome. . . . 'Partership' is a better term for this than 'contract'. 'Joint adventurers' in curing or in investigation is better still." (Ramsey, "The Ethics of a Cottage Industry in an Age of Community and Research Medicine," 284 *New England Journal of Medicine* 700 at 705 (Apr. 1, 1971).)

While there is much to be said for Dr. Ramsey's view of the matter, and while perhaps it even comes closer to why we regard consent as so important despite all the defects of properly engineering consent, it is worth noticing again how dangerous glib generalizations can be. As another writer experienced in medical research has pointed out, "The patient usually will not act counter to what he perceives to be the desire of his doctor-investigator. This, of course, brings us to the generally regarded optimum of the partnership between investigator and the experimental subject." However, of necessity, he then goes on to add, "Is it not possible to motivate the patient to volunteer to a sense of partnership that may actually impair his ability to judge what is best for him?" (Morris, "Guidelines For Accepting Volunteers: Consent, Ethical Implications, and the Function of a Peer Review," 13 *Clinical Pharmacology and Therapeutics* 782 at 786 (1972).)

It would seem that we are compelled to admit that no matter where we turn there are no easy answers to what shall count as "legally adequate consent;" rather there seem to be questions of ever escalating complexity and each answer seems to generate greater difficulty. The problem of the over-motivated "partner" is in some ways at the core of our concern with the involuntarily committed patient. We must confront the reality of the involuntarily detained patient who, even if he does not view himself as a "partner," has been subjected to behavior control procedures which do diminish the ago autonomy necessary if even acquiescence, let alone consent, is to be of any significance. But in analyzing this problem it is important to bear in mind that any contact between two human beings constitutes behavior control and that there is always the problem of trying to discover whether conduct is voluntary or involuntary in light of, or despite, the behavior control which has been exercised. There is always coercion in the doctor-subject relationship and it will always be the case that after "adequate" coercion the patient or subject will, as one writer put it, "testify for the defense. . . . "

Perhaps we can draw the following tentative conclusions about some of the general problems regarding "legally adequate consent." (1) Consent must be tailored to fit the individual patient, and what he is told, how he is told and by whom, and under what circumstances, are likely to be more important in determining whether consent is legally adequate than is any talismanic reference to information as the criteria for valid consent. (2) Even if consent is symbolic and unrealistic in almost every case, it is nonetheless important in showing the kind of respect which is necessary to preserve the essential humanity of a person regardless of the position or status in which he finds himself, be it that of a voluntarily hospitalized patient or one committed involuntarily. (3) Perhaps most important, we must recognize that any judgments made about legally adequate consent are essentially inadequate unless we have previously undertaken the task which neither courts, nor commentators, nor philosophers, nor psychiatrists have yet done for us. And that is, to have the kind of information we need about the nature of man. Or as Jay Katz has said: "Any meaningful discussion of 'informed consent' . . . would first have to be grounded in a detailed examination of our assumptions about the nature of men. . . . " (Katz, "Who is to Keep Guard Over the Guards Themselves?," 23 *Fertility and Sterility* 604 at 608 (1972).)

In addition to the matters already raised, it is extremely important to recognize that in question number one, as with the problem of John Doe and the original Agression Study proposal, the question was not consent for an intervention designed to save life. Instead we confront the even more subtle question of consent for an experimental intervention, one which was intended to be therapeutic, but therapeutic in a way which would affect not the maintenance, but the *quality* of life. This is seen to be an exceedingly important difference once we begin to ask: (1) what should the doctor-investigator say about the possible changes in life style which are expected to flow from the therapeutic intervention?; (2) should he say anything about life style, or is he properly restricted to discussing only the "anatomical and biochemical" changes which are expected?; (3) should he refuse to answer questions, let alone volunteer information, about life style changes that can be expected if the probable, hoped for biochemical changes are attained?; (4) are these questions more subtle or important where the therapeutic intervention is with the brain rather than with, say, the kidneys, despite the growing literature to support the belief that renal transplants generate very important psychological problems for both donor and recipient? (Many renal transplant teams include a psychiatrist.) Not only are there no obvious answers to any of the above questions, one reasonably wonders if these are even appropriate questions!

Acting not entirely out of frivolity, nor to minimize the difference between a quality of life intervention and one which is for life maintenance, we set out below a consent form for another surgical intervention on an area of the body somewhat lower than the brain. It is set out in part to illustrate the futility of believing that there are litmus paper tests available for determining what constitutes legally adequate consent even in "easy" cases.

Consent Form for Hernia Patients

I, __________, being about to be subjected to a surgical operation said to be for repair of what my doctor thinks is a hernia (rupture or loss of belly stuff—intestines—out of the belly through a hole in the muscles), do hereby give said doctor permission to cut into me and do duly swear that I am giving my informed consent, based upon the following information:

Operative procedure is as follows: The doctor first cuts through the skin by a four-inch gash in the lower abdomen. He then slashes through the other things—fascia (a tough layer over the muscles) and layers of muscle—until he sees the cord (tube that brings the sperm from testicle to outside) with all its arteries and veins. The doctor then tears the hernia (thin sac of bowels and things) from the cord and ties off the sac with a string. He then pushes the testicle back into the scrotum and sews everything together, trying not to sew up the big arteries and veins that nourish the leg.

Possible complications are as follows:

1) Large artery may be cut and I may bleed to death.
2) Large vein may be cut and I may bleed to death.
3) Tube from testicle may be cut. I will then be sterile on that side.
4) Artery or veins to testicles may be cut—same result.
5) Opening around cord in muscles may be made too tight.
6) Clot may develop in these veins which will loosen when I get out of bed and hit my lungs, killing me.
7) Clot may develop in one or both legs which may cripple me, lead to loss of one or both legs, go to my lungs, or make my veins no good for life.
8) I may develop a horrible infection that may kill me.
9) The hernia may come back again after it has been operated on.
10) I may die from general anesthesia.
11) I may be paralyzed if spinal anesthesia is used.
12) If ether is used, it could explode inside me.
13) I may slip in hospital bathroom.
14) I may be run over going to the hospital.
15) The hospital may burn down.

I understand: the anatomy of the body, the pathology of the development of hernia, the surgical technique that will be used to repair the hernia, the physiology of wound healing, the dietetic chemistry of the foods that I must eat to cause healing, the chemistry of body repair, and the course which my physician will take in treating any of the complications that can occur as a sequela of repairing an otherwise simple hernia.

____
Patient

____
Lawyer for Patient

____
Lawyer for Doctor

____
Lawyer for Hospital

____
Lawyer for Anesthesiologist

____
Mother-in-Law

____
Notary Public

Perhaps one of the best balanced statements about the concerns we have been examining is found in a discussion by the distinguised legal theorist Paul Freund, who wrote: "The concept of consent has been much derided as unrealistic and artificial, and of course it embraces a range of responses that differ in their degree of autonomy and understanding. The psychological constraints or compulsions that operate on a seriously ill patient are different from those that affect a person attracted to an experiment through an advertisement. Nevertheless a requirement of 'voluntary, informed consent' does have values beyond the symbolic one of respect for individual autonomy and personality. It is far from the be-all and end-all of legal and ethical safeguards, but it is a valuable ultimate check, reminding one of Keynes' rationale for the gold standard: that it is a safeguard in case the managers of the currency should all go mad at once." (Freund, "Legal Frameworks For Human Experimentation," *Daedalus* 314 at 323 (Spring 1969).)

D. Duress-Submission-Acquiescence-Consent: The "Voluntariness" of Consent. Anyone who has ever been treated by a doctor for any relatively serious illness, let alone anyone who has been hospitalized for a serious illness, is likely to acknowledge that a competent doctor can get almost any patient to consent to almost anything. This is so for a number a reasons. First, the patients do not want to make decisions about complex medical matters and recognize that any amount of information furnished to them for the decision is likely to be inadequate and partial. In addition, there is the general tendency to avoid making decisions in stress situations characteristic of all human beings, a characteristic which was referred to above, quoting from Fromm, as "the dizziness of freedom." "The desire to involve the patient in the decision-making process in regard to details of medical care implies that there should be fuller and franker discussion about the use of everything from drugs to surgical techniques. Whether the public wants this is a matter for debate; I personally doubt it. In my own experience as a physician and investigator, not only are patients usually incapable of making the decisions in question (which is not surprising) but they are usually not desirous of making such decisions. . . . In many complex decision-making situations in medicine, the patient is really more in the position of being on an airplane that has defective landing gear, is running out of gas, and whose pilot has to make some sort of landing in one of several alternate places than in the position of a passenger who is asked whether he wishes to board a plane whose pilot indicates that he is about to fly for the first time with his eyes closed and 'no hands'." (Lasagna, "Some Ethical Problems In Clinical Investigation," in Mendelsohn, Swazey and Tanis, *Human Aspects of Biomedical Innovation* 98 at 106 (1971).)

Equally to the point are the remarks of Dr. Barnes of the Rockefeller Foundation. Writing for the Symposium on Ethical and Scientific Problems in Human Experimentation, he observes in connection with the stilbestrol matter: "Having reviewed the early reports on the stilbestrol study, the writer has been unable to pursuade himself that 'Informed Patient Consent' would have provided any protection whatsoever. All patients except those who are constitutionally drug nihilists would have signed such a form." (Barnes, "Clinical Studies in the Human: The Ethical and Scientific Problem," 23 *Fertility and Sterility* 593 at 595 (1972).)

In addition to the fact that generally patients do not wish to make decisions about complex medical matters, and apart from the fact that a competent doctor is likely to be able to get his patient to consent to almost anything, it is also important to bear in mind that when a patient enters a hospital situation he almost always suffers regression and feelings of helplessness (see the discussion by Payne in Katz at 650). It is almost unnecessary to add what Dr. Anna Freud said to medical students about the doctor-patient relationship: "You can understand where all the irrational attitudes of your adult patients toward their health and toward their bodies come from. It is true you deal with adults, but every adult who is ill, who has fever, who is in pain, or who expects an operation, returns to childhood in some way. He feels small and helpless and due to the ease with which he transfers his feelings on the past onto you, you become the parent, you own his body.'' (Quoted from Anna Freud in Katz at 636). The same view is advanced by Dr. Paul Schilder. ''Sooner or later the patient will have to add faith to his relation to the physician if he wants to get a sufficient amount of consolation out of his relationship. . . . When faith enters the relation, the superior-inferior relation between physician and patient is obviously still more emphasized. . . . The relation becomes similar to that between the adult and the child. . . . From this relation to the complete surrender of the patient to the physician is only a short step. The physician does not only become a father, but he also becomes a father endowed with magic powers. . . . Since the physician is so far superior in this relation, reasoning obviously becomes unnecessary and the physician has to direct the faith of his patient.'' (Quoted from Schilder in Katz at 637.) In view of this almost inevitable feature of the doctor-patient relationship, and in view of the psychodynamics out of which this relationship arises, one must wonder about the allegation found in the testimony, particularly of Drs. Lowinger and Watson, that the institutional structure compels committed patients to accept any recommendation made by the doctor. Indeed, in view of the testimony of these doctors that there are few physicians available, and that the patients seldom see doctors, it may well be the case that the distance between the patients and their doctors makes it easier for them to resist the psychodynamic relationship which compels a patient into seeing a doctor as his father-savior. That is, the involuntarily committed patient may be in a *better* position to avoid being caught up into the doctor-faith-healer relationship than is the private voluntary patient. Perhaps this helps compensate for other coercive aspects which obtain in the situation of an involuntarily committed patient. On balance it may well be the case that the coercive character of the detention is less compelling, less overwhelming, than is the faith-in-my-doctor-healer-savior syndrome which characteristically emerges in the private, ''voluntary,'' doctor-patient relationship.

In any event, any effort so finely to balance the coercive features which affect consent is likely to be unproductive. It is sufficient to recognize that the patient is always under duress when hospitalized and that in the hospital or institutional setting there is no such thing as a volunteer. The question then is: What degree of alleged voluntariness is requisite for consent for some purpose, as compared to the degree of voluntariness required to find acquiescence for other purposes, and as compared again to submission and perhaps even duress?

What then are the realities about ''informed consent?'' (1) Informed consent, let alone legally adequate consent, is at best a goal which one strives for but which is almost never achieved in an ideal form. (2) Consent, even if informed, is almost never educated. (3) Many important medical ''decisions'' made by patients are regarded as legally adequate despite the absence of relevant information. (The experience with kidney donors is particularly revealing in this respect. See Katz at 619–21.) (4) Patients are likely to consent to almost anything a competent doctor wants once the psychodynamics of the doctor-patient relationship become operative. (5) Patients are often so anxious to consent to an innovative procedure that the doctor's main problem is to make these patients view the risks realistically rather than seek out the risks in some frantic hope of cure or improvement.

In light of these realities it is perfectly clear that legally adequate consent involves the effort to secure that optimal balancing by the doctor and the patient, but particularly by the doctor, of the fears of the patient, the ambitions of the doctor, and the often exaggerted hopes which patients have about the utility of the medical intervention. Thus, what a doctor tells a patient and how he acts with him are more likely to determine the quality of the consent than is any amount of information furnished to the patient on a piece of paper. For this reason, review committees which concern themselves only with what the doctor and patient each write down about what was said are likely to be gestures no more significant than the symbolism involved in the usual mechanical informed consent procedure. The psychodynamics of what constitutes an intelligent, adequate consent that should count for legally adequate consent is thus a function, as Dr. Yudashkin so carefully explained is his testimony in this court, of the personality of the patient and the personality of the doctor. (See transcript at page 32–A9 ft.) The situation in which a patient finds himself surely affects how the patient behaves, but it does not decide the personality of the patient. Those patients who come to the situation with an aggressive, questioning, hostile attitude do not suddenly lose it by being hospitalized, either involuntarily or otherwise. And those patients whose docility has characterized them prior to the hospitalization will not suddenly become aggressive, inquiring, curious people because they are put into an institutional setting.

Confronting realities in the consent situation may not lead to any clear or even clearly helpful answers. But it does make one thing clear: What is legally adequate consent cannot be determined by category or status but only by evaluation on an individual basis in terms of what the doctor said, what he did, and how he did it, to which patient and under what circumstances, and for what purpose. To think that all voluntary patients can give legally adequate consent (or that no involuntary patients can) is to play an Alice in Wonderland game where the cost of the game will be borne both by patients and medical research as well as by those compromised human rights which are adversely affected whenever crude yes-or-no generalizations are thought adequate for questions only answerable by the most subtle, cautious, judicious, careful, individual evaluation of cases. To answer the consent question which is before this court by a blanket "No" is to say that no involuntarily committed patient could, under any circumstances, either by himself or in concert with his legal representative, ever give legally adequate consent for a procedure of the kind outlined in the question. But to so hold would be logically equivalent to holding that the *status* of having been committed destroys the individual personality and situation of the committed person. Making such a substitution of status for person is morally abhorrent and contrary to the most basic philosphical and political principles of democracy. It is also contrary to minimal standards for the practice of medicine which require that each patient be treated as an individual human being.

E. The Use of Volunteers for Medical Experimentation. A number of witnesses in this judicial proceeding have suggested that in order to avoid the stultification of medical research which might follow were an entire class of potential subjects to be denied the possibility of ever giving legally adequate consent, volunteers alone should be used for such experiments as were deemed necessary. We shall try to show this gesture is futile because it does not avoid the need to deal with the core problem of identifying standards for determining legally adequate consent regardless of the category of person with whom we are concerned. In other words, we shall suggest here that regardless of whether we are concerned with voluntary mental patients, or involuntarily committed mental patients, or voluntarily hospitalized patients, or patients hospitalized under circumstances of some coercion, or whether we are dealing with so-called voluntary subjects for medical experimentation, the core problem of consent simply does not go away—it stays with us and it is the same problem.

In short, it is not the category or status of the subject-patient which determines the adequacy of consent, but rather the individual and his personality. To think that it is somehow more democratic or more socially just to permit only volunteers to serve as subjects for medical experimentation is to be blind to the reality that we all have our drives and that volunteers are but volunteers in one sense only. Inviting volunteers rather than permitting a certain class of persons to be considered as potential participants in medical investigations, particularly when the research is believed to be thereapeutic for the participant, is to play upon the needs of the so-called volunteers. If a volunteer comes forward out of neurotic desire to satisfy masochistic drives to subject himself to pain or discomfort, or if the volunteer comes forward because of other psychological compulsions, is it appropriate to call such a person a volunteer? Nor is it but a wild shot in the dark to think that there are such motives for volunteering. "Regardless of age, sex, education, intelligence and geographic location of a volunteer, the reasons for offering to participate in a research study are essentially the same. So, too, are the personality types of the volunteer, most of whom are obsessional or schizoid. Likewise, the incidence of psychopathology among volunteers is remarkably similar everywhere. On the basis of psychologic tests administered to a group of college student volunteers participating in drug response studies, Lasagna and von Felsinger found that 50 per cent were severly maladjusted psychologically. Pollin and Perlin, in a clinical study at the National Institute of Mental Health, discovered 'significant psychopathology' in 52 per cent of volunteers. They defined 'significant psychopathology' as the presence of symptoms, but of an order or number insuffient for the diagnosis of a syndrome. Esecover, Malitz, and Wilkens reported a high incidence of psychopathology in paid normal volunteers for hallucinogenic drug studies. Psychiatric diagnoses were made on almost 50 per cent of their group. More than one third of the group were rated as 'needing psychiatric treatment,' and one fifth of the group were or had been in psychiatric treatment. In my survey, the prevalence of psychopathology corresponds closely to the findings of these investigators. An individual's decision to volunteer for a research project may be indicative of personality deviation or psychopathology in varying degrees. The more severe the psychopathology of the volunteer, the more related are the motives to this and the more unrealistic are the reasons for volunteering." (Ayd, "Motivations and Rewards for Volunteering to be an Experimental Subject," 13 *Clinical Pharmacology and Therapeutics* 771 at 774 (1972).)

In one of the studies Dr. Ayd refers to, the authors report: "Our study dealt with clinical psychiatric evaluations for 56 subjects volunteering for hallucinogen studies. . . . Our focus in this work was on motivations for volunteering, incidents and types of psychopathology, relationship between psychopathology and motivations, and personality patterns. The sample was composed of 46 males and 10 females. . . . All subjects had some college and 46 had varying degrees of post-graduate training. Volunteers were recruited by posting an announcement." They conclude by saying, "Although diagnostic categories are admittedly rough estimations of psychopathology, they can be exceedingly useful. On the basis of our clinical impressions, the prevalence of psychopathology in the volunteer group seemed quite high. Psychiatric diagnoses were made on almost 50 per cent of the group. More than one-third of the group were rated as 'needing psychiatric treatment,' and one-fifth of the group were or had been in psychiatric treatment." (Esecover, Malitz, and Wilkens, reported in part in Katz at 622–23.)

If so-called volunteers so frequently act out of what might, for present purposes, be called irrational motives, does the question as to legally adequate consent really get solved by inviting such so-called volunteers? Nor should it be thought that the irrationality of the motives of volunteers is something experienced only occasionally. Apparently, the contrary is the case, as is shown, for example, by kidney donor studies. "Fellner and Marschall . . . studied 12 renal homotransplant donors and found that they made their decision to donate a kidney 'in a split second,' 'instantaneously,' or 'right away,' when the subject of kidney transplant was first mentioned to them. The decision to be a donor occurred before they inquired into the possible consequences for themselves, before they sought reassurance as to the eventual benefits for the recipient, and before the transplant team presented all the relevant information and statistics and asked them to decide." (Ayd, *supra* at 772–73.)

Cognizant of the fact that the use of so-called volunteers is at best a mechanism for assuaging guilt feelings, but no real solution to the problem of legally adequate consent dealt with on an individual basis, some have sought to compromise reality and necessity with token idealism, by concluding that prison inmates ought not be permitted to volunteer since they (unlike "free" volunteers) would almost always be doing so for motives which were irrational. Because we are in this case especially concerned with involuntarily committed mental patients, the analogy to prisoners is especially illuminating. And it is interesting to note that while those for whom doctrinaire slogans suffice as a substitute for investigation and analysis often conclude that prisoners may not volunteer, those who have investigated the matter more carefully often come to a different conclusion. Thus Ayd, in the article previously cited, first presents what are "the most oft-cited reasons for a prisoner's willingness to be an experimental subject." After identifying some eleven such reasons, he concludes: "These motives of a prisoner in volunteering to be a research subject (with the exception of the hope for a reduction of sentence) are identical to those listed for 'normal' nonprisoner volunteers. . . . " Ayd then lists the several research studies which have been done in this area. (Ayd, *supra* at 773.) Lasagna, whose empirical research on volunteering has already been referred to, considered the subject again in an article entitled "Special Subjects in Human Experimentation," where he concludes that whether one is speaking of prisoners, children, the mentally incompetent, students, or other special categories, the issue would appear to be the same. He writes, "There is, unfortunately, a tendency for people to moralize about the ethical problems in human research in terms of black-and-white categorical imperatives. I much prefer John Fletcher's statement: 'It is far easier to act on the basis on an abstract principle than it is to make a fitting response to new situations on the basis of concrete and immediate responsibility.' Absolutist doctrines seem no more defensible in this area than in others. What sometimes passes for ethical profundity may, in fact, be only shallowness and an irresponsible or arrogant failure to appreciate the richness of the moral alternatives and the subtlety of the ethical issues. . . . It would seem preferable to avoid dogma, codes, pontifical stands, and the temptation to talk in capital letters. . . . " (*Daedalus* at 459–60 (Spring 1969).)

The same concern with avoiding doctrinaire, sloganeering, cliched approaches to the solution of subtle ethical problems is found in the conclusion of a distinguished Harvard law professor who, in writing about this problem, says: "Both law and morals disapprove of the use of certain tactics in securing consent—such as falsification, failure to state crucial facts, and undue pressure. What is 'undue' is a function of the situation. We can decide (as, for the most part, we have) that to seek the consent of a prisoner is not undue despite the presence of pressures absent in the case of the citizen at large. He must not, however, be threatened with adverse consequences if he refuses, and for this reason his refusal should not be of record. Let us admit that problems arise in part because there are disturbing contradictions in the prison situation itself. But that statement characterizes almost any life situation, and for that reason it may be the path of wisdom to focus on the simplicities. Experimentation on prisoners offers advantages to the experimenter, to the prisoner, and to the public. It offends, I believe, only a very few persons. Similar considerations may govern the use of the aged and the derelict, persons whose interests are drastically narrowed and whose life is one of dull, inescapable monotony. To become involved in a vital experiment, to become socially useful, may provide a fillip to their lives. I would conclude with Dr. Lasagna that 'the motivation for volunteering is highly complex and not easily discernible; we are all captive to certain drives. . . . I would hope that we might not be doctrinaire in our approaches toward different volunteer groups.' " (Jaffe, "Law As a System of Control," *Daedalus* 406 at 424–25 (Spring 1969).) A similarly balanced nondoctrinaire approach is recommended by Paul Freund, one of the most respected scholars in America, who in the Introduction to the special *Daedalus* issue to which so many references have been made, suggests: "The special problems arise with classes that are under some disability or constraint—children and prisoners. If the experiment may be of direct benefit to the child, the consent of the parent or guardian should be enough. . . . Prisoners . . . present another controversial group. The basic standard ought to be that their will should not be overborne either by threats of punishment or by promises of reward. Within those limits, although some investigators rule out prisoners as subjects, there seems to be no good reasons for depriving this group of the satisfactions of participation on an informed basis, satisfactions that to them are often great indeed, bolstering their self-esteem and furnishing links to the general community and its values." (Freund, "Introduction to the Issue 'Ethical Aspects of Experimentation With Human Subjects'," *Daedalus* xii (Spring 1969).) In connection with Freund's suggestion that prisoner involvement in experimental projects may be of direct benefit to the prisoner, Ayd points out: "Contrary to the surmise that prisoners because of personality maladjustment, are likely to be unreliable adherents to the rules of a research project, they are usually most cooperative when serving as experimental subjects. . . . Most prisoner-volunteers enjoy being a member of a group doing something for the benefit of others. As McDonald has pointed out, they develop a genuine *esprit de corps*. This can and has led to a marked improvement in behavior, independently of drug effects. . . . The improved conduct noted by many investigators who have worked with inmate volunteers indicates that participation in the research project can and does benefit them. This is true even if they are not paid. . . . Thus, being a research subject whether prisoner or nonprisoner, affords an opportunity to participate actively in a pursuit that can change modes of behavior and the ability to relate to others . . . I consider it a fundamental privilege of a prisoner to be able to have whatever psychologic and spiritual benefits can be derived from being a research subject for the welfare of others. . . . " (Ayd, *supra* at 775 and 777).)

We have spent this much time dealing with the question of prisoners because of the possible relevance to the matter of consent for involuntarily committed mental patients. But there are two important distinctions which must be borne in mind. First, throughout this discussion we have been talking of consent for medical experimentation, not consent for therpaeutic intervention. Secondly, the question of a prison environment, while comparable in some of its coercive features to any other detention, is necessarily different from that of a mental institution. In addition, just as mental institutions vary greatly one from another, so too do prisons, and therefore any generalization about prisoners is subject first to the reservation necessary for institutionalized persons generally and then to the further reservation as to how comparable prisons and institutions for the mentally incompetent really are. However, it was thought that there was sufficient relevance to warrant the discussion and indeed the relevance is supported by other work which suggests a close connection between even voluntary patients and prisoners. Dr. Calabresi, Professor of Medical Science at Brown, in commenting upon Ayd's paper, points out that although his own experience has been limited almost exclusively to patients with cancer and other severe medical disorders, he was led to say: "It struck me that there were some impressive similarities between patients with cancer and prison volunteers, which can be conveyed by the following four words: *captivity, futility, monotony,* and *dependency.*" Referring to the two categories, prisoners and cancer patients, he says further: "Both . . . are very restricted and subjugated, each by his respective predicament. Neither can readily escape from the consequences of his captivity. For example, their way of life is altered so that they can no longer plan freely for the future. . . . A sense of futility envelopes both groups. There is a loss of purpose to life and a lack of a purposeful goal or ability to anticipate meaningful accomplishments. . . ." He then discusses the similar senses of boredom in both classes of persons and the intense sense of fear and guilt which is found in both prisoners and seriously ill patients. (Calabresi, "Discussion," 13 *Clinical Pharmacology and Therapeutics* 779 (1972).)

The discussion of so-called volunteers for medical experimentation was undertaken to show how unrealistic it is to believe that the problem of consent can be solved through this mechanism. Persons volunteer who are often neurotic, if not psychotic, and the percentage of psychiatric disorders in volunteers is extraordinarily high. In addition, persons volunteer for a multiplicity of reasons; these reasons range from the desire to do good, to the desire to escape boredom, to the need for money, to the desire to establish family transfer relations with the investigator. There are all sorts of reasons, some of which we would clearly have to discount as grossly irrational. Thus it follows that asking for volunteers for human experimentation in no way avoids the ultimate difficulties of case-by-case analysis in terms of whether the consent given is legally adequate. If then this is the posture in which we find ourselves, is not the advice of so many scholars who have studied this matter the preferable, indeed the necessary, common law way of handling the matter? Avoid doctrinaire, yes-no, light switch responses to matters so subtle as those with which we are concerned in determining whether there is legally adequate consent. Instead of categorically proposing that no prisoners can consent, or that all college students can consent, or that no mentally incompetent can consent, are we not necessarily driven to the much more difficult but nonetheless unavoidable task of examining each individual on the case-by-case basis? Particularly does this counsel of wisdom become imperative when we realize that the problem with which we are concerned in this case is not consent to an experiment but consent to an experimental *but therapeutic* intervention. Indeed, the even more difficult problem which we confront is that we are here concerned with therapeutic intervention which is not designed to serve or maintain life, but to affect the quality of life. To argue that a mechanical light switch answer is available to a question of this complexity constitutes, at best, abandonment of the field to the forces of irrationality and make-believe. For surely there is no obviously rational, attractive decisional mechanism available by which the entire category of human beings who happen to have a particular status should be held to be disenfranchised from the possibility of a therapeutic intervention, even if experimental, when responsible physicians reasonably believe that that intervention may significantly and favorably affect the quality of their lives.

F. Legally adequate consent and mental incompetence. Now we will consider in greater detail the consequences of the doctrinaire application of unexamined and often irrelevant generalizations which produce quick and easy, light switch kinds of answers to the subtle problems of law, medicine, and ethics. That approach results in slogans like "voluntary patients can consent," "children can never consent," "mentally incompetent can never consent," and "involuntarily detained can never consent." We have already considered some of the inadequacies which flow from it, and some of the reasons for the rejection of any such doctrinaire appraoch. We will now consider more fully the problem in connection with the mentally incompetent person involuntarily detained at a facility within the jurisdiction of the State Department of Mental Health.

At the outset, it is important to bear in mind the careful testimony of the only witness heard in this matter who has had any significant amount of experience with patients involuntarily detained on grounds of mental incompetence. Dr. Yudashkin, it will be recalled, went into great detail to indicate that there was a wide range of differences in the personalities of persons confined in mental institutions and that the range of reactions among this spectrum of persons is not different from that which might be expected from any cross-section of the population. There are those who will submit, let alone consent, to almost anything. As Dr. Yudashkin pointed out, and as one might expect, persons are sometimes involuntarily committed because they are so overly aggressive and hostile that they fall within the statutory standard for commitment. With such personality types it is not unexpected that they will deny consent even for a therapeutic intervention which any "relatively normal" individual might welcome were the opportunity available for the correction of an abnormality which was impairing his life or its quality. In addition, we must remember that considerable support is rendered for this view as to the diversity of personality types in mental institutions by the fact that thirteen of the C.S.P.'s at Ionia, of their own accord and without any intervention, did advise petitioner in this matter that they would not under any circumstances consent. Did this not demonstrate that even within a single institution, let alone among different ones, there will be a range of reactions to the opportunity to make oneself available for an experimental therapeutic procedure? How can one argue, as did Lowinger and Watson, that the coercive environment of the institutional setting is itself enough to require the doctrinaire approach which produces a slogan such as: "Involuntarily committed persons cannot consent"? Such an approach makes sense only for a politically radical psychiatrist who takes the view that persons involuntarily detained are always so detained because of the political-social structure which led to their commitment. On such a theory, all detained persons are political prisoners, and what requires therapeutic intervention are not these "victims" of society but society itself. Lowinger, in describing the radicals' role in psychiatry, a role with which he identifies himself, says after detailing what the radical psychiatrists have been doing: "What does all this mean to psychiatry? This is a public attack on the belief in the psychiatrist, the mental hospital, the university department and community mental health centre. It is being said that these are not the authority and should no longer be believed at face value. This is also an attack on the oppression caused by many of the traditional systems of psychiatry, the use of drugs, diagnosis, commitment, individual therapy and so on. It is a recognition of psychiatry as a sedative-tranquillizing force, helping the survival of the social order, and it is a challenge to psychiatry to become a liberating force in a radical and new conception of society. . . . In any event, what are the goals of the Radical Caucus? The most important goal is the destruction of the American Psychiatric Association, which is the psychological branch of the American Medical Association. This is necessary but not sufficient if the American people are to build a new mental health system within a new health system which is community controlled, without cost to the recipient and engaged in liberating rather than imprisoning people." (Lowinger, "Radicals in Psychiatry," 17 *Canad. Psychiatric Assoc. J.*, Special Supp. II, 193 at 195 (1972).) Thus, considering the position of radicalism from which he speaks, one can at least understand the social and political motives for Dr. Lowinger's doctrinaire, radical extremism.

But if one can understand the politics of the radical psychiatrist's argument that no involuntarily detained, mentally incompetent person can consent, how does one explain the same doctrinaire approach and slogan for a psychiatrist who apparently is not a political radical? The absurdity of this doctrinaire approach is illustrated by the John Doe situation itself. On the one hand, Dr. Watson was arguing vigorously, indeed even aggressively, that John Doe was ready for release and that he was normal enough to be released, despite the history of the atrocious crimes which he had committed and despite the psychiatric literature which suggests that necrophilism is evidence of a most serious psychiatric disorder. But on the other hand, the same Dr. Watson argued with equal vigor that even the month before John Doe was normal enough to be released, he was not normal enough to give legally adequate consent. For Watson, John Doe was normal enough to change his mind, but a month earlier he was not normal enough to consent. That these contradictory postures could be argued, and argued with equal vigor, surely is a testament to Watson's intellectual and professional "flexibility." How can an individual be human enough, and endowed with a sufficiently healthy will and with adequate ego autonomy to be releasable, but at the same time so abnormal and deficient in will and ego strength that he must be denied even the *right* to consent to an experimental therapeutic intervention?

If one is tempted to lump together all persons who have in common the status of having been involuntarily detained on grounds of mental incompetence, Dr. Yudashkin's testimony should be recalled wherein he carefully distinguished several very different categories of detained persons. He pointed out, for example, that among the 16,000 in the State of Michigan, there are at least 1,000 who are satisfied with their condition, who do not wish to improve, who do not wish to leave the institution. Now, so far as concerns the consent question, ought these people be regarded as subject to so coercive an environment that they are therefore, by definition, declared to be so nonhuman that they are incapable of consenting for innovative or experimental therapeutic procedures? How can this group of a thousand human beings be "disposed of" on some such grounds, even if there are some in the institution who ought not be permitted to consent because their personalities are such that they would submit or acquiesce to almost anything? Those who are inclined to regard involuntary commitment on grounds of mental incompetence as an automatic veto on any possibility of giving legally adequate consent are fond of quoting a slogan used by Dr. Willard Gaylin which appears to offer them support. This is not to suggest that Rev. Burke adopted the extremist position, "No involuntary patient can consent." On the contrary, although he felt that consent would be very difficult in the case of persons committed on grounds of mental incompetence (a position which no rational person could deny), the whole tenor of his testimony was in opposition to the kind of irrational extremism which concludes, "No involuntary patient can consent." But nonetheless, it was in cross-examination of Rev. Burke that we encountered Gaylin's "aphorism," so frequently used to avoid the analysis which would otherwise be appropriate on the question of consent for those committed because of mental incompetence.

"The damaged organ is the organ of consent"—this is the aphorism attributed to Dr. Gaylin, which is supposed inevitably to lead to the conclusion that mentally incompetent persons (voluntarily detained or not) are incapable of giving legally adequate consent. The theory here is that since the brain is itself the organ which is crucial for the decision on consent, and since by definition (since mentally incompetent) that organ is diseased, that diseased organ cannot give consent. At first blush, there is a certain facile logic which seems to make this argument attractive. But, as is almost always the case in matters of morals, slogans confuse more than they illuminate and this slogan is no exception. If the brain is diseased, and therefore cannot consent, how may one come to the conclusion that the same diseased organ can *deny* consent? It surely must be true that if there is a disease of the organ which diminishes its cognitive or emotional capacities, then the disease must be symmetrical. If the brain is too diseased to consent, how can it not be too diseased to deny consent? If consent is construed as a process which is largely cognitive, and if the organs or system of organs are so diseased that they are cognitively or emotionally impaired to the degree which makes it impossible for them to provide meaningful consent, then is it not necessarily the case that that organ is also so impaired that it canot furnish meaningful denial of consent?

If we do then attach real signigicance to the idea that "the damaged organ is the organ of consent," what consequences follow as regards consent? There would seem to be two plausible possibilities: (1) any person who is declared mentally incompetent, and who is therefore presumed to have a "damaged organ," is treated like those lower, nonhuman animals who, because they are "lower" animals, are presumed incapable of either consenting or not; and (2) each mentally incompetent person is not therefore stripped of his humanity, but is instead made the beneficiary of special protections because he may, because of his incompetence, suffer from a "damaged organ" or from an organ which is damaged in different ways. The point here (again) is the need to avoid treating the status (mental incompetency) as the only relevant criterion for so crucial and subtle a matter as legally adequate consent. And treating "damaged organ" as the litmus paper test is surely no improvement whatsoever.

There is a further aspect of the "damaged organ" approach which requires attention. Those who take the view that mental incompetence necessarily implies the impossibility of securing legally adequate consent (and ignoring here the possibilities for consent by legal represetation) often conclude that because the individual cannot give consent he must be presumed to deny consent. We have already noted the logical defect in this argument and here call attention to a further defect. Even if it were accepted as persuasive that inability to give legally adequate consent necessarily implied denial of consent, and therefore rejection of the experimental therapeutic intervention, does not attaching this consequence to the "action" of the "damaged organ" violate the very hypothesis which underlies the "damaged organ" argument? Is not that hypothesis the belief that because the organ is damaged the organ ought not be permitted to make important decisions? Yet, is not the continuation of the patient in his present condition (because the experimental intervention is rejected) just such an important decision? The point here is that doing nothing is doing something! And allowing the individual to remain as he is is a serious decision and one which has enormous consequences for that individual. Consequently, if there is any strength to the "damaged organ" hypothesis it compels acceptance *not* of the conclusion that nothing should be done with the subject (because he cannot consent), but rather of the conclusion that, whatever decision is made about what should be done, it is a decision in which the "damaged organ" is *not* the *crucial* factor!

Most clinical investigators, and certainly the doctors in this case, reject the "diseased organ" hypothesis, not because it is entirely inadequate, but rather because it leads, and leads logically, to a conclusion which is unacceptable. It is the conclusion which would require the doctor to subject the mentally incompetent person to an experimental procedure despite the objections of that person. Yet most clinicians, and certainly the doctors in this case, would be personally unwilling to subject a person to any experimental therapeutic procedure if that person objected and even if that person were a very serious mental incompetent of very low I.Q. What is more, most doctors, and certainly those involved in this case, would be unwilling to carry out a therapeutic experimental procedure under the above circumstances even if there had been legally adequate consent by the legal representatives. Surely there may be cases which will push this problem to the limit (e.g., a self-mutilating, mentally retarded, dangerously aggressive patient who, despite an I.Q. of 20, while incapable of speech, nonetheless resists efforts at subjecting him to an innovative therapeutic intervention which it is believed will significantly improve his condition). Fortunately, this is not the case before this court and we need not decide even more difficult hypothetical cases in order to decide the sufficiently difficult one now before us.

The further defect in the "diseased organ cannot consent" argument is the failure to appreciate that the doctrine of consent has not just one but, as previously pointed out, two different functions. The doctrine functions to recognize and protect the essential dignity of the human personality and to acknowledge the fact that we deal with a human being and not an experimental animal. It is important that this symbolic function of consent not be suppressed even when there is primary concern with the other (medical-legal) concern with consent. However, on the other hand, one can argue that there can be no therapeutic intervention when the consenting organ is damaged only if one takes the extremist position that the symbolic function of consent is more important than the therapeutic function. But here again we see the danger of rushing into an extremist blind alley rather than proceeding carefully to make the necessary cost-benefit analysis which is required if we are to avoid unnecessary irrationalities. On such a cost-benefit analysis, the Gaylin slogan is highly suspicious, at least in a case such as the one now before this court where the individual is offered the possibility of an experimental procedure which is therapeutic for him. What is more, the therapy is directed at the very organ which is admittedly damaged. Thus to use the "diseased organ cannot consent" argument in the case of innovative or experimental *therapy* is entirely inconsistent with the reasons for the doctrine of consent, which is both to protect the dignity of the individual *and* to assure that only those therapies will be utilized which are appropriate for the given individual case. The doctrine of consent functions to individualize therapy and not to make individuals either subject to or immune from a therapeutic modality just because of their status as members of a certain class. The "diseased organ cannot consent" argument on the other hand, does just the opposite: it makes status as members of a class the exclusive criterion for exclusion from a whole range of therapy modalities.

Professor Jaffe of the Harvard Law School extends this argument even further and applies it also to the case of nontherapeutic experimentation. He writes: "In the search for rules as opposed to general standards, there is a disposition to conclude that certain classes of persons are not proper subjects of experimentation. Thus it may be said that children, the feeble-minded, the aged, and prisoners should never be the subjects of experimentation. These conclusions may rest—in the cases of children, the feeble-minded, or the aged—on the notion that such persons are not in a position to understand the risks involved or the nature of the experiment and thus cannot give a meaningful consent. In the case of prisoners, the objections are more obscure, but they rest, perhaps, on the notion that prisoners are under pressures to give consent which put them to unfair advantage or which are inconsistent with the aims of the criminal law. Reasoning of this sort, I would suggest, improperly makes consent an ultimate or absolute value irrespective of the interest that consent is designed to protect. A rule forbidding experimentation on a given class of persons may exclude experimentation of value to that class. Even where that is not the case, to prohibit the use of an available source of subjects may unnecessarily hobble experimentation and deprive members of a given class of an opportunity to participate that they might welcome." (Jaffe, *supra* at 423.)

There is a further reason for questioning the "diseased organ cannot consent" argument. Much of the strength of this argument would seem to be drawn from the belief that, since the organ is diseased, it ought not be subject to any coercion—an idea which at first seems highly commendable and consistent with the development of the emerging law as to adhesion contracts where gross disparities in bargaining power may be the basis for judicial intervention to protect overreaching. However, in applying this kind of thinking to our present problem, there are two distinguishing considerations that need be borne in mind. First, while the law seeks to protect the weaker party from overreaching by the stronger party, it does not deny the weaker party the possibility for contracting. (See the discussion on this point by Dawson in Katz at 560 and after.) In addition, the adhesion contract argument applied to the mentally incompetent is in one important respect seriously misleading. In the economic contract area the doctrines of adhesion and duress make considerable good sense. Leaving the weaker party where he was before the contract by refusing to enforce the contract probably leaves him no worse than he would be if he were made to perform the contract. But the same cannot be said for the mentally incompetent individual who if denied the possibility of "contracting" will indeed be left in his original position. However, that position is not one which is at all comparable to the position which the incompetent might occupy where he permitted to "contract" for the experimental therapeutic intervention. In other words, leaving parties where they were before the alleged adhesion contract was signed may make some sense in the domain of economic contracting but it does not have equal applicability in the area with which we are here concerned because leaving the diseased organ where it was (because it is diseased) is precisely to defeat the very reason for the therapeutic intervention.

This last argument is also applicable to some situations where a mentally incompetent person is permitted to "consent" to a nontherapeutic medical experiment because the knowledge to be gained from the experiment might lead to a therapeutic intervention. However, we are here defending only the propriety of permitting consent for the therapeutic interventions. In such cases it is impossible to deny that, if one argues that the mentally incompetent, involuntarily detained person can neither consent nor deny consent, then he surely is left in his original position. In addition, as is the case with the argument about coercion, so too with the "damaged organ" theory. If it is concluded that the person cannot consent, this conclusion is functionally equivalent to holding that he can deny consent. And the pragmatic consequence of *attributing* a denial of consent to the patient (who is said to be legally incapable of consenting) is *not* to protect the patient from coercion, but rather to subject him to a different coercion. Now he is coerced into remaining in his original (abnormal) condition. He is legally denied the possibility of "consenting" to the procedure which could improve his condition. He is denied the one possibility which is thought to hold out a hope for his therapeutic improvement. Therefore, if the basis for the belief that mentally incompetent, involuntarily detained patients should be unable to consent is either the damaged organ or institutional coercion hypothesis, it is perfectly clear that the best interests of the mentally incompetent detained person are compromised because he is anyway coerced, but now he is coerced into staying just as he is. In addition, it is important to remember that doing nothing always means doing something in medicine, and doing nothing may be just as much, if not more, of an experiment than doing something. So that by denying the patient any chance to consent he is anyway being coercively treated, and, what is more, he is being treated in a negative way which may be highly experimental and, by definition, he is not being given the treatment of choice from the medical point of view. We are compelled to recognize that there is no way to escape from the coercion problem. And sometimes doing something is less experimental than doing nothing. All of us, whether institutionalized or not, are subject to coercion all the time. Hence the problems for the law are how to minimize the adverse effects of improper coercion and how to structure institutional relationships so as to insure the maximum degree of freedom from coercion consistent with the legitimate demands of society and of the individual.

The problem of consent for mentally incompetent persons is not one which is either new or novel. On the contrary, the common law of England has long recognized, as does the common law in the United States, that when an individual lacks capacity to act for himself because of incompetence, then someone else may, in appropriate cases, act for the benefit of that individual. (For example, see *Crippen v. Pulliam,* 61 Wash. 2d 725, 380 P.2d 475 (1963).) In addition, there are decisions which recognize that an individual may be legally capable of giving consent for some purposes but not for all. (For example, see *Lacey v. Laid,* 166 Ohio St. 12, 139 N.E. 2d 25 (1956).) In addition, American decisions recognize that in the case of children who because of age lack competence to consent, their parents may grant consent for medically appropriate treatment. (See, for example, *People v. Pierson,* 196 N.Y. 201, 68 N.E. 243 (1903).) However, parental consent might not be permitted if the child were to be exposed to greater danger than necessary. (See, for example, *Mitchell v. Davis,* 205 S.W. 2d 812, (Tex. Civ. App. 1947).)

There is thus well-established precedent for granting to someone other than the individual patient the power to consent where the patient lacks capacity for any one of several reasons, and in addition there is the well-established practice in medicine of telling the patient's family or friends things which are not told to the patient himself so that the doctor may feel more readily justified in acting where the family or friends concur in the proposed therapeutic intervention. This surrogate "informed consent" is especially common where life-threatening procedures are thought necessary for therapeutic purposes. Indeed, there are decisions which hold that in exceptional circumstances standard medical practice would warrant the physician in withholding details from the patient when to do so is thought to be in the best interest of the patient, even though good medical practice in such situations would warrant disclosure to the patient's family or friends. (See, for example, *Kennedy v. Parrott,* 243 N.C. 355, 90 S.E.2d 754 (1956); *Natanson v. Kline,* 186 Kan. 393, 350 P.2d 1093, *aff'd on rehearing,* 187 Kan. 186, 354 P.2d 670 (1960).) Even the policy statement of the FDA regarding consent for use of investigational new drugs provides that "regulations on use of investigational new drugs on humans shall impose the condition that investigators obtain the consent of the such human beings *or their representatives* except where they deem it not feasible or in their professional judgment contrary to the best interest of such human beings." (Quoted in Katz at 573.) Thus not only does the FDA permit a legal representative to grant consent, but also nondisclosure is permitted in exceptional circumstances. As might be expected, the provision which permits the use of a new drug even without consent "in exceptional circumstances" has generated considerable controversy and has been the source of much difficulty in the literature and in practice. Dr. Francis Kelsey, who was then chief of the FDA's Investigational Drug Branch, Division of New Drugs, stated in what is probably the most authoritative statement on the matter: "In the final analysis the law is clear in that the basic rule is that the patient consent must be obtained except where a conscientious professional judgment is made that this is not feasible or is contrary to the best interest of the patient." (Quoted in Curran, *supra* at 559, with citation to the original source.) It is interesting to notice that when pressed to the wall, the standard relied upon by Kelsey was "conscientious professional judgment" and that the FDA, although so concerned with the regulation of new drugs, was unable to provide any more manageable standard than one which ultimately rested on such professional judgment. It is also worth observing that not only does the FDA permit nondisclosure and consent by relatives or friends, but also that the same practice is observed in Veterans' Administration programs. Writing about the VA procedure, Shaw and Chalmers say: "The success of a program of therapy depends to a consdierable degree upon the confidence and mutual trust between the patient and the physician. Excessively detailed informed consent can seriously disrupt this relationship. Thus, while 'informed consent' is a required feature of VA clinical studies, in practice the degree of informing is scaled to fit the needs of the patient, with due regard to his physical and emotional health and his capacity to comprehend in more or less detail the alternative therapies. In the case of the critically ill patient, thorough cataloging of the pros and cons of the alternative forms of therapy may be considered to be against the best interest of the patient. In such a circumstance and in the case of the mentally incompetent patient, the nearest relative must give his consent and be kept informed. Thus, varying degrees of compromise are adopted in accordance with the physician's judgment of what is in the best interest for the patient's welfare. The peer review committees are charged with reviewing and approving the propriety of the technique of obtaining informed consent as a safeguard for the patient's welfare and a check on the physician's judgment." (Shaw and Chalmers, "Ethics in Cooperative Clinical Trials," 169 *Annals of New York Academy of Sciences* 487 at 492 (1970).) Not only to the FDA and the VA permit nondisclosure and consent by a "legal representative," but also Dr. Leo Alexander, who was consultant for the Nuremberg Trials, and whose memorandum on medical experimentation to the War Crimes Court became the basis for the so-called Nuremberg Code, specificaly permits mentally ill patients to consent for medical experimentation through their next of kin or legal guardian, when they themselves are incapacitated, or as he puts it, "delirious or confused." (See Alexander, "Psychiatry: Methods and Processes for Investigation of Drugs," 169 *New York Academy of Science Annals* 344 at 349 (1970).) (Neither his proposal nor his memorandum to the War Crimes Court was limited to the experimental use of drugs.) In addition, Alexander is talking about experimentation, although he limited it to "experiments concerning the nature and treatment of nervous and mental illness or related subjects." It is nonetheless still experimentation, whereas our problem, as has been stressed, is not experimentation but consent for innovative or experimental therapy. Pope Pius XII, in a statement to the First International Congress of Neuropathology, on the moral limits of medical research and treatment, said: "What we say here must be extended to the *legal representatives* of the person incapable of caring for himself and his affairs; children below the age of reason, the feeble-minded and the insane. These legal representatives, authorized by private decision or public authority have no other rights over the body and life of those they represent than those people would have themselves if they were capable. And they have those rights to the same extent. They cannot, therefore, give the doctor permission to dispose of them outside those limits." (Katz 549 at 551.)

In light of the above, we must conclude that as regards permitting the legal representative to furnish legally adequate consent for one lacking the capacity himself there is both ample legal precedent and persuasive moral authority. Perhaps the matter has been well summed up by Maurice Visscher, an exceptionally distinguished medical researcher, who takes an even more extreme view than that which is here under consideration, if one remembers that he is talking about experimentation and not merely about innovative or experimental therapy. He says: "The dilemma which I have outlined confronting the ethical investigator is, stated simply: 'What is one's moral obligation when a problem of social significance is under study, and the only subjects that can be studied are unable, because of their age or physical condition, to give 'uncoerced informed consent'? One school of thought says only that it is unfortunate for society, and perhaps for the patient himself, but the principle of requiring individual informed consent is so important that it must never be abrogated. Another school, to which I belong, says that no principle ever stands alone as paramount, but that rather an entire situation must be evaluated before an ethical judgment can be reached. I have come to the conclusion that when some benefit can reasonably be expected to accrue to individuals who are incompetent to give meaningful consent, either because of their age or their disease state, and when proper previous studies and consultation give the assurance that Percival required, there is justification for eliminating the individual consent requirement. This does not mean that parents or guardians of children should not retain the right to refuse consent, nor that relatives should not have such rights in the case of the unconscious or disoriented adult, but it does mean that failure to obtain the informed consent of the individual subject is not *ipso facto* a breach of ethics." (Visscher, "The Two Sides of the Coin and the Regulation of Experimental Medicine," 169 *New York Academy of Sciences Annals* 319 at 324 (1970).)

From the above discussion it would seem that the following are the primary areas of concern: (1) if anyone can ever give legally adequate consent, what is the unsurmountable barrier which would warrant denying to all involuntarily detained patients or their legal representatives the opportunity to consent?; (2) is it more degrading or less degrading to say that the right to consent is denied to committed persons and their legal representatives?; (3) is it more humane or less humane to permit consent by those detained or by those acting on their behalf, when the consent is for innovative or experimental medical therapy?; (4) do we accord greater respect to the essential human dignity of detained persons by permitting them to remain unchanged in their existing condition or by permitting someone to act for them, if they cannot themselves, in a situation where there is hope for improving their condition?; and finally, and most important, (5) may it not be argued that the only time consent is more than symbolic for *any* person confronted with a serious medical decision, is when there is an adequate legal representative available, who is not under the coercion of the confinement, be it allegedly voluntary or allegedly involuntary, and who is not under the disability either of brain or other bodily abnormality which adversely affects free will? Consequently, perhaps the most impressive argument for permitting consent, no matter what one may say about the subject himself, may be made when the consent is given by a legal representative.

We cannot pretend that there are clear and obvious answers for each or any of these questions. On the contrary, as has been suggeted above, that which strikes one as obvious is likely to be misleading in matters as subtle as these. But we do think it appropriate to ask whether the law and society come out better on moral, social, or medical grounds if the law adopts the doctrinaire, light switch approach and holds that no involuntarily detained person nor his legal representative may ever consent to a therapeutic intervention if it is experimental or innovative. Or need we rather proceed as the common law characteristically does and avoid the status question in favor of rules which accomodate cases on an individual basis? Where issues as subtle as these need be decided, and where the relevant social policies are so complex, it would seem that as a minimum, the court ought not to adopt an approach which in effect treats committed persons as less than human. Despite the "civil rights" posture alleged to be advanced by those who maintain that no involuntarily committed person should ever be able to consent to an experimental or innovative medical therapy, their position strikes us quite the contrary because in reality it is antithetical to even the minimum human rights of committed people. By denying them the possibility to consent their humanity is denied, and then to add gratuitous injury to undeserved offense, we deny that anyone can even act to preserve whatever humanity is left to him. Not only are these committed persons deprived of their liberty (for reasons which may vary from very good to very poor), but because they are deprived of their liberty, we shall also deprive them of their humanity. If they are incapable of consenting, and no one is capable of consenting on their behalf, what does it mean to say that they are still human beings?

The reasoning which requires that a legal representative be permitted to furnish legally adequate consent when the subject himself lacks capacity in no way diminishes the duty to inform the subject himself to whatever extent he is capable of comprehending the problem. Nor do we have a clear answer to the problem of whether an experimental therapeutic procedure should be carried out if the subject denies consent (despite his diminished capacity) when his legal representative does consent. Of course, there is considerable disagreement on this matter and there are interesting precedents for deciding either way. Probably most doctors, and certainly those involved in this case, take the view that if the subject himself does not consent, even if his legal representative does consent, the procedure ought not be initiated. However, this question is peripheral to the most crucial matter before this court and therefore will not here be pursued any further.

It does not require much imagination to recognize that the issue the court needs to consider here is but the tip to the iceberg of a much larger, and indeed overwhelming, philosophical problem. To what extent, and how, may the law continue properly to protect the freedom of individuals against the threat of manipulation of human behavior by scientific technologies? Obviously, this is not the place to pursue this philosophical matter in depth; perhaps it will suffice to suggest that the law does surely have a role, as it always has had in the regulation of human conduct, and that the place for the law here, as it characteristically has been in the common law, is to avoid sweeping the problem under the moral rug by adoption of a doctrinaire solution which hides the problem rather than deals with it. In addition, we need to recognize that even though experimental medical interventions may control human behavior, it does not follow that failure to permit the intervention means that the behavior of the subject will not be controlled. Rather it means only that the behavior will be controlled differently. Permitting the mentally incompetent subject to remain in his existing condition is also behavior control; permitting him and/or his representative to consent to a procedure which is intended to change his behavior (i.e., the procedure is therapeutic) is also behavior control, as is *anything* else done to or with the person. So the problem of freedom versus behavior control is in no way avoided if the court were to hold that mentally incompetent people involuntarily detained can never consent. It would only mean that the field is abandoned to irrational forces, irrational because this group believes that freedom is preserved against those who would manipulate the behavior of the patient by denying the patient or his representative all freedom—freedom to consent. The point here is that there is always manipulation of behavior and the question is how best to construct institutional mechanisms for the proper protection of freedom while accommodating other legitimate social objectives. The point is *not* how can the courts best avoid the issue! The issue is unavoidable!

As Roger Ulrich said at the 1967 Harvard conference on behavior control technologies: "The thought that some day human behavior might be brought under scientific control in the same manner that other natural events have been is repugnant to some because it seems to imply a corresponding loss of freedom of choice that human beings are supposed to possess. Another basis of apprehension is the tendency to think of behavioral control in terms of *Brave New World* or *1984*; that is, in terms of control by coercion, punishment, or restriction, technically called, 'aversive stimulus control.' A third general basis for concern is the fear that people will lose individuality or dignity. Ostensibly these are all legitimate concerns; but let us examine them more closely. When we visit a mental hospital and observe the despair of patients for whom reality is so unpleasant that they can no longer respond to it, can we honestly say that these people would be deprived of dignity if their environments were controlled in such a way as to make their lives meaningful? When we read daily of youngsters who, for reasons beyond their control—accident of birth, cultural deprivation, and so on—drop out of school or commit delinquent or criminal acts, is it meaningful to say that we have deprived them of freedom of choice if we can manipulate their environment in such a way as to make them more productive citizens? Does it make sense to become preoccupied with what may be pseudo-problems of dignity and self-determination when we consider what might be done for the millions of so-called mentally retarded children presently destined to live in institutions as 'vegetables'? . . . Although the potential dangers of behavorial control certainly require careful consideration, the majority of debates about behaviorly control actually miss the point. Too much time is consumed by the question of whether behavioral control can or should be effected. Men *can* and *do* control the behavior of other men. Our culture must accept the assumption that man is an organism which obeys certain laws of behavior and that the control of human nature is a ubiquitous fact. Questions of goals, methods, and choice of practitioners are of extreme importance, but are premature if used as arguments against the implementation of behavioral control. . . . If we refuse to apply our knowledge of behavior we are not simply taking a neutral position. Rather, we are endorsing other forms of control that gain in potency as we withhold the competition offered by our methods." (Mendelsohn, Swazey, and Taviss, "The Harvard Conference on Behavior Control in Human Aspects of Biomedical Innovation," in Mendelsohn, Swazey, and Taviss, *Human Aspects of Biomedical Innovation* 111 at 116–17 (1971).)

What respondents are here urging to the court is that it not abandon all mentally incompetent committed persons to the forces of irrationality, that it not blind itself to the fact that if such persons or their representatives can or cannot consent, such persons will in either event be subject to behavior control technologies. It is simply a question of which kind of technologies and by whom they shall be employed. Such committed persons will be controlled in any event, as are we all, and therefore the real issue is how the court can best protect the proper freedom of such committed persons. It is our contention that this is not done by abandoning them to the forces of irrationality which would treat memebership in a class (the involuntarily committed) as a sufficient reason for destroying what is left of the humanity and individuality of persons who have been unfortunate enough already to requre institutionalization.

In our analysis of the consent problem we have thus far deliberately avoided interjecting the further element of consent for a particular type of innovative or experimental procedure and specifically for the type which is concerned with surgery on the brain. It is our view that only if one takes some metaphysical and irrational position about the mind can there be any reason for differentiating the brain from other organs of the human system. Only if one is prepared to follow Dr. Breggin's metphysics into the realm of mystical speculation might one conclude that there is something about the mind which constitutes the seat of the soul or that there is something about the mind, as distinguised from the brain, which requires that the mind and/or brain never be touched, no matter what it means for the rest of the operating human system. Such a view, bordering as it does on almost medieval metaphysical obscurities, can only serve to confuse an already difficult matter. Surely we gain no illumination on the subtle problems with which we are concerned if we begin from a position of irrationality, a position for which there is no demonstrable evidence, a position for which not even faith provides much help, for there is surely no reason to believe on the basis of faith or feeling that a mind exists apart from the brain housed in our bodies. To think that the brain may not be touched no matter what it means for the rest of the operating organism involves the most crude kind of philosophical speculation about mind-body problems.

To correct a tumor is apparently permissible, but to correct a lesion which is destroying the effective operation of the brain is somehow magically wrong. It is difficult to draw any line of this kind in theory, let alone in practice, and a theoretical argument which maintains such a view is entirely inconsistent with any medically or philosphically rational conceptualization of the relationship of mind and body. Only by some kind of magic could one be led to the belief that the brain should not be touched to correct a physical lesion, but could be touched to correct a tumor, and that only when a tumor is involved does the somatic condition of the rest of the body warrant the intervention. The hypothesis which underlines this magical kind of thinking is so extreme that it is difficult to deal with it cogently in argument. Perhaps it will suffice to suggest that the arguments built on the sanctity of the mind are internally inconsistent if they permit tumors to be removed from the brain but do not permit other surgical interventions, and even more glaringly inconsistent when they permit a temporal lobectomy for the control of epileptic behavior but deny other surgical procedures, much less drastic than temporal lobectomy, when these latter procedures are for the control of paraepileptic behavior. In addition, the "mind is sacred" thesis does not even have the status of a religious argument of the kind which could be made for a Jehovah's Witness who did not wish to have a blood transfusion. While one could cogently argue in support of a Jehovah's Witness's right to die rather than have his religious belief suppressed in favor of a medical intervention, there is no comparable argument which can be made for the sacred mind thesis. Or if this thesis is a religious article of faith, then let the law protect those who hold this faith from neurosurgical or psychosurgical procedures, but let not the law impose the religious commitment upon all of society any more than it imposes the Witness's objection to blood transfusion upon all of society! To argue, as did Breggin, that a self-mutilating, dying mental incompetent may not consent or have anyone consent on his behalf to surgical procedures on the brain because there is something special, unique, or magical about the brain is to capitulate to the forces of irrationality and to deprive modern medicine of any plausible scientific basis. Such a view would move medicine back beyond the dark ages and require that we try to comfort the self-mutilating, dying person by advising him that the magic of his brain has not been interfered with and that he will die with that magic intact. We must say we find little comfort in this position, and were we the self-mutilating mentally incompetent, we should hope that some more realistic comfort would be accorded us than to advise us that the magic of our diseased brain will be permitted to remain intact.

It has been mentioned before, but merits stressing, that we are here concerned in this declaratory action not with the question of legally adequate consent for an experimental procedure, but rather with the question of consent in the instance of an individual who is mentally incompetent but who is considered a suitable subject for an innovative or experimental medical procedure which is believed to be therapeutic. It is to be noticed that in the hypothetical question the parameters of decision make it quite clear that existing modalities have not succeeded, and that in the event that the procedure proposed involves surgery on the brain, there need first be demonstrable organicity in the brain, and further, that the procedure is believed to be one which will correct the abnormal condition attributable to that organicity. While one may argue the medical questions, it is important to notice the question presented to the court does not require for its answer the answers which are given to these medical questions. On the contrary, it is presumed by the question that the modalities of treatment available have failed, that there is organicity, that the procedure is designed to relieve the abnormality attributable to that organicity, and that the abnormality is tormenting to the individual or so disruptive that he cannot live safely or live safely with others. What we need to stress is that, while these elements are treated by us below, the problem for decision by the court in this declaratory action is not dependent upon the answers to these medical or scientific or philosphical questions. Rather the question for the court, as put by the hypothetical case, presupposes that the fact pattern is the one indicated; namely, should an involuntarily detained person or his representative be denied the opportunity to participate with the rest of humanity in a cure which is believed to be available, just because that individual is either incompetent or detained? We find no basis in reason, justice, law, or medicine for concluding that because an individual has been committed on grounds of insanity or incompetency he therefore ceases to be human and may therefore be deprived of the rights of his humanity. On the contrary, it is our view that it is precisely because he has already been subjected by the forces of nature, accident, birth, or society to a condition which requires his involuntary detention that he ought to be placed first in the line to receive potentially curative medical therapy rather than being denied even the possibility of getting into line.

G. The Right to Treatment and the Problem of Consent. It is precisely considerations such as those last mentioned which bring us to the topic of present concern: are not persons who are involuntarily committed deserving of more than detention? Is this not what the right to treatment is all about? Have not courts constructed the right to treatment out of an awareness of the fact that persons involuntarily committed are deserving of more than custodial care? Does not the right to treatment carry with it a duty on the part of the state to make available to committed persons modern medical therapy?

The one question which no right to treatment case has yet confronted, let alone answered, is whether an individual may be continaully detained once properly committed because there is no treatment modality available for his cure or improvement. The problem will be the same no matter whether the standard be that of *Rouse,* "treatment which is adequate in light of present knowledge," or that of Judge Bazelan (writing in a law review), "therapy which recognizes psychiatric opinion generally regards as falling within the range of acceptable alternatives," or the *Nason* suggestion of "therapy determined by competent doctors in their best judgment within the limits of permissable practice." No matter to which criterion we appeal, there will remain the problem of whether, even if there is a right to treatment, an individual may be detained involuntarily at a mental facility because having once been properly committed there is now no known treatment modality which satisfies any of these tests. If to this we add the complexity which would follow from the proposal that would deny involuntarily detained persons or their legal representatives the possibility of consenting to innovative or experimental medical procedures which were intended to be therapeutic, we are left with an even worse dilemma. Now we have the problem of a patient involuntarily committed, and therefore the beneficiary of the right to treatment, and a treatment modality being offered which may lead to release, but the patient is not even capable of being considered for the procedure because neither he nor his representative can give legally adequate consent. We find it unthinkable that there might be a proper "right to treatment" but no right to an available treatment for which consent is required, even though in the opinion of the medical experts the treatment may lead to release or significant improvement.

There are two extremes in connection with this right to treatment issue; in our view both are unattractive and legally untenable. There are those who argue on the basis of vaccination cases such as *Jacobson v. Massachusetts,* 197 U.S. 11 (1904), that if there is a right to treatment then those persons who have that right are subject to the duty of submitting to treatment which is deemed to be appropriate. There are at the other extreme those who would say that even if there is an appropriate treatment, nonetheless neither the involuntarily committed patient nor his representative can consent to such treatment. We find both of these extremist positions defective for three reasons: (1) both are inconsistent with basic human rights; (2) both are contrary to the principles of reasonable management of committed patients; and (3) both are incompatible with the legitimate interest of society and with the protection of freedom which the courts are supposed to insure. It is rather our view that if there is a right to treatment then the right requires that the benficiary of the right or his legal representative be permitted to consent to an innovative or experimental medical procedure on the brain or elsewhere, if such treatment is deemed appropriate for the cure of improvement of the abnormality which requires the involuntary detention of that individual.

In short then, we urge the court to recognize that if there is a right to treatment which protects involuntarily committed mental patients, of necessity there must be no effort made to preclude at least the possibility that such persons, or those acting on their behalf, are given the opportunity to consider and to consent to innovative or experimental medical procedures designed to be therapeutic. To hold that there is a right to treatment but that no involuntarily committed patient may under any circumstances consent to such innovative or experimental therapy is both inconsistent and evidence of the kind of irrational extremism which is contrary to the common law way of dealing with problems concerning the protection of human freedoms. The common law method for dealing with human freedom questions is on a case-by-case basis, and this method stands in contrast to those who think all actual or imagined threats to freedom can be dealt with by sweeping legislation.

Respondents have urged the court to confront the realities of the consent situation and to recognize that, if not always at least characteristically, consent for medical intervention is at best symbolic, and even though we might not wish to require that a legal representative always consent to a medical procedure which involved risk, at least for cases involving involuntarily committed persons there is both good precedent and good reason for urging such a measure. However, we do not wish to create the impression that it is our view that consent by the subject and consent by a legal guardian are of themselves the most important source of protection for the human and medical rights of persons involuntarily detained who are considered for a surgical intervention on the brain which might be innovative or experimental, even though therapeutic. Rather, we believe that this is but one useful element in protecting human rights and turn next to the more general problem of balancing the various relevant interests and to the further question of what kinds of institutional mechanisms can best effect that balance.

II. The Possibility of a Prohibition Upon Therapeutic Interventions Because Innovative or Experimental.

A. The Price of Safety. Important as is the question of legally adequate consent for one involuntarily detained, even more important is the matter which the court need now consider, and furthermore it is exceedingly important to bear in mind that, despite all the discussion about experimentation and investigation, such is not the problem before this Court. This must be stressed again and again. This Court is confronted with the significantly different issue of whether or not there should be judicial determination that a particular procedure is to be prohibited in the State of Michigan, even though it is recognized as being regarded as therapeutic by the doctors concerned with the case, even though the doctor intends the procedure to be therapeutic, and even though the motive of the doctor in undertaking the work is to provide therapy and not merely investigative experimentation. Whether that therapeutic intervention should nonetheless be subject to some prohibition because it is experimental or innovative is the sole issue this Court needs to decide in connection with the second so-called hypothetical before the Court. It is extraordinarily difficult to deal with this matter not because the intellectual issues themselves are difficult—that is quite enough—but rather because there has never been a decision in a common law country, nor to our knowledge in a civil law country, where a court has acted to impose a prohibition upon a therapeutic intervention in some general category of cases. Rather, as is characteristic of the common law method, the courts have been willing to use the traditional mechanism of liability for medical malpractice when the case concerned a therapeutic intervention which was experimental. In these cases, though there has been consent and even though the consent has been informed, when the intervention was "too experimental," or to use more traditional language, was not warranted by the standards applicable to the situation as it confronted the doctor, the patient, and ultimately the court, then there might be a basis for a malpractice action. Consequently, in terms of the existing common law there is absolutely no precedent whatsoever, either in the decisional law or in practice, for a court-imposed prohibition upon a medical intervention for a whole class of cases because of some theoretical objection to the procedure per se.

At this point we pass over any discussion of the alleged objectionableness of the specific procedure considered in this matter, and are concerned here only in pointing out that there is not a single precedent of any kind applicable to the decision which this Court is being asked to make. Nor is it by accident that there is an absence of precedent in this area, for there are perfectly good reasons, and indeed in our opinion overwhelming reasons, why no court has been willing to accept responsiblity for prohibiting medical interventions in whole classes of cases when in the opinion of the treating doctor and those concerned with the medical welfare of the individual, there was good reason to believe that the medical intervention was appropriate.

It is perfectly true that absolute safety in medical research could be attained, safety in the sense that no one would ever suffer any experimental risk. It is simply that the price may be one we are unwilling to pay. It is also perfectly clear that the price we are willing to pay is determined by the conventional cost-benefit mechanism where we let the market control the choice between risks and human suffering. (See the discussion on this point and the analogy to accident prevention with automobiles in Calabresi, "Reflections on Medical Experimentation in Humans," *Daedalus* 387 (Spring 1969).) We do not wish to suggest, nor does Calabresi in his analogy with automobile accidents, that the lives selected on a rather individual basis for risks in medicine are comparable to the lives lost through accident in the use of automobiles. However, it is perfectly clear that we do make decisions in both domains knowing perfectly well that lives and the quality of life will be affected by the decisions made. We do not suggest that the sacrifice of human life or the risk to human life is made more acceptable by calling it an inevitable "social cost" of medical research. Rather, we wish to stress here that if the goal is zero risk in medical research and in the practice of medicine, then it is simply the case that medical research would have to be terminated. But it is equally clear that such an alternative may ultimately extract an even higher price than the price we now pay.

As of this date in the history of the development of medicine, it is reasonably clear that in excess of a hundred people die each year from aspirin alone, that probably something like 300 babies a year die from vaccination, and that probably as many as a thousand persons a year die from penicillin. Yet we continue to permit the use of all these (nonexperimental?) treatment modalities and make that decision because the risk is balanced against the benefit. (See Barnes, "Clinical Studies in the Human: Ethical and Scientific Problems," at 23 *Fertility and Sterility* 593 (1972); and Howard, "The Stagnation of Therapeutic Progress," 14 *Psychosomatics* 12 (1973).) In the last cited article it is pointed out that as the result of the rigid requirements for drug use and development in the United States, "between 1963 and 1970, Americans discovered 133 new drugs; the French, 137; West Germans, 82; Swiss, 39. In the same period there were only 35 new drugs introduced in the United States, but 156 were introduced in France and 118 in West Germany. In other words, we introduced only 1 out of 4 new drugs discovered in the United States. . . . In less than a decade, the United States has slipped from world leadership in pharmaceutical development to position 5." (Howard, *supra* at 12.) It is necessary to recognize that our decision to risk an almost zero risk rate for drug progress has been in part a reaction to the thalidomide disaster and that the decision to prevent the introduction of new drugs has extracted a price in the availability of drugs in the United States. It is also perfectly clear that we have been unwilling to accept a comparable zero or near zero risk for other important predictable areas of human loss. For example, we are prepared to tolerate something in the range of 250,000 deaths per year from cigarette addiction, over 50,000 from automobile accidents, and probably in excess of 2,000 from firearms. We need to recognize that in any domain where risk is an element, the price of zero risk is likely to be zero progress or the loss of some other benefit.

In the field of medicine it is certainly reasonable to recognize that there are all kinds of subtle factors at work in deciding whether or not an experimental procedure ought be persued. But in the domain of therapy this problem is even more complicated. For example, had the efforts of Senator Thaler in New York been successful in prohibiting pediatric research of all kinds, would we today have the polio vaccine available? Had the emotionalism, irrationalism, and anti-intellectualism encountered in connection with psychosurgery been equally evident, and had these forces led to judicial action against the early heart surgery work, would we now have the knowledge and possibilities available for cardiac therapy? "Even physicians were in a sense intellectually and emotionally unprepared for the earliest triumphs of cardiac surgery. What, then, would have been the layman's reaction to a full exposition of the problems involved in the original Blalock-Taussing shunts? And what of cardiac catheterization? The benefits of this technique have, quite appropriately, won Nobel Prizes for three of the physicians who pioneered in its use, but is it difficult to imagine lay journalists dubbing the early experimentation of these men barbaric and Nazi-like? ("And then, dear readers, these monsters have the temerity to thrust a tube down the length of one's arm into the very chambers of the human heart! The mind of anyone not completely brutalized by prolonged immersion in the bloody charnel houses of Science boggles at the thought!") (Lasagna, "Some Ethical Problems in Clinical Investigation," in Mendelsohn, Swazey, and Taviss, *Human Aspects of Biomedical Innovation* 105 (1971).) As Jay Katz has pointed out in a similar context: "When Werner Forssmann was awarded the Nobel Prize for his pioneering work on cardiac catheterization the Royal Committee noted: '[Forssmann's] later disappointment must have been all the more bitter. [He was] subjected to criticism of such exaggerated severity that it robbed him of any inclination to continue. This criticism was based on the unsubstantiated belief in the danger of the intervention, thus affording proof that, even in our enlightened times—a valuable suggestion may remain unexploited on the grounds of a preconceived opinion.'" (Katz, "Who Is To Keep Guard Over the Guards Themselves?," 23 *Fertility and Sterility* 604 at 605 (1972).)

The list of irrational, exaggerated "popular" reactions to medical research could surely be extended, but would serve no purpose. It is sufficiently clear that any decision to be made must be made only within the context of answers to the following questions: (1) is the Court the proper institutional source from whence to derive decisions about progress in medical therapy?; (2) if the Court does deem itself the appropriate agency for such decisions, can it get the kind of information necessary for such decisions? Does it have the personnel with the appropriate technical knowledge? Can it get the personnel to make the requisite decisions?; (3) if the Court cannot have available the requisite decision-making resources, ought the Court to play some role other than primary decision maker?; (4) if the Court ought to play a role other than primary decision maker, has this case been one in which the Court finds that it has had the facilities, background, information, and competence to play the role of secondary decision maker?; (5) if the Court recognizes that it does not have the personnel, technique, training, or resources for playing decision maker at primary or secondary levels, what are the alternatives which are available?

NOTES

Chapter 1

1. V. Mark and F. Ervin, *Violence and the Brain* (1970).

2. See P. Rennick, E. Rodin, T. Keiser, and C. Rim, "Psychotropic Effects of Tegretol: A Double Blind Study," 16 *Epilepsia* 198 (1975).

3. See H. Steadman, "Implications from the Baxtrom Experience," 1 *Bulletin of the American Academy of Psychiatry and Law* 189 (1973).

4. Fortner v. Koch, 272 Mich. 273, 261 N.W. 762 (1935).

5. Trap v. United States, 356 U.S. 86 (1958).

6. Roe v. Wade, 410 U.S. 113 (1973).

7. D. Stafford-Clark and F. Taylor, "Clinical and Electroencephalographic Studies of Prisoners Charged with Murder," 12 *Journal of Neurology, Neurosurgery, and Psychiatry* 325 (1949).

Chapter 2

1. C. Offir, "Psychosurgery and the Law: The Movement to Pull Out the Electrodes," 7 *Psychology Today* 69 (May 1974).

2. V. Mark and F. Ervin, *Violence and the Brain* (1970).

3. V. Mark and R. Neville, "Brain Surgery in Agressive Epileptics," 226 *Journal of the American Medical Association* 765 at 766 (Nov. 12, 1973).

4. R. Neville, "Pots and Black Kettles: A Philospher's Perspective on Psychosurgery," 54 *Boston University Law Review* 340 at 346 (1974).

5. G. Annas and L. Glantz, "Psychosurgery: The Law's Response," 54 *Boston University Law Review* 249 (1974). Emphasis added.

6. S. Chorover, "Psychosurgery: A Neuropsychological Perspective," 54 *Boston University Law Review* 231 (1974). Emphasis added.

7. Hearings on S. 974, S. 878, and S. J. Res. 71 before the Subcommittee on Health of the Senate Committe on Labor and Public Welfare, 93d Cong., 1st Sess., pt. 2., at 339 (1973). Emphasis added.

8. *Id.* at 359.

9. V. Mark, "Psychosurgery Versus Anti-Psychiatry," 54 *Boston University Law Review* 217 (1974); also see V. Mark, "A Psychosurgeon's Case *For* Psychosurgery," 8 *Psychology Today* 28 at 30 (July 1974).

10. National Research Service Award Act of 1974, P.L. 93–348, 88 Stat. 342, § 202 (c) (1974).

11. Ch. 616, § 1(6) [1973 Ore. Reg. Sess.] (S. Bill 298), *amending* Ore. Rev. Stat. 677.190 (1971).

12. See C. Atkins and A. Lauriat, "Psychosurgery and The Role of Legislation," 54 *Boston University Law Review* 288 (1974); Note, "Kaimowitz v. Department of Mental Health: A Right to Be Free From Experimental Psychosurgery?," 54 *Boston University Law Review* 301 at 338, n. 200 (1974).

13. H.R. 5371, 93d Cong., 1st Sess. § 1 (1973).

14. Mass. S. 660 (1974); see Atkins and Lauriat, *supra* note 12.

15. M. Shapiro, "Legislating the Control of Behavior Control: Autonomy and the Coercive Use of Organic Therapies," 47 *Southern California Law Review* 237 (1974). An extract from the article is printed as Appendix A.

16. *Id.* at 240. Shapiro defines mentation: "*Mentation* refers to cognition, understanding, perception, emotion—loosely, any mental functioning or activity." *Id.* at 246, n. 14.

17. Calif. Assembly Bill 2296. See Shapiro, *supra* note 15 at 339.

18. Kaimowitz v. Dept. of Mental Health, Civil Action N. 73-19434-AW (Cir. Ct. Wayne Co., Mich., July 10, 1973), *summarized* at 42 U.S.L.W. 2063 (July 31, 1973). References are to the slip opinion.

19. B. Brown, L. Wienckowski, and L. Bivens, *Psychosurgery: Perspective on a Current Issue* 1 (HEW Pub. No. (HSM) 73–9119, 1973). Hereafter referred to as the NIMH definition.

20. *Id.* at 6. Emphasis added.

21. Quoted in Chorover, "The Pacification of the Brain," 7 *Psychology Today* 59 at 64 (May 1974).

22. *Psychosurgery: Perspective on a Current Issue, supra* note 19 at 6. Emphasis added.

23. V. Mark, W. Sweet, and F. Ervin, "The Effect of Amygdalotomy on Violent Behavior in Patients With Temporal Lobe Epilepsy," in E. Hitchcock, L. Laitinen, and K. Vaernet, eds., *Psychosurgery* 139 (1972).

24. Shapiro, *supra* note 15 at 242.

25. *Id.*

26. *Id.* at 240, n. 5.

27. *Id.* at 286.

28. *Id.,* n. 166.

29. J. Hospers, *An Introduction to Philosophical Analysis* 608 (2d ed., 1967); Shapiro, *supra* note 15 at 286.

30. Shapiro, *supra* note 15 at 286–87.

31. *Id.* at 286, n. 166.

32. *Id.* at 246.

33. My colleague, Dr. Ernst Rodin, who is board-certified and experienced in some of the medical specialties particularly relevant to this discussion, read this chapter. After making a number of helpful suggestions, he added:

    Not being a lawyer or philosopher, I do have difficulties with the definitions proposed, all of them as a matter of fact and I have a feeling that your operational definition may also be taken apart by the adversary system. The main problem that I see is "evidence of diseased tissue" which is "causally related to some symptoms." I don't know if the following comments help you any, but the problem is again one of definitions which cannot be overcome at our current level of knowledge. For instance, what constitutes evidence of diseased tissue? Is it an abnormality apparent to the naked eye of the surgeon? Is it a microscopic slide which shows the stained cells but not their processes (the single most common histological method to determine abnormalities)? Is it a microscopic slide which shows the cell processes rather than cell bodies (the technique has been available for over 100 years but is hardly used because it is complex)? Or is it a histochemical analysis which shows the absence or excess of certain amino acids or neurohumors? If you compound this problem with the fact that all of these forms of disease cannot be diagnosed without intrusive procedures, like biopsy samples, because death alters the biochemical properties to an extent that it makes any conclusion for the in vivo state impossible, then one must admit that any meaningful research on mental illness dealing with the organ of the illness, i.e. the brain, can at this time not be done and, therefore, any cause between mental symptoms and brain disease will remain undiscovered. I have come to the facetious but currently true conclusion that the human brain is unwilling to yield its secrets as to how it functions and will protect itself against any and all meaningful attempts to do so, even if it has to resort to the hiring of lawyers to protect itself from science.

Louis P. Wienckowski, Ph.D., director of the Extramural Research Programs at HEW, was also kind enough to read a draft of this chapter. In addition to making a number of important suggestions, he added:

I would not take strong exception to your definition since virtually all of the clear examples of psychosurgery that I can think of do not deal with diseased brain. However, it does seem to me that your exhaustive development of this definition creates a large loophole by setting up the condition that the presence of diseased brain tissue, or at least evidence that there is tissue disease or damage, exempts any brain surgery from the psychosurgery label. The same sort of detailed reasoning that you devote to taking apart the NIMH and Shapiro definitions could also be devoted to defining diseased brain tissue. With the current imprecision of clinical testing, and the lack of clearly established norms, the existence of brain disease or damage is frequently inferred and often cannot be confirmed or disconfirmed until the brain is actually examined, and even when actual specimens of brain tissue are available, the diagnosis of diseased or healthy tissue is frequently difficult. How would you define "demonstrable evidence of diseased brain tissue"?

Chapter 3

1. "Scientific medicine has always emphasized that its scientific knowledge is tied closely to the structure and function of the physical organism. Suppose we knew how to block a certain kind of behavior by neurosurgical means, whether or not the cause of that behavior were some brain abnormality; although the 'cure' is physiological, our knowledge of the cause of the behavior does not live up to the model of scientific medicine. It might be objected that medicine uses many procedures, aspirin, for one, whose mechanisms are not understood to treat conditions whose cause is not understood. Our answer is that medicine generally does not, and in fact ought not, use procedures in these circumstances that are as drastic, irreversible, and experimental as psychosurgery."

V. Mark and R. Neville, "Brain Surgery In Aggressive Epileptics," 226 *Journal of the American Medical Association* 765 at 767 (Nov. 12, 1973).

2. P. Steinfels, "Confronting the Other Drug Problem," 2 *Hastings Center Report* 4 at 6 (Nov. 1972).

3. B. Brown, L. Wienckowski, and L. Bivens, *Psychosurgery: Perspective on a Current Issue,* HEW Pub. No. (HSM) 73–9119 (1973).

4. V. Mark and F. Ervin, *Violence and the Brain* 16, 24, 26, 31, and 147 (1970). And see J. Hodson, "Reflections Concerning Violence and the Brain," 9 *Criminal Law Bulletin* 684 at 692 (1973).

5. V. Mark, "Brain Surgery in Aggressive Epileptics," 3 *Hastings Center Report* 1 at 2 (Feb. 1973).

6. *Id.* at 3. Emphasis added.

7. *Id.* at 2. Emphasis added.

8. Mark and Neville, *supra* note 1 at 768. Emphasis added.

9. *Id.* at 766. Emphasis added.

10. *Id.* at 765. Emphasis added.

11. L. Wittgenstein, *Philosophical Investigations,* Sec. 66 at 32e (Oxford: 1958, third ed. 1967).

12. Mark and Neville, *supra* note 1 at 766; also see Mark, *supra* note 5 at 1.

13. Mark, *supra* note 5 at 3.

14. See Hodson, *supra* note 4.

15. Mark and Neville, *supra* note 1 at 766.

16. *Id.* at 767.

17. *Id.*

18. W. Scoville, "'Only as a Last Resort . . . '," 3 *Hastings Center Report* 5 (Feb. 1973). Emphasis added.

19. S. Chorover, "The Pacification of the Brain," 7 *Psychology Today* 59 (May 1974).

20. *Id.* Emphasis added.

21. See J. Staddon, "On the Notion of Cause, With Applications to Behaviorism," 1 *Behaviorism* 25 (1973).

22. Hodson, *supra* note 4 at 694.

23. Mark and Neville, *supra* note 1 at 767.

24. Hodson, *supra* note 4 at 694–98.

25. E. Valenstein, *Brain Control* 266–67 (1973), quoting from G. Burckhardt, "Über Rinenexcisionen, als Bertrag zur Operativen Therapie der Psychosen," 47 *Allgemeinen Zeitschrift für Psychiatrie* 463 (1891).

26. A. Storr, "A Linking of Disciplines," 41 *Encounter* 85 at 88 (Nov. 1973).

27. Staddon, *supra* note 21 at 30.

28. *Id.* at 27. And see the citation there.

29. *Id.* at 32.

30. Chorover, *supra* note 19 at 63–64. At another point in this article the author claims that "the fact remains that from the start, prefrontal lobotomy could be justified only by ignoring the evidence from animal experiments" (60). However, the "fact" also remains that animal work is not automatically or necessarily applicable to humans. See the text to note 31.

31. Valenstein, *supra* note 25 at 219.

32. I think of Luria's account of his patient Zasetsky, who lost nearly his entire memory after a bullet damaged his left parietal, occipital, and temporal lobes. See A. Luria, *The Man With a Shattered World* (1972); also see A. Luria, *The Working Brain* (1973).

33. Chorover, *supra* note 19 at 69.

34. L. Wittgenstein, *The Blue and Brown Books* 24–25 (Harper Torchbook ed. of 1965, based on Blackwell ed., 1958).

35. C. Chihara and J. Fodor, "Operationalism and Ordinary Language: A Critique of Wittgenstein," in G. Pritcher, ed., *Wittgenstein: The Philosophical Investigations* 384 (1966). Reprinted from 2 *American Philosophical Quarterly* 281 (1965).

36. *Id.* at 393.

37. R. Albritton, "On Wittgenstein's Use of the Term 'Criterion'," in Pritcher, *supra* note 35 at 236. Reprinted from 56 *Journal of Philosophy* 845 (1959).

38. *Id.* at 236.

39. *Id.* at 233.

40. *Id.* at 233.

41. *Id.* at 244.

42. A. Quinton, "Contemporary British Philosophy," in Pritcher, *supra* note 35 at 11. Reprinted from D. O'Connor, ed., *A Critical History of Western Philosophy* 535 (1964).

43. Wittgenstein, *supra* note 11; Sec. 569 at 151e, Sec. 199 at 81e, Sec. 432 at 128e.

44. *Id.*, Sec. 19 at 8e, Part II (XI) at 226e, Part II (XI) at 220e.

45. *Id.*, Sec. 654 at 167e.

46. Quinton, *supra* note 42 at 13–20.

47. P. Strawson, "Review of Wittgenstein's *Philosophical Investigations*," in Pritcher, *supra* note 35 at 35. Reprinted from 63 *Mind* 70 (1954).

48. *Id.* at 37.

49. Wittgenstein, *supra* note 11, Sec. 325 at 106e.

50. *Id.*, Sec. 654 at 167e.

51. *Id.*, Sec. 656 at 167e.

52. "Variants on 'use' in Wittgenstein are 'purpose' 'function' 'role' 'part' 'application'." Strawson, *supra* note 47 at 25.

53. Wittgenstein, *supra* note 11, Sec. 583 at 153e.

54. Staddon, *supra* note 21 at 31.

55. *Id.* at 27.

56. F. Freemon, "Letter to the Editor," 15 *Perspectives in Biology and Medicine* 311–12 (1972).

57. Compare this example to the following statement in M. Roth, "Psychiatry and Its Critics," 122 *British Journal of Psychiatry* 373 at 378 (1973): "When the whole repertoire of criticisms and recommendations of anti-psychiatry are analysed, we find moral condemnation in place of scientific search for causes; social determinism in place of unbiased evaluation of the relative contributions

made by biological, experiential, familial and social factors . . . prejucial denunciation . . . and dogmatic assertions."

58. Quoted from R. Dubos in R. Marston, "Medical Science, the Clinical Trial, and Society," 3 *Hastings Center Report* 1 (April 1973).

59. A. Bernstein and H. Lennard, "Drugs, Doctors, and Junkies," 10 *Transaction* 14 at 24 (May—June 1973).

60. Quoted from a statement issued by "The Boston Area Medical Challenge Clubs composed of members and friends of the Revolutionary Communist Progressive Labor Party." See H. Ballantine, 1 *Medical Opinion* 46 (July 1972).

61. R. Veatch, "The Medical Model: Its Nature and Problems," 1 *Hastings Center Studies* 59 at 67 (1973).

62. *Id.* at 68.

63. *Id.* at 68–70.

64. *Id.* at 70.

65. *Id.* at 76.

66. D. Hamburg and H. Brodie, "Psychological Research on Human Agressiveness," 23 *Impact of Science on Society* 181 at 190–91 (1973).

67. *See* L. Levi, ed., *Society, Stress, and Disease* (1971). In this volume see especially the contributions by A. Kagan at 36–48, R. Lazarus at 53–58, K.-E. Fichtelius at 61–69, and E. Fabricius at 71–78. Kagan opens by urging: "The purpose of these symposia is to establish whether psychosocial stimuli cause disease through the mediation of stress," and quickly adds, "there is little doubt that psychosocial factors bring about some of the psychological changes of stress" (36).

Chapter 4

1. O. Ødegård, "Season of Birth in the General Population and in Patients with Mental Disorder in Norway," 125 *British Journal of Psychiatry* 297 (1974); P. Dalen, *Season of Birth: A Study of Schizophrenia and Other Mental Disorders* (1975); O. Hagnell and N. Kreitman, "Mental Illness in Married Pairs in a Total Population," 125 *British Journal of Psychiatry* 293 (1974).

2. See T. Kuhn, *The Structure of Scientific Revolution* (1962).

3. S. Peltzman, *Regulation of Pharmaceutical Innovation: The 1962 Amendments* (1974), and also the more detailed work of the same author in R. Landau, ed., *Regulating New Drugs* (1973).

4. Dr. Breggin acknowledged this purpose when I questioned him in connection with his testimony in the Detroit psychosurgery case. There is nothing secretive about Dr. Breggin's purpose, for he makes no effort to conceal that he wants to reach political (not scientific) decision makers.

Chapter 5

1. Hearings on S. 974, S. 878, and S. J. Res. 71 before the Subcommittee on Health of the Senate Committee on Labor and Public Welfare, 93d Cong., 1st Sess., pt. 2 at 338.

2. *Id.* at 358.

3. *Id.* at 351–52. Dr. Andy did concede that the patient and his relatives have a role. He said: "The ethics for the diagnosis and treatment of the behavioral illness should remain in the hands of the treating physicians who are qualified to treat the illness, and the patient, the relatives and designated friends who are vitally interested in the patient's illness and well being" (*Id.*).

4. T. Szasz, *The Myth of Mental Illness* (1961); *Law, Liberty, and Psychiatry* (1963).

5. B. Brown, L. Wienckowski, and L. Bivens, *Psychosurgery: Perspective on a Current Issure* 9, HEW Pub. No. (HSM) 73–9119 (1973).

6. Senator Kennedy questioned Dr. Robert G. Heath of Tulane about his work with implanted electrodes and asked him, "How are we to know that [this technique is] always going to be used constructively, positively?"

Dr. Heath:	For one thing, about a million dollars worth of equipment is required for our studies, as well as a large number of highly skilled personnel.
Senator Kennedy:	What about in five years or so? Is it that complex from an engineering viewpoint?
Dr. Heath:	I think it is probably too complex. I do not think you will have to worry about too many being done. By these technics, we can work with one or two patients a year at the most. I cannot conceive of it being done off the cuff

	simply and quickly. I hope we can come up with less complex procedures in the future.
Senator Kennedy:	Should we not be concerned about mass application?
Dr. Heath:	I do not see any cause for concern of mass application of such technics. I think drugs do have marked effects and they are readily available. I think they will continue to be a problem unless their use can be effectively controlled.

Hearings, supra note 1 at 368.

7. Dr. Willard Gaylin, President of the Hastings Institute, in his appearance before the Kennedy subcommittee, began this way:

I think behavior control is an enormously serious problem that has not been attended to adequately; that it needs a kind of regulation that is not at present available, that some of these are legislative, and some of these are not legislative; some of them are already indicated and designed and some have still to be researched.

About three years ago the Hastings Institute began to be concerned about the prospects of behavioral control technology. It was seen as roughly analogous to the situation of ecology before that term was invented. In those days technologists were concerned about urban crowding, marine biologists were concerned about the rivers and waterways, etc., yet there was not an awareness that these isolated people were dealing with similar problems.

Behavior control is seen by many of us in the field as a problem arising in a similarly disparate way. Psychosurgeons are beginning to do more meticulous and detailed operations for purposes of behavior modification. There are new drugs becoming much more refined than the old ups and downs we used to have, and there is the increasing impact of television (with an estimate of 4 year olds watching 40 to 60 hours per week). Total institutions are shaping people; the nature of the response to Dr. Skinner's book with its recommendation for mass social engineering indicated the seriousness of the problem.

So we undertook a kind of research, beginning with what we thought was the simplest and narrowest form of behavior control—psychosurgery. I still feel psychosurgery is probably attended to much more than is warranted in terms of its real threat to manipulation of the population as compared with some of the other things. . . .

It seems unlikely, if there were some plot to take over the country by a totalitarian, to use some of the ideas suggested today that psychosurgery would be the method of choice. I doubt that they would find the most efficient technique for mass control would be planting electrodes on a population of 200 million, or psychosurgery, when they have access to a limited national television, and to schools with compulsory education, to psychological inputs and to drugs, all of which afford a more convenient, cheaper, economic mass method of manipulation.

Hearings, supra note 1 at 373–74.

8. *Id.* at 358.

9. R. Restak, "The Promise and Peril of Psychosurgery," *Saturday Review/World* 54 (Sept. 25, 1973).

10. An edited transcript of the discussion has been published as "Physical Manipulation of the Brain," *The Hastings Center Report,* Special Supplement 9 (May 1973). Hereafter cited as the *Hastings Report*.

11. *Id.*

12. *Id.* at 10–11.

13. *Id.* at 11.

14. *Id.* at 11.

15. *Hearings, supra* note 1 at 342.

16. *Hastings Report, supra* note 10 at 9.

17. Restak, *supra* note 9 at 54.

18. *Hearings, supra* note 1 at 342.

19. Testifying before the Kennedy subcommittee, Brown argued: "The surgical treatment of epilepsy, while in one sense a form of psychosurgery since behavioral symptoms are altered, should be excluded from this discussion when the disease can be clearly diagnosed and there is convincing evidence that epilepsy is caused by organic pathology in the brain." *Hearings, supra* note 1 at 335. The NIMH report about psychosurgery contains a similar suggestion: "The surgical treatment of epilepsy, while in one sense a form of psychosurgery since behavioral symptoms are altered, should be excluded from this discussion when the disease can be clearly diagnosed and there is convincing evidence that epilepsy is caused by organic pathology in the brain. Of course any other neurosurgical treatment to repair or remove damaged brain tissue, or to remove tumors, is not psychosurgery." *Psychosurgery: Perspective on a Cur-*

rent Issue, supra note 5 at 1. Even Dr. Breggin would permit brain surgery for the treatment of epilepsy:

Senator Kennedy:	Epilepsy?
Dr. Breggin:	That would not be psychosurgery. The definition of psychosurgery is to destroy normal brain tissue to control the emotions or behavior or, a diseased tissue when the disease has nothing to do with behavior . . . the man is trying to control. For example, some of Dr. Andy's patients may be brain damaged, but that is not what makes them violent. It is just a good excuse to mutilate further: damage, damage, damage, until you get the calming effect. So if you are operating on epilepsy, you are not talking about psychosurgery.

Hearings, supra note 1 at 359.

What is interesting about this unanimity of view is that it would be very difficult to differentiate, on the basis of available scientific hard data, surgically treatable epilepsy from some cases of paraepileptic phenomena. It would also be difficult to specify exactly the clinical syndrome or epilepsy which justifies a surgical intervention. But apparently some 2,000 temporal lobectomies (retroactively) bestow "scientific" credibility upon the existence of the requisiste syndrome.

20. Kaimowitz v. Dept. of Mental Health, Civil Action N. 73-19434-AW (Cir. Ct. Wayne Co., Mich., July 10, 1973), *summarized* at 42 U.S.L.W. 2063 (July 31, 1973). Trial transcript at A47-A49/28.

21. *Id.* at 31–32/29.

22. *Hearings, supra* note 1 at 359.

23. *Id.* at 362.

24. V. Potter, *Bioethics* (1971).

25. "We must somehow evolve a system of technology assessment whereby the state of knowledge can be assessed and its readiness for application can be addressed with the context of relevant social, human, and ethical issues. Such a system would assure the timely application of relevant technology and help prevent the premature use of those techniques not thoroughly explored for their human and social implications.

We believe that the answer to the dangerous use of knowledge is the creation of new knowledge, combined with a sensitive, rational, and humanitarian perspective on the applications of that knowledge. It is also important to broaden the training of scientists and practitioners to include such ethical issues and the humanities."

Psychosurgery: Perspective on a Current Issue, supra note 5 at 10–11.

Chapter 6

1. M. Shapiro, "Legislating the Control of Behavior Control: Autonomy and the Coercive Use of Organic Therapies," 47 *Southern California Law Review* 237 at 256–57 (1971). An extract from the article is printed as Appendix A.

2. *Id.* at 257.

3. *Id.* at 257, n. 53.

4. *Id.* at 258–59.

5. *Id.* at 259, n. 60.

6. See J. Swazye, "Phenylketonuria: A Case Study in Biomedical Legislation," 48 *Journal of Urban Law* 883 (1971).

7. See Shapiro, *supra* note 1, Appendix I, 339; see C. Atkins and A. Lauriat, "Psychosurgery and the Role of Legislation," 54 *Boston University Law Review* 288 (1974).

8. Shapiro, *supra* note 1 at 257, n. 53.

9. *Id.* at 253.

10. *Id.* at 335.

11. *Id.* at 336, n. 336.

12. *Id.* at 253.

13. *Id.* at 331.

14. *Id.* at 247.

15. V. Mark and F. Ervin, *Violence and the Brain* (1970). Three years after the publication of the book, Mark said it "was meant as an initial stimulus to the medical and scientific community for a discussion of these issues." V. Mark and R. Neville, "Brain Surgery in Aggressive Epileptics," 226 *Journal of the*

American Medical Association 756 at 768 (Nov. 12, 1973). For another example of the same kind of misuse of "science," see V. Mark, W. Sweet, and F. Ervin, "Role of Brain Disease in Riots and Urban Violence," 201 *Journal of the American Medical Association* 895 (Sept. 11, 1967).

16. R. Breggin, "The Return of Lobotomy and Psychosurgery," 118 *Congressional Record* E1602–E1612 (daily ed. Feb. 24, 1972); R. Breggin, "New Information in the Debate over Psychosurgery," 118 *Congressional Record* E3379–E3386 (daily ed. Mar. 29, 1972); R. Breggin, "Psychosurgery for the Control of Violence—Including a Critical Examination of the Work of Vernon Mark and Frank Ervin," 118 *Congressional Record* E3383–E3384 (daily ed. March 30, 1972).

17. Shapiro, *supra* note 1 at 329–30.

18. *Id.* at 257.

19. *Id.* at 327.

20. *Id.* at 333, n. 327.

21. *Id.* at 280, n. 147.

22. *Id.* at 337, n. 338.

23. *Id.* at 334.

24. *Id.*

25. *Id.* at 257, n. 53.

26. *Id.* at 260–61.

27. *Id.* at 262–63.

28. *Id.* at 267.

29. *Id.* at 297.

30. *Id.* at 297, n. 202.

31. *Id.* at 266.

32. See the text accompanying footnotes 34 to 52 in chapter 3.

33. L. Wittgenstein, *Philosophical Investigations,* Sec. 593 at 155 (1953).

Chapter 7

1. U. S. Dept. of Health, Education, and Welfare, Protection of Human Subjects, Proposed Policy, 39 Fed. Reg. 30649 (Aug. 23, 1974). Kaimowitz v. Dept. of Mental Health, Civil N. 73-19434-AW (Cir. Ct., Wayne Co., Mich., July 10, 1973), *summarized* at 42 U.S.L.W. 2063 (July 31, 1973), at 22 in slip opinion. All references are to the slip opinion. See R. Slovenko, *Psychiatry and Law* 259 and 270–73 (1973).

2. Note, "*Kaimowitz v. Department of Mental Health:* A Right to be Free from Experimental Psychosurgery?," 54 *Boston University Law Review* 301 at 325 (1974).

3. *Id.* at 315.

4. *Supra* note 1, §46.504(b), 39 Fed. Reg. 30655–30656.

5. Canterbury v. Spence, 464 F. 2d 772 (D.C. Cir. 1972), *cert. denied* 409 U.S. 1064 (1972); Cobbs v. Grant, 8 Cal. 3d 229, 502 P. 2d 1 (1972); Cooper v. Roberts, 220 Pa. Super. 260, 286 A. 2d 647 (1971); Wilkinson v. Vesey, 110 R.E. 606, 295 A. 2d 676 (1972); Fogal v. Genesse Hosp., 41 App. Div. 2d 468, 344 N.Y. S. 2d 552 (1973); Trogun v. Fruchtman, 58 Wis. 2d 469, 207 N.W. 2d 297 (1973). A recent case to the contrary is Tatro v. Lukin, 212 Kan. 606, 512 P. 2d 529 (1973).

6. Note, "Informed Consent—A Proposed Standard for Medical Disclosure," 48 *New York University Law Review* 548 at 553 (1973).

7. Canterbury v. Spence, *supra* note 5 at 783.

8. The case which grew out of this experiment is Hyman v. Jewish Chronic Disease Hospital, 42 Misc. 2d 427, 206 N.E. 2d 338 (1964). See E. Langer, "Cancer Studies Stir Public Debate," 143 *Science* 551 (1964); E. Langer, "Human Experimentation: N. Y. Verdict Affirms Patient's Rights," 151 *Science* 663 (1966).

9. See Langer (1964), *supra* note 8 at 552.

10. U. S. Dept. of Health, Education, and Welfare, *Protection of Human Subjects,* § 46.3(b), 39 Fed. Reg. 18913 at 18917 (1974).

11. See Langer (1964), *supra* note 8 at 551.

12. B. Mason, "Brain Surgery to Control Behavior," 28 *Ebony* 62 (Feb. 1973). The article carries the caption, "New Threat to Blacks," and has the subtitle, "Controversial Operations Are Coming Back As Violence Curbs." On page 68 of the article there is a half-page picture of a black psychiatrist, Dr. Alvin

Poussaint, Associate Professor of Psychiatry, Harvard University Medical School, who is quoted as saying: "These brain studies are racist. They say that black people are so animal and savage that whites have to carve on their brains to make them human beings. . . . " For an alternative view, see "2 Black Neurosurgeons Defend Behavior-Altering Operations," New York Times, Thurs., Jan. 8, 1976, p. 34.

13. In 1975 John Doe was apprehended while shoplifting ladies' underpants. He was wearing several pairs of such underpants when apprehended. It has been alleged that after being furnished the necessary "Miranda warnings," he again confessed to the murder and rape committed in 1954. In April 1976, the Detroit Free Press reported that Doe had been convicted of second degree murder and sentenced to life imprisonment. However, "Judge Boros noted [Doe] could be eligible for speedy parole because of credit for time served [at Ionia State Hospital]. But the Judge insisted parole officers consult him before deciding [Doe's] case. Boros contended that [Doe] is a 'clear and present danger to the community if not closely confined.'" Detroit Free Press, April 7, 1976, p. 4.

14. B. Brown, L. Wienckowski, and L. Bivens, *Psychosurgery: Perspective on a Current Issue* 2, HEW Pub. No. (HSM) 73–9119 (1973).

15. See S. Shuman, "Responsibility And Punishment: Why Criminal Law," 15 *American Journal of Jurisprudence* 25 (1970); S. Shuman, "The Placebo Cure For Criminality," 19 *Wayne Law Review* 847 (1973).

Chapter 8

1. B. Rensch, *Biophilosophy (1971)*. For an even more "extreme" view, see E. Chain, "Social Responsibility And The Scientist In Modern Western Society," *14 Perspectives In Biology and Medicine* 347 and 367 (1971):

> The main theory which has dominated thinking in the biological field for almost a century is that of the Darwin-Wallace concepts of evolution and natural selection through the survival of the fittest. This mechanistic concept of the phenomena of life in its infinite varieties of manifestations which purports to ascribe the origin and developments of all living species, animals, plants and microorganisms, to the haphazard blind interplay of the forces of nature in the pursuance of one aim only, namely, that for the living systems to survive, is a typical product of the naive 19th century euphoric attitude to the potentialities of science which spread the belief that there were no secrets of nature which could not be solved by the scientific approach given only sufficient time.

2. "At no stage of the process have the genetic changes occurred with the present or any future state in view; they came to pass exclusively because they were adaptive when and where they happened. There is one thing that natural selec-

tion cannot do: since it has no foresight, it cannot build genotypes that will be favorable not in the present but in some future environments. It is for this reason that evolution controlled by natural selection may end in maladaptation and extinction. A genetic endowment that makes a species well adapted today may be faulty in the future." T. Dobzhansky, "Darwinian Evolution and the Problem of Extraterrestrial Life," 15 *Perspectives in Biology and Medicine* 157 at 163 (1972). Also see I. Asimov, *The Wellsprings of Life* (1960).

3. T. Dobzhansky, "Unique Aspects of Man's Evolution," in J. Pringle, ed., *Biology and the Human Sciences* 121 at 123–25 (1972); also see G. Simpson, *This View of Life* (1964); G. Simpson, *Biology and Man* (1969).

4. V. Wynne-Edwards, "Ecology and the Evolution of Social Ethics," in Pringle, *supra* note 3, 49 at 51.

5. Dobzhansky, *supra* note 3 at 128–29.

6. A. Kroeber, *Anthropology* (1948).

7. G. Miller, "Linquistic Communication As a Biological Process," in Pringle, *supra* note 3 at 83–84.

8. E. Robin, "The Evolutionary Advantages of Being Stupid," 16 *Perspectives in Biology and Medicine* 369 (1973).

9. Miller, *supra* note at 7 at 73–74.

10. J. Rostand, *Can Man Be Modified?* (1959).

11. "Some forty years ago, in a short but well-know passage, Haldane . . . examined the logical possibilities of evolving altruistic behavior through natural selection in man. He said that, 'if any genes are common in mankind which promote conduct biologically disadvantageous to the individual in all types of society, but yet advantageous to society, they must have spread when man was divided into small endogenous groups. As many eugenists have pointed out, selection in large societies operates in the reverse direction'. Even so, such conditions appeared to him to be far from sufficient for the spread of inborn altruism, because self-sacrifice is bound to come off second best and the genes responsible for it consequently to diminish, in proportion to alternative alleles. He concluded with the comment that 'I find it difficult to suppose that many genes for absolute altruism are common to man." Wynne-Edwards, *supra* note 4 at 61, quoting from J. B. Haldane, *The Causes of Evolution* (1932). Also see R. Ardrey, *The Territorial Imperative* (1966). For a contrary view, see A. Montagu, *The Direction of Human Development* (1955); D. Daniels, M. Gilula, and F. Ochberg, eds., *Violence and the Struggle for Existence* (1970); G. Bach and H. Goldberg, *Creative Aggression* (1974).

12. E. Chargaff, "Bitter Fruits From the Tree of Knowledge: Remarks On The

Current Revulsion From Science," 16 *Perspectives in Biology and Medicine* 486 at 494 (1973).

13. S. Toulmin, "The Alexandrian Trap: Thoughts on 'The Eternal Scientist'," 42 *Encounter* 61 at 64 (Jan. 1974).

14. M. Martin, "The Scientist as Shaman," *Harper's* 54 at 57 (Mar. 1972).

15. *Id.* at 54. The word "scientist" was coined and first used in publicity about 135 years ago by Whewell in speaking to the British Association for the Advancement of Science. See Toulmin, *supra* note 13 at 61.

16. P. Medawar, *The Hope of Progress* (1973).

17. Medawar himself believes in the general possibility of finding technological solutions for technological ills, and among the reasons for his conviction that science can be controlled more closely than is usually thought he notes that there tends to be a wide gap between demonstrating the feasibility of something and realising that feasibility in practice. He concedes that "we cannot point to a single definitive solution of any one of the problems that confront us" in the political, economic, social or moral domains, but his defence is persuasive: "We are still beginners, and for that reason may hope to improve." R. Williams, "The Soluble is Pawn to the Possible: Science and Politics," 42 *Encounter* 77 (Jan. 1974).

18. D. Callahan, "Science: Limits and Prohibitions," 3 *Hastings Center Report* 5 at 6 (Nov. 1973).

19. *Id.*

20. B. Feld, "Human Values and the Technology of Weapons," 8 *Zygon* 48 at 57 (Mar. 1973).

21. Chargaff, *supra* note 12 at 494.

22. Callahan, *supra* note 18 at 6.

23. T. Parsons, *The System of Modern Societies* (1971).

24. C. Geertz, "Ideology as a Cultural System," in D. Apter, ed., *Ideology and Discontent* 62 (1946), quoted in B. Gustin, "Charisma, Recognition, and the Motivation of Scientists," 78 *American Journal of Sociology* 1119 at 1123 (1973).

25. As Claude Bernard said in one of the earliest works about experimental medicine, "Experimental method rests necessarily on feeling, reason, and experiment. Feeling gives rise to the experimental idea or hypothesis, i.e., the previsioned interpretation of natural phenomena. Reason or reasoning serves only

to deduce the consequences of this idea and to submit them to experiment. An anticipative idea or an hypothesis is, then, the necessary starting point for all experimental reasoning.'' *An Introduction to the Study of Experimental Medicine* 32 (1927).

26. R. Sperry, ''Science And The Problem of Values,'' 16 *Perspectives in Biology and Medicine* 115 (1973); M. Polyani, *Science, Faith, and Society* (1964).

27. *Manifesto: British Society For Social Responsibility* (1969), quoted in part in S. Rose and H. Rose, ''Can Science Be Neutral,'' 16 *Perspectives in Biology and Medicine* 605 (1973); 607–608.

28. 1 *Hastings Center Report* 4 (Sept. 1971).

29. J. Ravetz, *Scientific Knowledge and Its Social Problems* (1971).

30. A probably not atypical account is Sir Bernard Lovell's report on how the radiotelescope operation at Jodrell Bank was kept alive. B. Lovell, *Story of Jodrell Bank* (1968); B. Lovell, *Out of the Zenith* (1973).

31. Franklin Long, one-time Assistant Director of the U.S. Arms Control and Disarmament Agency, estimated in the Ciba symposium that in recent years some forty percent of the world's total research and development effort has been for military purposes. Science, he suggests, has become a major driving force for all technology, ''and notably so for military technology,'' while, at the same time, ''security'' has been given a ''military or quasi-military interpretation.'' Williams, *supra* note 17 at 78; also see J. Lederberg, ''The Freedoms and the Control of Science: Notes from the Ivory Tower,'' 45 *Southern California Law Review* 596 (1972), especially 603 and after.

32. K. Mendelssohn, *The World of Walter Nernst: The Rise and Fall of German Science* (1973).

33. J. Schoolar, *Science, Scientists, and Public Policy* 285 (1971).

34. Assistant Secretary for Health Charles C. Edwards and the scientists are quoted in ''NIH Scientists, Administration Official Trade Charges over Autonomy of Agency,'' The Chronicle of Higher Education 5, col. 1 (Mar. 4, 1974).

35. Quoted in B. Bursten, ''Psychiatric 'Expertise' and Social Values,'' 41 *Current Medical Dialog* 78 (Feb. 1974).

36. R. Veatch, ''Generalization of Expertise,'' 1 *Hastings Center Studies* 29 at 36 (1973).

37. H. Krebs, ''Some Facts of Life–Biology and Politics,'' 15 *Perspectives in Biology and Medicine* 491 at 491–95 (1972).

38. J. Naughton, "A Little Global Difficulty: Reflections on the Doomsday Debate," 42 *Encounter* 72 at 73 (Jan. 1974).

39. Martin, *supra* note 14 at 55–56.

40. F. von Hippel and J. Primack, "Public Interest Science," 177 *Science* 1166 at 1167 (Sept. 29, 1972).

41. L. Graham, *Science and Philosophy in the Soviet Union* (1974); also see J. Solomon, *Science and Politics: An Essay on the Scientific Situation in the Modern World* (1975).

42. For a discussion of the implications of this broad definition, see V. Sidel, "Medical Ethics and Socio-political Change," 2 *Hastings Center Report* 8 (Sept. 1972); also see D. Callahan, "The WHO Definition of 'Health', " 1 *Hastings Center Studies* 77 (Nov. 1973).

43. For example, when Judge Bazelon found that an involunatily institutionalized mental patient had a consitutional "right to treatment" and that courts could examine the treatment programs provided, the American Psychiatric Association insisted: "The definition of treatment and the appraisal of its adequacy are matters of medical determination." "Council of the A.P.A. Position Statement on the Question of Adequacy of Treatment," 123 *American Journal of Psychiatry* 1458 (1967); also see the discussion in A. Stone, "Psychiatry and the Law," 1 *Psychiatric Annals* 18 at 34 (Oct. 1971). Although surely present, self-serving motives are less obvious in this APA illustration than in the AMA instance. In addition, political and social considerations are less immediately identifiable in the APA case, although a little analysis will show that the adequacy of treatment in a state hospital is a matter of many considerations other than purely medical ones. The same is also true for "the definition of treatment," as will be made clearer below.

44. An excellent collection of articles is in 1 *Hastings Center Studies* (Nov. 3, 1973), an entire issue devoted to "The Concept of Health."

45. Some important works arranged chronologically are: T. Parsons, *The Social System,* especially Chap. 10 (1951); A. Lewis, "Health as a Social Concept," 4 *British Journal of Sociology* 109 (1953); B. Wootton, *Social Science and Social Pathology* (1959); M. Foucault, *Madness and Civilization (1956); D. Mechanic, Medical Sociology* (1968); R. Wilson, *The Sociology of Health* (1970); R. Dubos, *The Mirage of Health* (1971); E. Freidson, *Profession of Medicine* (1971).

46. T. Szasz, *The Myth of Mental Illness* (1961), *The Manufacture of Madness* (1970).

47. R. Laing, *The Divided Shelf* (1960), *Interpersonal Experience* (1966), *The Politics of Experience* (1967); E. Goffman, *Asylums* (1961), *Stigma* (1961); R. Leifer, *In the Name of Mental Illness* (1969).

48. P. Sedgwick, "Illness–Mental and Otherwise," 1 *Hastings Center Studies* 19 at 21 (1973).

49. " 'Positivism,' for the present discussion, may be taken to refer to an approach towards the investigation of human pathology which, modelling itself upon antecedents which it believes to be characteristic of the natural sciences, (a) postulates a radical separation between 'facts' and 'values' (declaring only the former to be the subject-matter of the professional investigator) and (b) suppresses the interactive relationship between the investigator and the 'facts' on which he works. The psychiatric labels which are catalogues in textbooks of medicine and clinical psychology are, on a positivist account, terms which represent, or at least approximate towards, existent processes inhabiting an objective structure within the individual: the structure may be his psyche, his autonomic nervous system, perhaps even in the last resort his brain, but it stands towards the investigator as the ultimate object of reference . . . " (*Id.* at 25).

50. For characteristics of the medical model, see R. Veatch, "The Medical Model: Its Nature and Problems," 1 *Hastings Center Studies* 59 (1973), especially 64 and after.

51. "[I]t is characteristic of the ill person that he no longer controls his world or destiny as he did before. He does not control, he is controlled. Here again, it is not difficult to see the similarity between aging and illness. Thus in both the aging and the sick there occurs: a disconnection from the larger world, a loss of the sense of personal invulnerability, loss of confidence in the completeness of reason, a loss of the feeling of control over the world and, with all this, the sinking into dependency." E. Cassell, "Is Aging a Disease?," 2 *Hastings Center Report* 4 (Apr. 1972).

52. E. Murphy, "The Normal, and the Perils of the Sylleptic Argument," 15 *Perspectives in Biology and Medicine* 566 at 576 (1972).

53. Sedgwick, *supra* note 48 at 32, *citing to* Mechanic, *supra* note 45 at 16. Also see the reference to A. Knutson, *The Individual, Society, and Health Behavior* (1965).

54. "According to Alcoholics Anonymous, the alcoholic is not to blame for having a physiologically peculiar reaction to alcohol. . . . All that the occupancy of the sick role can do for alcoholics at the present time is remove blame. . . . " M. Siegler and H. Osmond, "The 'Sick Role' Revisited," 1 *Hastings Center Studies* 41 at 47 (1973). In this article the authors examine the sick role, beginning with the four essential features of that role as identified by Parsons: (1) exemption from normal social responsibilities; (2) involuntariness; (3) expected desire for recovery; (4) expected seeking of help. See Parsons, *supra* note 45.

55. T. Parsons, "Definitions of Health and Illness In the Light of American Values and Social Structure," in E. Jaco, ed., *Patients, Pysicians, and Illness* (1958).

56. Freidson, *supra* note 45 at 5 and 252.

57. P. Steinfels, "The Concept of Health," 1 *Hastings Center Studies* 3 (1973). Steinfels refers to a case mentioned by Lewis (*supra* note 45 at 123) where in a certain area the prevalence of "psychopathic personality" dropped drastically once it was decided that unemployment was not a "symptom" of the disorder. Perhaps an even more dramatic illustration of "disease by ballot" is found in a recent action of the Board of Trustees of the American Psychiatric Association which "removed homosexuality from the automatic status of mental disorder," as reported under the headline, "A.P.A. Drops Stigma From Homosexuality," 2 *Clinical Psychiatry News* 1 (Jan. 1974).

58. "Another objection to the WHO definition is that, by implication, it makes the medical profession the gate-keeper for happiness and social well-being. . . . [O]bviously enough, matters get out of hand when all physical, mental, and communal disorders are put under the heading of "sickness," and all sufferers (all of us, in the end) placed in the blameless "sick role." Not only are the concepts of "sickness" and "illness" drained of all content, it also becomes impossible to ascribe any freedom or responsibility to those caught up in the throes of sickness. The whole world is sick, and no one is responsible any longer for anything. . . . For as soon as one treats all human disorders—war, crime, social unrest—as forms of illness, then one turns health into a normative concept, that which human beings must and ought to have if they are to live in peace with themselves and others. Health is no longer an optional matter, but the golden key to the relief of human misery. We *must* be well or we will all perish. "Health" can and must be imposed; there can be no room for the luxury of freedom when so much is at stake." Callahan, *supra* note 42 at 81–83.

59. Olmstead v. U.S., 277 U.S. 438 at 478 (1928).

60. Application of the President and Directors of Georgetown College, Inc., 331 F. 2d 1000 at 1015 (D.C. Cir. 1964).

61. It is by no means obvious that the legislative inquiry is necessarily less "prosecutorial" than cross-examination in court. For example, Senator Kennedy in questioning an essentially sympathetic scientific witness tried to push him beyond what he could say as a scientist in order to acquire a "fact" which might help the Senator in his legislative capacity.

Dr. Brown:	If one could pinpoint accurately the precise locus of the center in the brain that stimulates the abnormal behavior or the tract through which it is disseminated and then remove or destroy only that portion of the brain, the patient could be relieved of his pathology over which he had no control and be returned to the community as a functioning, responsible member of society.

Senator Kennedy:	Can you do that accurately?
Dr. Brown:	That is the basic issue—
Senator Kennedy:	Well, that is your conclusion?
Dr. Brown:	In many situations, it can. In the majority of situations, the very nature of the research is to determine if there is such a locus; and this is the dilemma we are faced with. It is not yet clear in a majority of instances that this can be accurately done for all cases.
Senator Kennedy:	Well, your testimony is that in a majority of cases, it cannot be?
Dr. Brown:	In the majority of cases where you have abnormal behavior without obvious brain pathology, you cannot accurately locate the brain locus reponsible.

Hearings on S. 974, S. 878, and S. J. Res. 71 before the Subcommittee on Health of the Senate Committee on Labor and Public Welfare; 93d Cong., 1st Sess., pt. 2 at 449.

62. Michigan Senate Bill No. 740; introduced June 25, 1973 by Senator Faxon.

63. One (S.2072) which attracted considerable attention was introduced in the Senate on June 26, 1973 by Senators Kennedy, Javits, Hathaway, Hughes, Pell, and Randolph.

64. For example, see the careful account of the legislation widely enacted to test for mental retardation in S. Bessman and J. Swazey, "Phenylketonuria: A Study of Biomedical Legislation," in E. Mendelsohn, J. Swazey, and I. Taviss, eds., *Human Aspects of Biomedical Innovation* 494 (1971).

65.

Senator Kennedy:	Let me ask you this: If a private doctor wants to practice psychosurgery is there any way that you can prohibit it?
Dr. Brown:	No. We only have direct control over those clinical and experimental procedures that are done under our research grant funds.
Senator Kennedy:	Do you know of every case, or every place where psychosurgery is performed in the country today?

Dr. Brown:	No, I do not. I would guess that somewhere from several hundred to perhaps a few thousand are performed. We do not have an overview or purview of all the clinical practice that is now taking place.
Senator Kennedy:	So these procedures are taking place in the numbers that you have mentioned and you have no way of knowing whether those are under the very carefully controlled conditions that you have outlined as being absolutely minimal at best?
Dr. Brown:	That is correct. We have no direct knowledge.

Hearings, supra note 61 at 343.

Later in his testimony Dr. Gaylin said:

There is a great need for greater regulation of surgical procedures. We should demand distinctions between therapeutic and experimental. Distinctions and clearly stated definitions.

We should know the kind of operations done, by whom, and for what purposes. The confusion demonstrated today about the number of cases of psychosurgery does not, I think, represent duplicity, but simple ignorance. It is time for a registry of surgical procedures performed.

Hearings, supra note 61 at 375.

R. Restak, "The Promise and Peril of Psychosurgery," *Saturday Review/World* 54 at 57 (Sept. 25, 1973), also points out: "At least one West Coast neurosurgeon . . . has taken to performing psychosurgery on children as an office procedure."

66. See B. Barker, J. Lally, J. Makatushka, and D. Sullivan, *Research on Human Subjects* (1973).

67. H. Schelsky, "A German Dilemma," 42 *Encounter* 76 at 80 (Feb. 1974).

68. For a discussion of these issues see S. Shuman, "Why Criminal Law? Paramaters for Evaluating Objectives and Response Alternatives," in J. Tapp and F. Levine, eds., *Law, Justice, and the Individual in Society* (Holt, Rinehart, Winston, forthcoming); S. Shuman, "Responsibility and Punishment: Why Criminal Law?," 15 *American Journal of Jurisprudence* 25 (1970); S. Shuman, "The Placebo Cure for Criminality," 19 *Wayne Law Review* 847 (1973).

Chapter 9

1. See N. Kittrie, *The Right to be Different: Deviance and Enforced Therapy* (1972).

2. P. Steinfels, "Values, Expertise, and Responsibility in the Life Sciences: An Introduction," 1 *Hastings Center Studies* 3 at 5 (1973).

3. P. Kurtz, "Medicine and the State: The First Amendment Violated, An Interview with Thomas Szasz," *The Humanist* 4 (Mar./Apr. 1973). Also see E. Freidson, *Profession of Medicine* (1970), which explains how "Medicine has displaced the law and the ministry from their once dominant positions" (xviii).

4. "Medicine is inherently moral. . . . 'Playing God'. . . . It becomes clearer and clearer what the phrase really means. *'Playing God' means making a non-technical decision—a moral decision.*" E. Cassell, "Making and Escaping Moral Decisions," 1 *Hastings Center Studies* at 53 and 57 (1973).

5. See M. Siegler and H. Osmond, "Aesculapian Authority," 1 *Hastings Center Studies* 41 (1973).

6. Although it is far more extreme than necessary, the recent case of cannibalism in the Andes following the crash of a plane illustrates this point. P. Read, *Alive: The Story of the Andes Survivors* (1974).

7. For an interesting discussion of this notion, see A. Kleinman, "Medicine's Symbolic Reality: On a Central Problem in the Philosophy of Medicine," 16 *Inquiry* 206 (1973).

8. K. Popper, *The Logic of Scientific Discovery* (1961); T. Kuhn, *The Structure of Scientific Revolution* (2nd ed., 1970); I. Lakatos and A. Musgrave, eds., *Criticism and the Growth of Knowledge* (1970).

9. Popper, *supra* note 8 at 93, also see 423 and after.

10. M. Lappé, "Genetic Knowledge and the Concept of Health," 3 *Hastings Center Report* 1 at 1, 2, and 3 (Sept. 1973).

11. J. Fletcher, "Indicators of Humanhood: A Tentative Profile of Man," 2 *Hastings Center Report* 1 (Nov. 1972).

12. J. Burtchaell, "Indicators of Humanhood: Raveled Syllogisms," 3 *Hastings Center Report* 13 (Feb. 1973).

13. Fletcher, *supra* note 11.

14. R. Sinsheimer, "Ambush or Opportunity," 2 *Hastings Center Report* 4 at 7 (Sept. 1972).

15. Application of the President and Directors of Georgetown College, Inc., 331 F. 2d 1000 (D.C. Cir. 1964).

16. See A. Sheldon, "Towards a General Theory of Disease and Medical Care," in A. Sheldon, F. Baker, and C. McLaughlin, eds., *Systems and Medical Care* (1971); H. Fabrega, "Concepts of Disease: Logical Features And Social Implications," 15 *Perspectives in Biology and Medicine* 583 (1972); H. Fabrega, *Disease and Social Behavior: An Interdisciplinary Perspective* (1974).

17. The distinction is dealt with in a number of articles in "The Concept of Health," 1 *Hastings Center Studies* (No. 3, 1973).

18. R. Lazarus, "The Concepts of Stress and Disease," in L. Levi, ed., *Society, Stress, and Disease* at 56 (1971).

19. Fabrega (1972), *supra* note 16 at 587–88; also see Kleinman, *supra* note 7 at 208–209, where he writes:

    A given medical system in its socio-cultural context does considerably more than name, classify, and respond to illness, however. In a real sense, it structures the experience of illness and, in part, creates the form disease takes. Disease occurs as a natural process. It works upon biophysical reality and/or psycological processes as the case may be. But the experience of illness is a cultural or symbolic reality. The experience of illness involves feelings, ideas, values, language and non-verbal communication, symbolic behavior, and the like. . . . We know a great deal today about typing and labeling of diseases, less so about symptom choice and culturally specified disease forms. . . . More than that, we know that symbolic communication forms a pathway of sorts between social and cultural events and psychophysiological reactions. . . . I do not mean merely that psychiatric disorders or psychosomatic diseases are in this sense symbolic phenomena, but any disease—smallpox, leprosy, syphilis, hypertension, cardiovascular disorders, cancer, etc.—is in part a cultural construct. Disease derives much of its form, the way it is expressed, the value it is given, the meaning it possesses, and the therapy appropriate to it in large measure from the governing system of symbolic meanings.

20. Fabrega (1972), *supra* note 16 at 588–90; also see D. Mechanic, "Health and Illness in Technological Societies," 1 *Hastings Center Studies* 7, especially 11 and after (1973); P. Sedgwick, "Illness—Mental and Otherwise," 1 *Hastings Center Studies* 19, especially 20–21 and 29 and after (1973).

21. For an exceptionally careful analysis of the MBD problem, see P. Wender, "The case of MBD," 2 *Hastings Center Studies* 94 (1974).

22. Sedgwick, *supra* note 20 at 30–31; also see R. Dubos, *The Mirage of Health* (1971).

23. Lazarus, *supra* note 18 at 56.

24. M. Friedman, S. St. George, S. Byers, and R. Rosenman, "Excretion of Catecholamines, 17 Ketosteroids, 17 OM Ketosteroids, and 5 Hydroxyindale in Men Exhibiting a Particular Behavior Pattern (A) Associated with High Incidence of Clinical Coronary Heart Disease," 39 *Journal of Clinical Investigation* 758 (1960); R. Rosenan, M. Friedman, R. Straus, M. Wurm, C. Jenkins, and H. Messenger, "Coronary Heart Disease in the Western Collaborative Group Study," 195 *Journal of the American Medical Association* 86 (1966).

25. J. S. Mill, *Utilitarianism, Liberty, and Representative Government* 72–73 (Everyman's Library, 1910).

26. P. Devlin, *The Enforcement of Morals* (1965); H. Hart, *Law, Liberty, and Morality* (1963). Devlin's book is based upon a lecture he gave in 1959.

27. Devlin, *id.* at 15.

28. See M. Moore, "Some Myths About 'Mental Illness'," 32 *Archives of General Psychiatry* 1483 (1975).

29. See J. Gottlieb and C. Frohman, "The Biochemistry of Schizophrenia," in S. Arieti, ed., *Handbook of Psychiatry* (2nd ed., 1974).

INDEX

Samuel I. Shuman is professor of law and professor of psychiatry, Wayne State University, and professor of forensic psychiatry, Lafayette Clinic. Born in Massachusetts, he received his Ph.D. degree from the University of Pennsylvania (1951), and graduated J.D. from the University of Michigan (1954) and S.J.D. from Harvard University (1959). The author or editor of five previous books and many articles, he is a member of the Michigan Bar Association, the American Law Institute, and the president of the American section of the International Association for Legal and Social Philosophy.

The manuscript was edited by Sherwyn T. Carr. The book was designed by Mary Primeau. The typeface for the text is Times Roman, designed by Stanley Morison about 1931. The display typeface is Futura Display, designed by Paul Renner about 1927–30.

The text is printed on Glatfelter paper, and the book is bound in Columbia Mills' Fictionette cloth over binder's boards. Manufactured in the United States of America.